T0372794

Ken Peake, DSW
Irwin Epstein, PhD
Daniel Medeiros, MD
Editors

Clinical and Research Uses of an Adolescent Mental Health Intake Questionnaire: What Kids Need to Talk About

Clinical and Research Uses of an Adolescent Mental Health Intake Questionnaire: What Kids Need to Talk About has been co-published simultaneously as *Social Work in Mental Health*, Volume 3, Numbers 1/2 2004 and Volume 3, Number 3 2005.

"I RECOMMEND THIS BOOK to all practitioners seeking to reinvigorate their practice and to all university professors with an interest in what their students are actually going to do after graduation. From the very first chapter, which eschews the more usual pathology perspective on adolescent mental health in favor of a developmental approach, every paper in this refreshing book challenges accepted wisdom in university circles about the nexus between research and practice. Central to the work is a distinction between 'research based practice' and 'practice based research,' with all of the contributors demon- strating the enormous potential of the latter approach for the helping professions. Following Peake and Epstein's seminal chapter on 'the reflective organization,' which provides the theoretical and philosophical underpinnings of the approach, the rest of the book shows how practice based research works, particularly in relation to the Adolescent Intake Questionnaire, from which the title of the book derives."

James Barber, PhD
Dean, Faculty of Social Work
University of Toronto

Clinical and Research Uses of an Adolescent Mental Health Intake Questionnaire: What Kids Need to Talk About

Clinical and Research Uses of an Adolescent Mental Health Intake Questionnaire: What Kids Need to Talk About has been co-published simultaneously as *Social Work in Mental Health*, Volume 3, Numbers 1/2 2004 and Volume 3, Number 3 2005.

Monographic Separates from *Social Work in Mental Health*

For additional information on these and other Haworth Press titles, including descriptions, tables of contents, reviews, and prices, use the QuickSearch catalog at http://www.HaworthPress.com.

Clinical and Research Uses of an Adolescent Mental Health Intake Questionnaire: What Kids Need to Talk About, edited by Ken Peake, DSW, Irwin Epstein, PhD, and Daniel Medeiros, MD (Vol. 3, Nos. 1/2, 2004, and Vol. 3, No. 3, 2005). *"Clinical and Research Uses of an Adolescent Mental Health Intake Questionnaire: What Kids Need to Talk About" explores the research on adolescent behavior culled from the answers to a clinician-designed intake questionnaire given to adolescent clients asking how they view their own risks, what they worry about, and what they wish to talk about. Respected authorities discuss the enlightening findings and present ways to reshape services, taking into account customer preference, risk and worry, and youth development (YD) perspectives while presenting practical clinical strategies to engage at-risk adolescents in mental health treatment.*

Social Work Approaches in Health and Mental Health from Around the Globe, edited by Anna Metteri, MSocSc, Teppo Kröger, PhD, Anneli Pohjola, PhD, and Pirkko-Liisa Rauhala, PhD (Vol. 2, No. 2/3, 2004). *"Broad-based and unique. . . . A much-needed publication for training and practice." (Charlene Laurence Carbonatto, DPhil, Senior Lecturer, Department of Social Work, University of Prestoria, South Africa)*

Psychiatric Medication Issues for Social Workers, Counselors, and Psychiatrists, edited by Kia J. Bentley, PhD, LCSW (Vol. 1, No. 4, 2003). *"Outstanding . . . . All social workers, counselors, and psychologists working in the mental health field would benefit from reading this outstanding book." (Deborah P. Valentine, PhD, MSSW, Professor and Director, School of Social Work, Colorado State University)*

Clinical and Research Uses of an Adolescent Mental Health Intake Questionnaire: What Kids Need to Talk About

Ken Peake, DSW
Irwin Epstein, PhD
Daniel Medeiros, MD
Editors

Gary Rosenberg, PhD
Andrew Weissman, PhD
Series Editors

Clinical and Research Uses of an Adolescent Mental Health Intake Questionnaire: What Kids Need to Talk About has been co-published simultaneously as *Social Work in Mental Health*, Volume 3, Numbers 1/2 2004 and Volume 3, Number 3 2005.

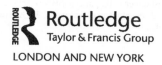

Routledge
Taylor & Francis Group

LONDON AND NEW YORK

Clinical and Research Uses of an Adolescent Mental Health Intake Questionnaire: What Kids Need to Talk About has been co-published simultaneously as *Journal of Social Work in Mental Health* Volume 3, Numbers 1/2 2004 and Volume 3, Number 3 2005.

First published 2005 by The Haworth Press, Inc.

2 Park Square, Milton Park, Abingdon, Oxfordshire OX14 4RN
605 Third Avenue, New York, NY 10017

Routledge is an imprint of the Taylor & Francis Group, an informa business

First issued in hardback 2020

Copyright © 2005 Taylor & Francis

All rights reserved. No part of this book may be reprinted or reproduced or utilised in any form or by any electronic, mechanical, or other means, now known or hereafter invented, including photocopying and recording, or in any information storage or retrieval system, without permission in writing from the publishers.

Notice:
Product or corporate names may be trademarks or registered trademarks, and are used only for identification and explanation without intent to infringe.

Cover design by Kerry E. Mack

Library of Congress Cataloging-in-Publication Data

Clinical and research uses of an adolescent mental health intake questionnaire: what kids need to talk about / Ken Peake, Irwin Epstein, Daniel Medeiros.
     p. cm.
     "Co-published simultaneously as Journal of social work in mental health, volume 3, numbers 1/2 2004 and volume 3 number 3 2005."
     Includes bibliographical references and index.
     ISBN 0-7890-2673-2 (hard cover : alk. paper)-ISBN 0-7890-2674-0 (soft cover : alk. paper)
     1. Adolescent psychiatry. 2. Psychiatric social work. 3. Questionnaires. I. Peake, Ken. II. Epstein, Irwin. III. Medeiros, Daniel.
  RJ503.C57 2005
  616.89'00835–dc22   2005001517

ISBN 978-0-7890-2673-6 (hbk)
ISBN 978-1-315-82118-4 (eISBN)

Indexing, Abstracting & Website/Internet Coverage

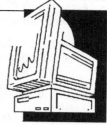

This section provides you with a list of major indexing & abstracting services and other tools for bibliographic access. That is to say, each service began covering this periodical during the year noted in the right column. Most Websites which are listed below have indicated that they will either post, disseminate, compile, archive, cite or alert their own Website users with research-based content from this work. (This list is as current as the copyright date of this publication.)

Abstracting, Website/Indexing Coverage . . . . Year When Coverage Began

- *Behavioral Medicine Abstracts (Annals of Behavioral Medicine)* . . . **2003**

- *CAB ABSTRACTS c/o CAB International/CAB ACCESS . . .*
  available in print, diskettes updated weekly, and on INTERNET.
  Providing full bibliographic listings, author affiliation, augmented
  keyword searching. <http://www.cabi.org> **2003**

- *CAB HEALTH c/o CAB International/CAB ACCESS . . . available*
  in print, diskettes updated weekly, and on Internet. Providing full
  bibliographic listings, author affiliation, augmented keyword
  searching. <http://www.cabi.org> **2003**

- *CareData: the database supporting social care management*
  and practice <http://www.elsc.org.uk/caredata/caredata.htm> **2001**

- *CINAHL (Cumulative Index to Nursing & Allied Health Literature),*
  in print, EBSCO, and SilverPlatter, Data-Star, and PaperChase.
  (Support materials include Subject Heading List, Database Search
  Guide, and instructional video.) <http://www.cinahl.com> **2003**

- *Criminal Justice Abstracts* **2003**

- *DH-Data (available via DataStar and in the HMIC*
  [Health Management Information Consortium] CD ROM) **2003**

- *e-psyche, LLC <http://www.e-psyche.net>* . . . . ***

(continued)

- *EBSCOhost Electronic Journals Service (EJS)*
  <http://ejournals.ebsco.com> 2003

- *Exceptional Child Education Resources (ECER),*
  (CD/ROM from SilverPlatter and hard copy)
  <http://www.ericec.org/ecer-db.html> 2003

- *Family & Society Studies Worldwide <http://www.nisc.com>* 2003

- *Family Index Database <http://www.familyscholar.com>* 2003

- *Family Violence & Sexual Assault Bulletin* 2004

- *Google <http://www.google.com>* 2004

- *Google Scholar <http://www.scholar.google.com>* 2004

- *Haworth Document Delivery Center*
  <http://www.HaworthPress.com/journals/dds.asp> 2004

- *IBZ International Bibliography of Periodical Literature*
  <http://www.saur.de> 2002

- *Index to Jewish Periodicals <http://www.jewishperiodicals.com>* 2003

- *Internationale Bibliographie der geistes- und*
  sozialwissenschaftlichen Zeitschriftenliteratur . . . See IBZ
  <http://www.saur.de> 2002

- *National Clearinghouse on Child Abuse & Neglect Information*
  Documents Database <http://www.nccanch.acf.hhs.gov> 2003

- *Psychological Abstracts (PsychINFO) <http://www.apa.org>* 2003

- *Referativnyi Zhurnal (Abstracts Journal of the All-Russian Institute*
  of Scientific and Technical Information–in Russian)
  <http://www.viniti.ru> 2003

- *Sexual Diversity Studies: Gay, Lesbian, Bisexual & Transgender*
  Abstracts (formerly Gay & Lesbian Abstracts) provides comprehensive &
  in-depth coverage of the world's GLBT literature compiled by
  NISC & published on the Internet & CD-ROM
  <http://www.nisc.com> 2003

- *Social Services Abstracts <http://www.csa.com>* 2003

- *Worldwide Political Science Abstracts (formerly: Political*
  Science & Government Abstracts) <http://www.csa.com> 2003

  * **Exact start date to come.**

(continued)

*Special Bibliographic Notes related to special journal issues
(separates) and indexing/abstracting:*

- indexing/abstracting services in this list will also cover material in any "separate" that is co-published simultaneously with Haworth's special thematic journal issue or DocuSerial. Indexing/abstracting usually covers material at the article/chapter level.
- monographic co-editions are intended for either non-subscribers or libraries which intend to purchase a second copy for their circulating collections.
- monographic co-editions are reported to all jobbers/wholesalers/approval plans. The source journal is listed as the "series" to assist the prevention of duplicate purchasing in the same manner utilized for books-in-series.
- to facilitate user/access services all indexing/abstracting services are encouraged to utilize the co-indexing entry note indicated at the bottom of the first page of each article/chapter/contribution.
- this is intended to assist a library user of any reference tool (whether print, electronic, online, or CD-ROM) to locate the monographic version if the library has purchased this version but not a subscription to the source journal.
- individual articles/chapters in any Haworth publication are also available through the Haworth Document Delivery Service (HDDS).

Clinical and Research Uses of an Adolescent Mental Health Intake Questionnaire: What Kids Need to Talk About

CONTENTS

PART I

Including At-Risk Adolescents in Their Own Health and Mental
  Health Care: A Youth Development Perspective   3
  Angela Diaz
  Ken Peake
  Michael Surko
  Kalpana Bhandarkar

Theoretical and Practical Imperatives for Reflective Social
  Work Organizations in Health and Mental Health:
  The Place of Practice-Based Research   23
  Ken Peake
  Irwin Epstein

Creating and Sustaining a Practice-Based Research Group
  in an Urban Adolescent Mental Health Program   39
  Ken Peake
  Diane Mirabito
  Irwin Epstein
  Vincent Giannone

Development and Utilization of a Practice-Based, Adolescent
  Intake Questionnaire (Adquest): Surveying Which Risks,
  Worries, and Concerns Urban Youth Want to Talk About   55
  Ken Peake
  Irwin Epstein
  Diane Mirabito
  Michael Surko

Clinical Uses of an Adolescent Intake Questionnaire: Adquest
  as a Bridge to Engagement   83
    Jennifer Elliott
    Michael Nembhard
    Vincent Giannone
    Michael Surko
    Daniel Medeiros
    Ken Peake

Which Adolescents Need to Talk About Safety and Violence?   103
    Michael Surko
    Dianne Ciro
    Erika Carlson
    Nyanda Labor
    Vincent Giannone
    Elizabeth Diaz-Cruz
    Ken Peake
    Irwin Epstein

Adolescents Seeking Mental Health Services: Self-Reported
  Health Risks and the Need to Talk   121
    Daniel Medeiros
    Leah Kramnick
    Elizabeth Diaz-Cruz
    Michael Surko
    Angela Diaz

Adolescents' Need to Talk About Sex and Sexuality in an Urban
  Mental Health Setting   135
    Nyanda Labor
    Daniel Medeiros
    Erika Carlson
    Nancimarie Pullo
    Mavis Seehaus
    Ken Peake
    Irwin Epstein

Adolescents' Need to Talk About School and Work in Mental
    Health Treatment   155
        Elizabeth Diaz-Cruz
        Daniel Medeiros
        Michael Surko
        Ruth Hoffman
        Irwin Epstein

Adolescents' Self-Reported Substance Risks and Need
    to Talk About Them in Mental Health Counseling   171
        Daniel Medeiros
        Erika Carlson
        Michael Surko
        Nicole Munoz
        Monique Castillo
        Irwin Epstein

Adolescents' Self-Reported Risk Factors and Desire to Talk
    About Family and Friends: Implications for Practice
    and Research   191
        Vincent Giannone
        Daniel Medeiros
        Jennifer Elliott
        Caroline Perez
        Erika Carlson
        Irwin Epstein

PART II

Lesbian, Gay, Bisexual, Sexual-Orientation Questioning
    Adolescents Seeking Mental Health Services: Risk Factors,
    Worries, and Desire to Talk About Them   213
        Dianne Ciro
        Michael Surko
        Kalpana Bhandarkar
        Nora Helfgott
        Ken Peake
        Irwin Epstein

Experience of Racism as a Correlate of Developmental
    and Health Outcomes Among Urban Adolescent Mental
    Health Clients   235
    Michael Surko
    Dianne Ciro
    Caryl Blackwood
    Michael Nembhard
    Ken Peake

Multiple Risks, Multiple Worries, and Adolescent Coping:
    What Clinicians Need to Ask About   261
    Michael Surko
    Ken Peake
    Irwin Epstein
    Daniel Medeiros

Data-Mining Client Concerns in Adolescent Mental Health
    Services: Clinical and Program Implications   287
    Ken Peake
    Michael Surko
    Irwin Epstein
    Daniel Medeiros

Collaborative Data-Mining in an Adolescent Mental Health
    Service: Clinicians Speak of Their Experience   305
    Dianne Ciro
    Michael Nembhard

Index   319

ABOUT THE EDITORS

Ken Peake, DSW, is Chief Operating Officer of the Mount Sinai Adolescent Health Center (AHC) in New York City, where he began as Director of Mental Health in 1990. Through this and his clinical experience, Dr. Peake has developed a range of programmatic and practice-based research initiatives that encourage clinicians and clients to participate in organizational learning. Dr. Peake stumbled into his career in 1972, when he volunteered as a youth worker on Manhattan's Lower East Side. For more than a decade, he worked as a youth worker, with homeless families, and with the children of abused women at the Henry Street Settlement in New York City. Following that experience and before coming to AHC, he spent ten years as a practitioner and clinical supervisor in community-based mental health in the South Bronx and in private practice.

Irwin Epstein, PhD, occupies the Helen Rehr Chair in Applied Social Work Research at Hunter College School of Social Work. Dr. Epstein has taught applied research courses and conducted practice-based research workshops at universities and social agencies in the United States, Australia, Europe, and Israel. He is co-author of several books and numerous articles on social worker professionalization and research utilization. He has provided consultation to a wide array of health, mental health, child welfare, and employee assistance programs in organizations as diverse as Mt. Sinai Hospital in New York, the Child Welfare Institute in Atlanta, Boysville of Michigan, Tel Hashomer Hospital in Tel Aviv, and the Royal Children's Hospital in Melbourne. He is currently co-evaluator of the Multidisciplinary Clinical Consultation Program of New York City's Administration for Children's Services. His most recent book, co-edited with Dr. Susan Blumenfield, is entitled *Clinical Data-Mining in Practice-Based Research: Social Work in Hospital Settings* (Haworth).

Daniel Medeiros, MD, has been working with adolescents since his senior year in college when he began working as a counselor at an adolescent crisis shelter in Boston. He continued his work by providing health education to teens in an outreach program while in medical school. The work for this book was based on his five-year experience at the Mount Sinai Adolescent Health Center (AHC), where he directed mental health services and worked directly with adolescents. In addition, Dr. Medeiros has coordinated a therapeutic adolescent after-school program, supervised an adolescent peer education program, and is currently directing an adolescent chemical dependency day program and a day program for teens with emotional issues at St. Luke's Roosevelt Hospital Center in New York City.

Clinical and Research Uses of an Adolescent Mental Health Intake Questionnaire: What Kids Need to Talk About

Clinical and Research Uses of an Adolescent Mental Health Intake Questionnaire: What Kids Need to Talk About has been co-published simultaneously as *Social Work in Mental Health*, Volume 3, Numbers 1/2 2004 and Volume 3, Number 3 2005.

ALL HAWORTH SOCIAL WORK PRACTICE PRESS
BOOKS AND JOURNALS ARE PRINTED ON
CERTIFIED ACID-FREE PAPER

PART I

Including At-Risk Adolescents in Their Own Health and Mental Health Care: A Youth Development Perspective

Angela Diaz
Ken Peake
Michael Surko
Kalpana Bhandarkar

SUMMARY. As urban adolescents encounter serious health and mental health risks, they present the allied health professions with important opportunities for health promotion and risk reduction interventions. However, the prevailing emphasis on adolescents' *risk behaviors* rather than on their *vulnerability* has limited our capacity to understand and serve them. Further limiting are the widely held myths that adolescents as a

Angela Diaz, MD, MPH, is Director, Mount Sinai Adolescent Health Center and Professor of Pediatrics and Chief of Adolescent Medicine, Mount Sinai School of Medicine. Ken Peake, DSW, is Assistant Director, Mount Sinai Adolescent Health Center. Michael Surko, PhD, is Coordinator, ACT for Youth Downstate Center for Excellence, Mount Sinai Adolescent Health Center. Kalpana Bhandarkar, BA, is Program Assistant, Downstate Center for Excellence. Mount Sinai Adolescent Health Center is located at 320 East 94th Street, New York, NY 10128.

[Haworth co-indexing entry note]: "Including At-Risk Adolescents in Their Own Health and Mental Health Care: A Youth Development Perspective." Diaz, Angela et al. Co-published simultaneously in *Social Work in Mental Health* (The Haworth Social Work Practice Press, an imprint of The Haworth Press, Inc.) Vol. 3, No. 1/2, 2004, pp. 3-22; and: *Clinical and Research Uses of an Adolescent Mental Health Intake Questionnaire: What Kids Need to Talk About* (ed: Ken Peake, Irwin Epstein, and Daniel Medeiros) The Haworth Social Work Practice Press, an imprint of The Haworth Press, Inc., 2005, pp. 3-22. Single or multiple copies of this article are available for a fee from The Haworth Document Delivery Service [1-800-HAWORTH, 9:00 a.m. - 5:00 p.m. (EST). E-mail address: docdelivery@haworthpress.com].

http://www.haworthpress.com/web/SWMH
© 2004 by The Haworth Press, Inc. All rights reserved.
Digital Object Identifier: 10.1300/J200v03n01_01

whole have few health problems and that they are poor judges of their own needs. This article presents an overview of current theories of adolescent risk and vulnerability and suggests *Youth Development* as an overarching framework for understanding both. Experience within a comprehensive, adolescent health and mental health center demonstrates how to meaningfully engage adolescents in their own health care from the start. *[Article copies available for a fee from The Haworth Document Delivery Service: 1-800-HAWORTH. E-mail address: <docdelivery@haworthpress.com> Website: <http://www.HaworthPress.com> © 2004 by The Haworth Press, Inc. All rights reserved.]*

KEYWORDS. Adolescent, youth development, vulnerability, risk, mental health, professional competencies

INTRODUCTION

This article presents an overview of current theories of adolescent risk and vulnerability and suggests *Youth Development* (Pittman, Irby, & Ferber, 2000) as an overarching framework for understanding both. Experience within a comprehensive, adolescent health and mental health center–the Mount Sinai Adolescent Health Center (AHC)–will be presented to demonstrate how to meaningfully engage adolescents in their own health care from the start. Embedded in the article is a discussion of commonly experienced barriers to implementing Youth Development (YD) principles and efforts undertaken at AHC to address them.

Despite popular images of adolescence as a period of mindless fun and self-absorption, adolescents present enormous challenges for health and mental health agencies and are classified as a "population at-risk" (U.S. General Accounting Office, 1996, p. 1). Experimentation and risk-taking put this group at particularly high risk for social morbidities such as unplanned pregnancy, alcohol and drug addiction, and HIV/AIDS, problems that often have lifelong impact and great social cost. Social and environmental factors influence the health risks of many adolescents. Lack of health insurance and access to health care, the easy availability of drugs, and the psychosocial sequela to violence in schools and communities combine with normative adolescent risk behaviors to produce an often-volatile mix.

By the millennium, there were already more than 39 million young people in the U.S. ages 10 to 19, with more than 35% belonging to racial and ethnic minorities (U.S. Bureau of the Census, 2001). The numbers of minority adolescents are growing at a faster rate than their white compeers, with greater concentrations of minority youth living in urban areas (National Adolescent Health Information Center, 2000). More than 25% of all adolescents live in poverty–a factor that exacerbates their health risks (Millstein, Irwin, & Brindis, 1991). More than 14% do not have health insurance of any kind (Newacheck, Brindis, Uhler, & Cart et al., 1999), and far fewer have coverage for mental health care, leaving many of their health and mental health needs unmet.

Uninsurance rates are higher in minority communities: black and Latino adolescents are much more likely than white adolescents to be uninsured (40% and 300%, respectively) (Newacheck et al., 1999). In addition to lack of insurance, poverty in inner cities brings many associated problems that further undermine the health of adolescents. These include economically depressed and dangerous neighborhoods, poor academic education, poor access to health care, lack of providers competent to address their specific health needs, and lack of opportunities that promote adolescents' healthy development (Blum, McNeely, & Nonnemaker, 2002).

MYTHS ABOUT ADOLESCENCE

The myth that adolescents don't need health care because they are a naturally robust population disguises the fact that adolescents as a group have serious health risks and lack access to needed medical and mental health care.

Adolescents are vulnerable for both health (Neinstein, 1996) and mental health problems (Burke, Burke, Regier, & Rae, 1991). One in five adolescents has a serious health problem and a much higher proportion has pressing health care needs, such as access to contraception, and one in five has a diagnosable mental health problem (Dougherty, 1993). Explanations for their vulnerability may be social as much as developmental (Blum et al., 2001; Eccles, Midgely, & Wigfield et al., 1993; Powers, Hauser, & Kilner, 1993). Furthermore, minority adolescents as a group are less healthy than white adolescents. Among white parents, 54% rated their adolescent's health as excellent, compared with 43% of Latino parents and only 39% of black parents (National Institutes of Health [NIH], 1997).

Despite this vulnerability, rates of physician visits for 11-21-year-olds are low. In 1994, for instance, adolescents made 9.1% of physician visits but represented 15.4% of the total population. Minority adolescents were significantly underrepresented relative to their percent of the population. Black adolescents made 8.3% of visits though they constituted 15.5% of the adolescent population. Latino adolescents made 9.3% of visits, though they constituted 13.6% of the adolescent population. By contrast, white adolescents accounted for 78.5% of physician visits, though they represented 67.6% of the total adolescent population (Ziv, Boulet, & Slap, 1999). Although 20% of adolescents have a diagnosable mental health disorder (Dougherty, 1993), only one fifth of these receive mental health care (Kerstenbaum, 2002).

Differential rates of health care access are not related to the greater health care needs of white adolescents but rather to barriers to care of minority adolescents (NIH,1997). These barriers include poverty, lack of health insurance, and lack of culturally competent health services. The absence of long-term and trusting relationships with health care providers suggests that the bio-psychosocial problems of many minority adolescents are never identified or addressed—unless they get into trouble of some kind. And, many do get into trouble.

So, for example, while 11% of all adolescents who enter high school leave before graduation, rates of high school dropout for blacks and Latinos are consistently higher than those for whites. Further, youth in low-income families are six times as likely as their peers in high-income families to drop out of school (National Center for Education Statistics, 2001). Although school dropout may not seem to be a health problem, it is a significant risk indicator and is correlated with poorer health outcomes both in the short-run and over the course of their lives (Millstein et al., 1991).

Dryfoos (1990) classifies over 25% of all U.S. teenagers as either *high risk* or *very high risk* of some kind. Within poor, inner-city communities, the normative risk-taking of adolescence is likely to have more serious and long-lasting negative consequences. Adolescents in these communities are more likely to engage in multiple, co-occurring risk behaviors, including use of drugs and alcohol, unprotected sex, violent activity, or school dropout.

UNDERSTANDING ADOLESCENT VULNERABILITY

The foregoing problems of urban minority adolescents require more effective health and mental health intervention strategies. More specifically, this means better engagement and assessment of individual adolescents at-risk and identification of broad risk groups. Yet, considerable ambiguity remains concerning identification of adolescents most at-risk and best practices in identification (Stanton, Fang, Li, Feigelman, Galbraith, & Ricardo, 1997). Moreover, the overarching term *at-risk* masks demographic vulnerabilities such as poverty, minority status and single parent households (Blum et al., 2001).

Furthermore, our understanding of adolescent vulnerability and its relation to risk has been hampered by the fragmentation of research on adolescent risk into specific problem areas such as violence, sexual activity, teen pregnancy, and substance abuse (Dougherty, 1993). Funding streams for services have been similarly fragmented, leading to intervention approaches that are more problem-focused than holistic.

Though recent theories of adolescent risk consider the interaction of risk factors, they continue to emphasize risk behaviors. *Gateway Theory* (Kandel & Yamaguchi, 1993) suggests that adolescents engage in escalating risk behaviors. It has been particularly influential in substance abuse prevention—for example smoking cessation can be viewed as a strategy for preventing escalation to other substance use. One area of interest that is evolving from this perspective is the study of risk antecedents and markers (Resnick & Burt, 1996).

Serial Risk Behavior Theory (Stanton et al., 1997) suggested by longitudinal studies of long-term risk behaviors has looked at the endurance of risk behaviors. This theory suggests that many adolescents shift from one risk behavior to another over time, with no apparent escalation in the total number of risk behaviors they engage in concurrently.

Together these theories have contributed much to our thinking about adolescent risk but raise as many questions as they answer, as they do not address the issue of *why* adolescents appear to take risks.

In contrast, *Problem Behavior Theory* (Blum et al., 2001; Donovan, Jessor, & Costa, 1985; Jessor, 1991) focuses on the co-occurrence of risk behaviors within *high-risk* groups and suggests that adolescents who are attracted to one risk behavior will be attracted to others. Its premise is that risk behavior is goal directed, rather than random *thrill seeking*, and that perceived risk is balanced against perceived and actual developmental benefits. Problem Behavior Theory suggests that adolescents who are attracted to one risk behavior will be attracted to others. Dryfoos (1990), in particular, suggests that risk behaviors co-occur in large numbers of adolescents, with the same high-risk groups engaging in multiple risk behaviors.

Concurrently, we need an increased understanding of how risk factors affect subsets of the adolescent population, particularly with respect to the influence of community and family contexts (Blum et al., 2001; Jessor, 1993; Mechanic, 1991). Adolescents who seem low-risk in their own behaviors might be at risk due to the behaviors of friends and associates (Bailey, 1992), or due to social factors rather than individual risk behaviors (Blum et al., 2001). Risk behaviors may also have different consequences for different subgroups, though this also has received little attention in research efforts (Shapiro & Seigel, 1998).

Clearly, too little is understood about social and environmental influences on adolescent risk and vulnerability (Eccles et al., 1993; Fahs, Smith, & Ata et al., 1999; Blum et al., 2001). Blum et al. (2001) build on Jessor's (1991) concept of adolescent risk as a product of five contributing domains: Biological/genetic factors, social environment, the environment as perceived by the adolescent, personality, and behavior. Blum and his colleagues suggest that in addition to these five domains, risk theory be built on an ecological systems model that incorporates study of childhood antecedents of risk behaviors, factors that contribute to positive health outcomes, and the influence of macrolevel factors such as politics, youth laws and policies, economics, and historical events. While this offers a promising framework for research, it is unlikely that at any time soon we will have an overarching theory that can be used to improve the efficacy of prevention and treatment programs.

EMPIRICAL KNOWLEDGE VERSUS CLINICAL LORE: THE MYTH OF ADOLESCENT SELF-PERCEIVED INVULNERABILITY

The myth that adolescents perceive themselves as invulnerable *prevents many clinicians from asking them directly about their health and mental health needs and from taking their responses seriously.*

Despite the increase in empirical theory-testing concerning adolescents (Zaslow & Takanishi, 1993), a dichotomy still exists between the clinical *construction* of adolescence, as a phase of life full of *sturm und drang*, and research findings (Quadrell, Fischoff, & Davis, 1993). Many clinicians regard adolescents' supposed *grandiosity* and feelings of *invulnerability* as defenses against the supposedly inevitable *storm and stress* of adolescence. Such ideas, though not supported empirically, can appear to provide compelling reasons why individual youth often appear to take risks without exploring their consequences (Offer & Schonert Reichl, 1992). However, many studies now question these popular ideas and suggest that they are *myths*.

Several studies suggest that adolescents can better assess the consequences of their behaviors and better understand their needs than has been generally assumed (Andrews, Garrison, & Jackson et al., 1992; Cohn, McFarlane, Yanez, & Imai, 1995; Durant, Seymore, & Jay, 1991; Kazdin, 1993; Offer & Schonert-Reichl, 1992; Quadrell et al., 1993). Moreover, an overemphasis on adolescence as unique because, in contrast to other periods of life, it is characterized by developmental *turmoil* might be one reason few studies actually compare adolescents with other age groups.

Based on the studies cited thus far, however, the authors propose the following conclusions: (1) many adolescents engage in activities that present serious risks to their health and safety resulting in a critical need for interventions, with 25% at high risk or very high risk; (2) there are extensive gaps in our knowledge about adolescent risk and vulnerability, particularly for minority adolescents; (3) there are extensive gaps in our knowledge about adolescent perceptions of their own health and mental health needs and in our *phenomenological* understanding of the meanings adolescents ascribe to their risk-taking (Zaslow & Takanishi, 1993); (4) clinicians overemphasize the theory of adolescent stress and self-perceived invulnerability as an explanation for adolescent risk-taking; and (5) explanatory theories of adolescent risk have underemphasized the contribution of social factors and institutional arrangements to adolescent vulnerability.

The emerging picture of *normal* adolescence and adolescent risk offers little comfort and clarity to direct service practitioners and program planners because it remains full of contradictions. Neither practice wisdom nor research studies alone provide an adequate basis for developing relevant, rigorous, comprehensive clinical intervention or needs assessments. Clinical risk assessment strategies, program design and ultimately funding strategies must be predicated on a better marriage of these knowledge areas and must be tested in the context of actual intervention.

ADOLESCENCE AS A PROFESSIONAL OPPORTUNITY

Although adolescents as a group embody serious health risks, they also present health systems with real opportunities for health-promotion and risk reduction strategies. Thus, they are characterized by the American Medical Association (1997) as a population developmentally at the "crossroads" of good and poor health (p. 1). On the positive side, adolescents are good consumers of information, especially as it relates to their own concerns, are eager to share their perspectives when they are asked, and are often intellectually and emotionally available. Each of these qualities offers openings for health-education and clinical counseling.

Many studies support this view (Offer & Schonert-Reichl, 1992; Quadrell et al., 1993; Weisz & Hawley, 2002). For example, there is evidence that when compared to adults, adolescents accurately assess the risks associated with their behaviors, but lack the necessary life-experience upon which to base good decision-making (Petersen, 1980). Further, inadequate fit between developmental stage needs of adolescents for increasing levels of personal autonomy in personal decision-making and meaningful roles in their social environment and actual opportunities for such participation, may also account for a significant portion of risk exposure in early adolescence (Eccles et al., 1993; Larson, 2002). This may be exacerbated by a lack of access to adolescent appropriate services (Pittman et al., 2000). Hence, preventive education and positive community supports are essential to reducing negative health outcomes for adolescents.

A YOUTH DEVELOPMENT PERSPECTIVE: BUILDING RESILIENCY THROUGH FAMILIES, COMMUNITIES, AND SOCIAL INSTITUTIONS

A Youth Development (YD) perspective (Pittman et al., 2000) offers theoretical opportunities for researchers and practitioners to better understand the contribution of social and institutional factors to adolescent vulnerability. YD is an approach that is enormously influential in the field of youth programming, but has still to gain traction in health and mental health professions. YD practice considers the fit between developmental needs and community characteristics, institutional factors, and opportunities necessary for healthy development of young people. At its most basic level, YD attests that healthy development requires meaningful involvement of adolescents in their communities, programs and institutions that serve them.

The YD approach begins from the axiom that for adolescents, even if it were possible or desirable to be free of problems, to be "problem-free is not [to be] fully prepared" for the future (Pittman et al., 2000, p. 20). In addition, for effective prevention and remediation of problems, those who engage young people need to provide opportunities for youth to build *personal and social assets* that will prepare them for a healthy and productive adulthood (Scales & Leffert, 1999). Examples of personal and social assets include motivation to master new skills; confidence in one's efficacy; a sense of autonomy and responsibility for self; good health risk management skills; critical thinking and reasoning skills; emotional self-regulation skills; perceived good relationships and trust with parents, peers, and some other adults; and, a sense of being connected and valued by larger social networks. Building such assets will also enable adolescents to be better prepared to cope with the inevitable problems of living.

To develop these assets, adolescents need increasing participation in decision-making and decreasing control from adults with whom they enjoy ongoing stable and supportive relationships (Eccles et al., 1993; Larson, 2002). In other words, adults must find ways to be able to allow adolescents gradual and increasing control over personal decision making while remaining available for advice and guidance when it is sought. Zimring (1982) has described this as a *learner's permit* approach to raising adolescents. This approach views adolescence as a period in which the learning process of development requires making mistakes, in addition to experiencing successes, if good decision-making skills are to be cultivated.

Similarly, services for adolescents should also encourage increasing participation and youth voice in their design and delivery as well as in broader civic engagement (Larson, 2002). Settings that grant responsibility, provide meaningful challenges to adolescents, and take their perspectives seriously therefore provide a good stage-environment fit for adolescents' developmental needs.

YD offers a conceptual framework to address a number of weaknesses in prior theories of adolescent risk. First, these theories have relied too much on the conception of adolescent development as a process of personal maturation through stages rather than an outcome of person-context interaction or stage-environment fit. Second, researchers have neglected the study of factors that lead to optimal functioning in adolescent development. Third, though evaluations of problem prevention programs are available, there still exists a need for increased applied and theoretical research integrated into prevention and treatment programs (Kazdin, 1993; Dougherty, 1993). Fourth, YD is consistent with Zaslow and Takanishi's (1993) observation that unless our research is predicated on an understanding of the meanings adolescents assign their own behaviors, we will fail to understand risk overall or serve them appropriately.

THE AHC EXPERIENCE:
HOW YOUTH DEVELOPMENT MIGHT WORK
IN HEALTH CARE

This paper was inspired, in part, by a conversation between its authors and the noted researcher on adolescents, Michael Resnick (personal communication, December 5, 2001). He posed a difficult challenge: "What might a youth development perspective look like in terms of mental health treatment for adolescents and how might it differ from current treatment that seems more pathology focused?" While we do not claim to answer that question completely here, we do believe that some of the experiences we have gained at the Mount Sinai Adolescent Health Center (AHC) provide a preliminary sketch of how YD is incorporated into health and mental health services.

For 35 years, AHC has provided comprehensive, holistic, confidential, and accessible health care to urban adolescents in the New York metropolitan area. AHC's organizational culture and persona combines elements of the academic medical center, of which it is a component, with a grassroots, community-based, high-volume service setting. Comprehensive medical, mental health and reproductive health services are provided in a freestanding facility to adolescents ages 10 through 21 years, who make more than 50,000 visits annually, with many more encounters occurring in school-based, college-based, and community-based settings.

AHC has no catchment area and serves adolescents from the entire New York metropolitan area. However, its *communities of concern* from which it draws most clients (i.e., East Harlem, Central Harlem, and the South Bronx) are classified as *Priority One Neighborhoods: Areas with severe health status problems* (Health Systems Agency, 1993). Such neighborhoods are characterized by extremely poor access to primary health and mental health care. Residents of these communities, mostly Latino and African-American, are three times more likely than the rest of New York City to be poor. Teen pregnancy rates are more than twice New York City averages. Sexually transmitted infection (STI) rates in these communities are more than twice the New York City average, with an even greater differential among teenagers. Adolescents from these communities experience high rates of early sexual activity, sexual activity with older partners, substance abuse, and family instability.

The latest AHC client census conveys a vivid profile of the vulnerable adolescents we engage. Ninety-nine percent are low-income, two-thirds are uninsured and most are of color (50% Latino, 43% African American, and 2% Asian). When routinely asked, of the female patients seen for a physical examination at AHC, 30% report a history of sexual abuse, incest, or sexual assault. Three-quarters of the male and female adolescents who receive AHC care are sexually active; 39% of females have a history of at least one pregnancy and 40% of those have been pregnant two or more times. Of adolescents seen at AHC, 65% have used alcohol, 54% have used marijuana or harder drugs, 49% report serious school problems, and 74% have witnessed significant violent events within their families or communities.

AHC PHILOSOPHY AND SERVICE DESIGN

AHC's philosophy drives its service design and programming. In an effort to promote accessibility, AHC tries to eliminate all barriers to service that might arise from a client's lack of health insurance, poor financial status, or judgment that using family health insurance will compromise his or her confidentiality. Services are easy to enter, and include an array of comprehensive health and mental health services that address adolescents' needs holistically. Because so many of our clients are poor, uninsured, or reluctant to use their parents' insurance, the Center's financial viability requires that a significant part of its effort be dedicated to fundraising and grant writing. Thus, services are offered for free to uninsured and underinsured adolescents who make up about 74% of AHC's clients.

This effort enables AHC to realize its mission of serving adolescents without regard for payment or insurance status. However, because grant funding can be categorical and can lead to a stratification of services–thus restricting the ability to address adolescents' needs in a holistic manner–AHC also strives to promote ongoing service review and redesign so that internal barriers between service specializations are minimized.

AHC is also a *safe place*, which requires staff to be clear about confidentiality guidelines and state laws protecting adolescent interests. Staff are trained to be comfortable with their ability to absorb and assess information about risky situations and behaviors and work with clients toward safe outcomes. Providing effective services for adolescents requires that practitioners be adept at dealing with parental concerns while maintaining confidentiality. For example, whereas only about half of the clients seeking mental health services choose initially to either inform or involve a parent, clinical staff are almost always able–over time–to bring parents into the picture in a manner that respects each adolescent's own pace and decision-making style.

Financial pressures and the demands of a busy clinic environment present significant barriers to maintaining the intensive supervision that is often required to enable practitioners to be comfortable in working confidentially with adolescents. Clinical supervision and consultation is an emphasis at AHC, and all practitioners participate in a variety of clinical support groups–which include a diverse mix of practitioners with a range of experience levels, specialties, and styles. Supervision groups are an effective way of creating adequate support–formal and informal–so that individual practitioners can maintain a balance between safely tolerating each adolescent's experimentation and working responsibly to ensure safety. In addition, every practitioner's *supervision package* is reviewed and redesigned annually, with many components being time-limited so that each clinician develops a wide range of core competencies over time.

Inevitably, AHC's mission includes advocacy at the federal, state, and local level, to increase adolescent access to care through policy change.

SERVICE APPROACH

AHC's approach is to collaboratively define client needs by asking clients directly and holistically about their health and mental health concerns and by assessing bio-psychosocial, cultural, and spiritual factors within the framework of developmental competence. Client needs are then addressed with a comprehensive range of services. In addition to physical, mental, and reproductive health, and health education, specialized services include HIV, rape, sexual abuse, dating violence, teen parenting, disordered eating, and more. AHC's services are designed to be adolescent friendly and culturally competent, with concerted outreach and coordinated follow-up that utilize family and community supports whenever possible.

Experience tells us that this requires time and some negotiation with clients who are hesitant to involve others. For mature teens aware of available services, this is less of a challenge than with highly vulnerable teens for whom systems navigation on their own is virtually impossible.

A PLACE TO TALK

Creating a safe place where adolescents can disclose their concerns requires providers to ask adolescents about their lives, as they need *permission to talk* about their own experiences. A national survey of adolescent girls (Schoen, Davis, Scott, & Collins et al., 1997) reveals that these girls wished their health care providers would ask about sensitive issues. In their experience, however, many providers had failed to do so. Even for teens who have access to care, the unresponsiveness and insensitivity of health and mental health systems to their developmental needs compromise care and limit *true* access. A recent study of adolescent risk-takers reports that 63% said they did not have the opportunity to speak with their health care providers about these risks, though many wished their providers were open to such discussions (Klein & Wilson, 2002).

More recently, research conducted at AHC reveals that clients who report, on an intake questionnaire, that they "don't know" whether they have been abused or raped or are in an abusive dating relationship are even more likely to want to talk about their safety with a counselor than those who can openly acknowledge this traumatic experience (Surko, Ciro, & Carlson et al., 2004). Clinical experience combined with empirical findings suggests that these adolescents are victims of trauma but are less equipped to deal with trauma than those who can more readily disclose that they have been traumatized. In other words, adolescents who state they are unsure if they have been forced to have sex are probably even more urgently in need of help than those who can clearly say they have been forced.

Weisz and Hawley (2002) have demonstrated the futility of simply extrapolating techniques from health and mental health services for adults for treatment with adolescents. The experience of the authors, and their colleagues at AHC, is consistent with this view. For example, Mirabito (2001) studied termination from AHC mental health services and found that, in contrast to theories derived from psychotherapy with adults, adolescents typically do not engage in a *termination process*. Instead, they simply stop coming. But by not formally acknowledging termination with their mental health provider, these adolescent clients say that they are *keeping the door open* for future service involvement. In their eyes, the therapeutic relationship remains open and continuously available to them.

At AHC, we have learned from our own research and from countless practice examples that to effectively serve adolescents they must feel they have permission to talk about their health concerns and that the meanings they ascribe to their experience will be respected. More generally, we have learned that we must be willing to set aside clinical lore that has been derived from work with adults and learn from what our clients tell us (and don't tell us).

Elsewhere Diaz and Manigat (1999) described an AHC practice begun in 1985, in which a physician interested in adolescent exposure to sexual abuse began asking clients directly about it during routine physical examinations. This approach disregarded theories that asking clients to self-disclose on first contact is ineffective because such experiences either are unavailable due to repression or would not be revealed because of the need to build a treatment relationship. Here again, theories derived from work with adults proved inapplicable to AHC clients. Thus, a one-year documentation of this practice during their annual physical produced a 23% disclosure rate.

Also discussed later in this volume is AHC's practice of routinely asking mental health clients at intake if they have experienced racism (Surko, Ciro, & Carlson et al., 2004). In a YD context, we view exposure to racism as highly relevant to client mental health and well-being. Rates of self-report of having experienced racism are as high as 40% and effective counseling with minority adolescents must take these experiences into account. Unfortunately however, few mental health providers who work with clients of color explore this issue directly and routinely from the start.

SETTING WIDE MARGINS

YD principles emphasize involving adolescents in decisions regarding their own services and respecting the uniqueness of their process. Involving young people in their health and mental health care in a way that builds their competence–a goal of all intervention–requires setting wide margins when assessing their behavioral risks. For example, this often involves respecting a client's desire not to address an issue at first even though the issue seems highly urgent to the practitioner. The practitioner must find comfortable ways of keeping the issue on the table and returning to it. How clinicians achieve this is discussed in detail elsewhere (Elliott, Nembhard, & Giannone et al., 2004). At the same time, involving young people in their health care decisions means making clear the ground rules such as when the clinician has to break confidentiality to ensure safety or acknowledging the clinician's feelings about important issues to address such as heavy substance use.

Most important is for practitioners to find ways to talk directly with young people about their concerns, and our concerns about them, while maintaining treatment where the client is rather than where the practitioner would like to be. This is in line with Zimring's (1982) learner's permit approach to work with adolescents, discussed earlier.

CLIENT INVOLVEMENT IN PROGRAMMING

YD framework urges that adolescents be involved in determining their service needs and planning their own programs. However, as part of a large academic medical center, AHC is not self-governing, disallowing adolescents to be formally involved in governance functions. The hierarchical and bureaucratic organizational culture of academic medical centers presents significant barriers to involving young people in governance. Nonetheless, creative ways are found to involve them–through program advisory boards that include consumers and focus groups concerning key initiatives.

One of the most significant ways that AHC involves adolescents in its organizational life is through its peer education program, now in its 16th year. Adolescents are recruited from the client population, trained in an 80-hour curriculum and paid to provide peer-to-peer community and school-based outreach, risk reduction education, health education and case finding. Though these 16-20 adolescents are paid for their work, they are considered clients. They attend individual therapy and a weekly support group, as well as ongoing training and supervision. This is necessary not only because they have the same levels of exposure to trauma and risk as our general client population, but also because other teens make disclosures, including serious risk exposure, to them. This can be highly stressful and requires ongoing support and professional guidance.

INNOVATIVE PROGRAMMING
AND ORGANIZATIONAL REFLECTIVITY

Remaining responsive to the needs of adolescents requires flexible programming that can use organizational reflection (Peake & Epstein, 2004) to learn and adapt. At times, AHC has been challenged in its attempt to maintain these *principles* in its practice. Flexible programming represents a major challenge for any organization, and more so for programs within large academic medical centers, which are often slow to change. It is an additional challenge in the face of severe budget constraints currently affecting such institutions, in which other constituencies may view a holistic approach to serving adolescents as a luxury beyond the proper scope of the institution and as an unnecessary financial drain. Innovation also requires organizational reflection and learning, which are best supported by organizational structures that are sufficiently flexible and open to identify new program needs and to incorporate into new practices into existing programs (Morgan, 1986). This, too, is in sharp contrast to conventional, bureaucratized organizational structures of academic medical centers.

How is reflection encouraged? At AHC, Practice-Based Research (PBR)–which engages practitioners in research but emphasizes practice relevance and client perspectives over research rigor (Epstein, 2001; Peake & Epstein, 2004)–is utilized alongside more conventional academic research methods more common in the medical field (Peake, Mirabito, Epstein, & Giannone, 2004). This volume is dedicated to exemplars of PBR in action, but other efforts at *reflection-in-action* (Schon, 1983) conducted over the years have included program design and innovation through client participation in focus groups, practitioner-designed assessment instruments, consumer feedback surveys, etc.

Finally, at AHC, having a director and management team that places considerable effort in obtaining both institutional buy-in and grant funding has resulted in a program that has considerable flexibility in structuring its services systems, short and long-term planning, operational decision-making, and budgeting. However, this requires a continuous re-commitment of energy and resources, and it can easily be overlooked in the course of daily administration. AHC addresses this potential barrier through periodic reevaluation, which includes an annual evaluation of the work environment and clinical support network by mental health program staff.

IMPLICATIONS FOR STAFFING

Serving vulnerable adolescents means recruiting, developing, and maintaining expert staff who are able to tolerate the ambiguities and challenges that are associated with clinical practice with this population. Practitioners need to be encouraged to innovate based on their practice experience and organizational support and resources must be made available to support reflection and innovation. Involving staff requires flexible and responsive decision-making structures. Mental health practitioners at AHC annually evaluate their practice environment, and this feedback is used in a continued redesign process. All AHC practitioners are expected, as they advance from beginner status, to develop expertise in a specialized area of adolescent care such as substance abuse, dating violence, rape, and incest, and are expected to participate in pro-

gram development. In addition to their general clinical practice, all practitioners are expected to develop a *portfolio* of responsibilities that includes administrative assignments. This model tends to reduce the potential for dichotomization of direct and administrative practice and allows faster, more effective
communication between practice and management.

Since mental health practitioners are expected to become adept at varying
aspects of work with adolescents, AHC management have developed written,
adolescent-specific, professional practice standards and competencies, along
with criteria for evaluating practitioner performance. These competencies–
which iterate the core skills required of practitioners, and performance evaluation standards and methods–are designed to embody the challenges of clinical
practice with urban adolescents. Core domains include patient evaluation,
professional and ethical practices, teamwork, ongoing clinical treatment, and
program development. Practitioners are expected to develop competency in
practice-based research (Epstein, 2001; Peake & Epstein, 2004), program development, and knowledge dissemination, within a culture in which practitioners are expected to be highly autonomous.

While this paper precludes the inclusion of this document a small sampling
illustrates how professional standards are codified and evaluated. For example, one core competency that requires that practitioners acquire *program development skills* is worded as follows:

> Adolescents . . . require creative approaches to service delivery. Integral
> to clinical practice with adolescents and their families is assessing and
> evaluating programmatic needs with the patient population, service area
> and communities served. The social worker must be able to initiate, plan
> and implement programmatic ideas to meet the needs of the program
> area and patient population; . . . demonstrate ability to develop program,
> and to use practice-based research and other evaluative approaches, in
> accordance with [professional and departmental] standards and program
> area needs and responsibilities.

Accompanying skills required include:

> [I]nterdisciplinary and community collaboration . . . ability to identify
> unmet psychosocial needs in the client population . . . engage and partic-
> ipate in practice research activities . . . the education and development of
> other staff members and patient populations . . . take initiative for [iden-
> tifying and addressing one's] own professional learning needs . . .

[U]tilizing in-house supervision, consultation, and educational resources both inside and outside of the institution.

As described elsewhere (Peake & Mirabito et al., 2004), practitioners were as instrumental in initiating and shaping this project as they are in defining the practice challenges they face every day.

A VISION FOR HEALTHY ADOLESCENT DEVELOPMENT

To promote the healthy development of urban adolescents, health systems need a multi-pronged approach. Adolescent-specific health services must be easily accessible. Practitioners must be trained in providing age-appropriate and culturally competent care. Staff must possess knowledge about health risks and risk management so that each adolescent served develops skills in problem solving and is capable of maintaining control over her or his own development. From the start, providers need to be able to get adolescents talking, keep them talking, and keep them thinking about their own risk behavior and development. Hence, the practitioner's role is to engage the client where she or he is, and make certain that any and all relevant issues are on the table, allowing adolescents permission to talk or not talk about any issue. Ultimately, the door to services must remain open, as adolescents should be able to return when they choose.

For healthy development of adolescents, Eccles et al. (1993) propose harmonizing adolescents' needs and opportunities for participation in decision-making. At AHC, our approach to promoting healthy behavior and development among adolescents is twofold: Fostering engagement in a therapeutic relationship so adolescents have a safe place to talk and building autonomy so that they can develop skills to manage their own risk behavior and development.

Clearly, in serving urban adolescents, medical, and mental health programs must be prepared to embrace difficult paradoxes and be simultaneously challenged and rewarded by working with this population. On the one hand, urban adolescents are high risk because of their experimentation, lack of experience in negotiating risky situations, and uncertainty with talking about their experiences with adults. Yet, they are also engaging, inquisitive, willing to learn new behaviors and able to participate in decisions about their services, health and mental health care, and about their future. The starting point for their participation is openly asking them about their lives and paying serious attention to their answers. That's what this volume is all about.

REFERENCES

American Medical Association. (1997). *American Medical Association: Guidelines for Adolescents Preventive Services.* Chicago, IL: American Medical Association.

Andrews, C.V., Garrison, C.Z., Jackson, K.L., Addy, C.L., & McKeown, R.E. (1992). Mother-adolescent agreement on the symptoms and diagnoses of adolescent depression and conduct disorders. *Journal of the American Academy of Child & Adolescent Psychiatry, 32,* 732-738.

Bailey, G.W. (1992). Children, adolescents, and substance abuse. *Journal of the American Academy of Child Adolescent Psychiatry, 31*(6), 1015-1018.

Blum, R., McNeely, C., & Nonnemaker, J. (2001). Vulnerability, risk, and protection. *Journal of Adolescent Health, 3,* 28-39.

Burke, K., Burke, J., Regier, D., & Rae, D. (1991). Comparing age onset of major depression and other psychiatric disorders by birth cohorts in five U.S. communities. *Archives of General Psychiatry, 47,* 511-518.

Cohn, I.D., McFarlane, S., Yanez, C., & Imai, W.K. (1995). Risk-perception: Differences between adolescents and adults. *Health Psychology, 14*(3), 217-222.

Diaz, A., & Manigat, N. (1999). The health care provider's role in the disclosure of sexual abuse: The medical interview as a gateway to disclosure. *Children's Health Care Journal, 28*(2), 141-149.

Dougherty, D.M. (1993). Adolescent health: Reflections on a report to the U.S. Congress. *American Psychologist, 48*(2), 193-201.

Dryfoos, J.G. (1990). *Adolescents at Risk.* New York: Oxford University Press.

Durant, R.H., Seymore, C., & Jay, M.S. (1991). Adolescent compliance with therapeutic regimens. In W.R. Hendee (Ed.), *The Health of Adolescents.* San Francisco: American Medical Association–Jossey Bass Publishers.

Eccles, J.S., Midgely, C., Wigfield, A., Buchanan, C.M., Reuman, D., Flangan, C., & MacIver, D. (1993). Development during adolescence: The impact of stage-environment fit on young adolescents' experiences in schools and in families. *American Psychologist, 48*(2), 90-101.

Elliott, J., Nembhard, M., Giannone, V., Surko, M., Medeiros, D., & Peake, K. (2004). Clinical Uses of an Adolescent Intake Questionnaire: Adquest as a bridge to engagement. *Social Work in Mental Health, 3*(1/2), 83-102.

Epstein, I. (2001). Using available clinical information in practice-based research: Mining for silver while dreaming of gold. *Social Work in Health Care, 33*(3/4), 15-32.

Fahs, P.S., Smith, B.E., Ata, A.S., Britt, M.X., Collins, M.S., Morgan, L.S., & Spencer, G.A. (1999). Integrative research review of risk behaviors among adolescents in rural, suburban and urban areas. *Journal of Adolescent Health, 24*(4), 230-243.

Health Systems Agency. (1993). *Framework for Primary Care Needs Assessment,* Health Systems Agency, New York City.

Hendee, W.R. (Ed.) (1991). *The Health of Adolescents.* San Francisco: American Medical Association–Jossey Bass Publishers.

Jessor, R.M. (1991). Risk behavior in adolescence: A framework for understanding and action. *Journal of Adolescent Health, 12*(8), 597-605.

Kandel, D., & Yamaguchi, K. (1993). From beer to crack: Developmental patterns of drug involvement. *American Journal of Public Health, 83*(3), 852-855.

Kazdin, A.E. (1993). Adolescent mental health: Prevention and treatment programs. *American Psychologist, 48*(2), 127-141.

Kerstenbaum, C. (2002). How shall we treat the children in the 21st Century. *Journal of the American Academy of Child & Adolescent Psychiatry, 39*, 1-10.

Klein, J., & Wilson, K. (2002). Delivering quality care: Adolescents' discussion of health risks with their providers. *Journal of Adolescent Health, 30*, 190-195.

Larson, R. W. (2002). Toward a psychology of positive youth development. *American Psychologist, 55* (1), 170-183.

MacKenzie, R.G. (1991). Adolescent substance abuse. In W.R. Hendee (Ed.), *The Health of Adolescents*. San Francisco: American Medical Association–Jossey Bass Publishers.

Mechanic, D. (1991). Adolescents at risk: New directions. *Journal of Adolescent Health, 12*(8), 638-643.

Millstein, S.G., Irwin, C.E., & Brindis, C.D. (1991). Sociodemographic trends in the adolescent population. In W.R. Hendee (Ed.), *The Health of Adolescents*. San Francisco: American Medical Association–Jossey Bass Publishers.

Mirabito, D.M. (2001). Mining treatment termination data in an adolescent mental health service: A quantitative study. *Social Work in Health Care, 33*(3/4), 71-90.

Morgan, G. (1986). *Images of Organization*. California: Sage Publications.

National Adolescent Health Information Center. (2000). Fact Sheet on Adolescent Demographics. National Adolescent Health Information Center. University of California, San Francisco. Retrieved August 25, 2002 from *http://youth.ucsf.edu/nahic/img/Demographics.pdf*

National Center for Education Statistics. (2001). Statistical Analysis Report: Dropout Rates in the U.S. 2000. U.S. Department of Education. Retrieved August 25, 2002 from *http://nces.ed.gov/pubs2002/2002114.pdf*

National Institutes of Health. (1997). *Women of Color Health Data Book*. Department of Health and Human Services. Office of Research on Women's Health. NIH Publication no. 02-4247.

National Research Council and Institute of Medicine. Committee on Community-Level Programs for Youth. Board on Children, Youth, and Families, Division of Behavioral and Social Sciences and Education. (2002). J. Eccles, & J.A. Gootman (Eds.), *Community Programs to Promote Youth Development*. Washington, DC: National Academy Press.

Neinstein, L. (1996). Vital Statistics and Injuries. In L. Neinstein (Ed.), *Adolescent Health Care a Practical Guide, 3rd Edition*. Baltimore: Williams and Wilkin.

Newacheck, P., Brindis, C., Uhler Cart, C., Marchi, K., & Irwin, C. (1999). Adolescent health insurance coverage: Recent changes and access to care. *Pediatrics, 104*(2), 195-202.

Offer, D., & Schonert-Reichl, K.A. (1992). Debunking the myths of adolescence: Findings from recent research. *Journal of the American Academy of Child & Adolescent Psychiatry, 31*(6), 1002-1014.

Peake, K., & Epstein, I. (2004). Theoretical and practical imperatives for reflective social work Organizations in health and mental health: The place of practice-based research. *Social Work in Mental Health, 3*(1/2), 23-37.

Peake, K., Mirabito, D., Epstein, I., & Giannone, V., (2004). Creating and sustaining a practice-based research group in an urban adolescent mental health program. *Social Work in Mental Health, 3*(1/2), 39-54.

Petersen, A. C. (1980). Developmental issues in adolescent health. In T.J. Coates, A. C. Petersen, and C. Perry (Eds.), *Promoting Adolescent Health: A Dialog Between Research and Practice*. New York: Academic Press.

Pittman, K., Irby, M., & Ferber, T. (2000). Unfinished business: Further reflections on a decade of promoting youth development. In *Youth Development: Issues, Challenges, and Directions*. Philadelphia, PA: Public/Private Ventures.

Powers, S.I., Hauser, S.T., & Kilner, L.A. (1989). Adolescent mental health. *American Psychologist, 44*(2), 200-208.

Quadrel, M.J., Fischoff, B., & Davis, W. (1993). Adolescent (In)vulnerability. *American Psychologist, 48*(2), 102-116.

Resnick, G., & Burt, M.R. (1996). Youth at risk: Definitions and implications for service delivery. *American Journal of Orthopsychiatry, 66*(2), 172-188.

Sarri, R., & Sarri, C. (1992). Organizational and community change through participatory action research. *Administration in Social Work, 16*(3-4), 99-122.

Scales, P.C., & Leffert, N. (1999). *Developmental Assets: A Synthesis of the Scientific Research on Adolescent Development*. Minneapolis, MN: Search Institute.

Schoen, C., Davis, K., Scott Collins, K., Greenberg, L., Des Roches, C., & Abrams, M. (1997). The Commonwealth Fund Survey of the Health of Adolescent Girls. New York: The Commonwealth Fund. Retrieved on August 18, 2002 from *http://www.cmwf.org/programs/women/adoleshl.asp#GIRLS*

Schon, D. (1983). *The Reflective Practitioner: How Professionals Think in Action*. New York: Basic Books.

Shapiro, R., & Seigel, A.W. (1998). Risk-taking patterns of female adolescents. *Journal of Adolescence, 21*(2), 143-159.

Stanton, B.F., Fang, X., Li, X., Feigelman, S., Galbraith, J., & Ricardo, I. (1997). Evolution of risk behaviors over 2 years among a cohort of urban African American children. *Archives of Pediatric Medicine, 151*, 398-406.

Surko, M., Ciro, D., Carlson, E., Labor, N., Giannone, V., Diaz-Cruz, E., Peake, K., & Epstein, I. (2004). Which adolescents need to talk about safety and violence? *Social Work in Mental Health, 3*(1/2), 103-119.

U.S. Bureau of the Census. (2001). Resident Population Estimates of the United States by Age and Sex. Population Estimates Program, Population Division, U.S. Census Bureau, Washington, DC.

U.S. General Accounting Office. (1996). At Risk and Delinquent Youth, Multiple Federal Programs Raise Efficiency Programs. GAO-HEHS. 96-34: Washington, DC: U.S. General Accounting Office.

Weisz, J.R., & Hawley, K.M. (2002). Developmental factors in the treatment of adolescents. *Journal of Consulting and Clinical Psychology, 7*(1), 21-43.

Zaslow, M.J., & Takanishi, R. (1993). Priorities for research on adolescent development. *American Psychologist, 48*(2), 185-192.

Zimring, F.E. (1982). *The Changing Legal World of Adolescence*. New York: Free Press.

Ziv, A., Boulet, J.R., & Slap, G.B. (1999). Utilization of physician offices by adolescents in the United States. *Pediatrics, 104*(1), 35-42.

Theoretical and Practical Imperatives for Reflective Social Work Organizations in Health and Mental Health: The Place of Practice-Based Research

Ken Peake
Irwin Epstein

SUMMARY. This article describes the common challenges to health and mental health organizations that require these agencies to become more "reflective" in their culture and structures. This necessitates integrating practice and research at all organizational levels. Schon's concept of *reflective practice* to health and mental health organizations is extended to develop the construct of a *reflective organization*, in which direct practitioners are integral to organizational learning through ongoing service evaluation and redesign. The theoretical and practical reasons why social work administrators and clinicians alike are obliged to integrate practice and research are discussed. University-based models of prac-

---

Ken Peake, DSW, is Assistant Director, Mount Sinai Adolescent Health Center, 320 East 94th Street, New York, NY 10128. Irwin Epstein, PhD, is Helen Rehr Professor of Applied Social Work Research in Health, Hunter College School of Social Work, 129 East 79th Street, New York, NY 10021.

[Haworth co-indexing entry note]: "Theoretical and Practical Imperatives for Reflective Social Work Organizations in Health and Mental Health: The Place of Practice-Based Research." Peake, Ken, and Irwin Epstein. Co-published simultaneously in *Social Work in Mental Health* (The Haworth Social Work Practice Press, an imprint of The Haworth Press, Inc.) Vol. 3, No. 1/2, 2004, pp. 23-37; and: *Clinical and Research Uses of an Adolescent Mental Health Intake Questionnaire: What Kids Need to Talk About* (ed: Ken Peake, Irwin Epstein, and Daniel Medeiros) The Haworth Social Work Practice Press, an imprint of The Haworth Press, Inc., 2005, pp. 23-37. Single or multiple copies of this article are available for a fee from The Haworth Document Delivery Service [1-800-HAWORTH, 9:00 a.m. - 5:00 p.m. (EST). E-mail address: docdelivery@haworthpress.com].

http://www.haworthpress.com/web/SWMH
© 2004 by The Haworth Press, Inc. All rights reserved.
Digital Object Identifier: 10.1300/J200v03n01_02

tice-research integration impede this process; Epstein's *Practice-Based Research* approach facilitates it. *[Article copies available for a fee from The Haworth Document Delivery Service: 1-800-HAWORTH. E-mail address: <docdelivery@haworthpress.com> Website: <http://www.HaworthPress.com> © 2004 by The Haworth Press, Inc. All rights reserved.]*

KEYWORDS. Reflective practice, reflective organization, organizational learning, practice-based research, practitioner research

WHY CREATE A REFLECTIVE CULTURE? EXTERNAL CHALLENGES TO HEALTH AND MENTAL HEALTH ORGANIZATIONS

A turbulent environment of fiscal constraint, managed care, shrinking resources and political ill will toward social work programs is shaping direct service and management practice. Both direct practitioners and managers must do more with less (Almgren, 1998; Carpenter & Platt, 1997; Globerman, 1999; Segal, 1999). Sound decisions about resource use and the ability to show positive client outcomes are critical. In health care settings, where psychosocial services may not be considered mission critical/core activities, trends in the financing and organization of care increasingly necessitate the justification of services in terms of the financial "bottom line" (Martin & Kettner, 1997). Even in mental health services, where social work may be valued as mission critical and cost effective, there is a trend toward "evidence-based practice" principles (Gambrill, 1999). As a result, familiarity with research principles and ability to navigate the historical divide between practice and research will be essential skills if practice wisdom is to be given voice in defining best practices.

While managing with reduced resources, being accountable, and justifying services, social work programs must simultaneously build capacity in the face of increased interorganizational competition for dollars and, for social workers in host settings, intra-organizational competition. Accordingly, the concept of accountability is expanding exponentially to include compliance with legal, professional, credentialing and funding mandates, consumer satisfaction and performance measurement–in terms of effective outcomes and cost containment (Martin & Kettner, 1997). The expansion of the concept of accountability to incorporate effectiveness and value for money spent on services has been termed *effects management* (Grasso & Epstein, 1987). As a result, we are challenged to integrate information-gathering and evaluative methodologies into all aspects of organizational practice. Paradoxically, this comes at a time when practitioners have less time and opportunity to assimilate research than ever before (Motenko, Allen, Angelos, Block, & DeVito et al., 1995; Reid, 1997; Strom & Gingerich, 1993).

At the service level, clinicians face additional paradoxes. Siporin (1992) notes that scarcity requires innovative service approaches, which are best achieved when clinician and manager roles are flexible and when time for reflection is available. Yet difficult times often exacerbate strains between practitioners and managers regarding professional autonomy versus organizational control (Grasso & Epstein, 1987; Patti, 1983).

For direct service workers, the result is an incremental but substantial expansion of roles and, often, less autonomy in decisions regarding their interventions. Simultaneously, clinicians now are asked to participate widely in accountability and evaluative systems, program development, and other organizational processes once considered purely management functions (Carpenter & Platt, 1997; Segal, 1999). Meenaghan (1998) succinctly summarizes the challenge saying that contemporary practitioners must become "program actors in a policy environment." How professionally prepared and organizationally supported they are for these changing roles is an open question.

Strom and Gingerich (1993, p. 79) point out that "The forces influencing service delivery are numerous and varied. They do not lend themselves to linear cause-and-effect explanations. Rather these issues, individually and in concert with others, help to shape the auspices under which services are provided, who may deliver and who may receive them and the conditions under which services may occur." Their organizational consequences–both positive and negative–are complex, interrelated, and multi-causal.

Though some authors cited earlier (Globerman, 1999; Woodrow & Ginsberg, 1997) have suggested that social workers may be well suited to cope with these sweeping changes in the practice environment, there are many indications that direct practitioners are experiencing severe strains to their professional identities as result (Carpenter & Platt, 1997; Chernus, 1999; Galambos, 1999; Gibelman & Whiting, 1999). Several effects of change have been documented in the literature.

In both the for-profit and nonprofit sectors, the pressure to reduce service costs has led to a tendency for clinical judgments to be replaced by treatment time limits (Borenstein, 1990). With managed care, the prescription of set lengths of service for different problem diagnoses may result in clients being "under-treated." This is one result of the "limitations of placing complex problems, often with systematic causes, into narrow individual diagnoses" (Strom & Gingerich, 1993, p. 80).

As a result, social workers are often caught between competing priorities–the needs of the individual client versus service limitations due to financial auspices and institutional pressures. Such conditions limit professional autonomy, clinical judgment, and the ability of practitioners to respond to the *whole person* in the context of the social environment. These limits conflict with core service values of the profession. With reduced supervisory staff social work managers must develop innovative ways to provide support to direct service practitioners and create appropriate vehicles to address these practice dilemmas.

Unlike clinicians, most social work managers recognize applied research and evaluation methodologies as central to their daily work (Weinbach, 1985). Practitioners on the other hand, have been described historically as wary of research, unskilled in it, and as not seeing its relevance to practice (Adler, Alfs, Greeman, Manske, & McClellan et al., 1993; Epstein, 1996; Sidell, Barnhart, Bowman, Fitzpatrick, & Full et al., 1996; Subramian, Siegel, & Garcia, 1994; Pruett, Shea, Zimmerman, & Parish, 1991). Longstanding fissures between practice and evaluation, research and accountability, have led to the characterization in social work literature of a "continuing crisis" between social work practice and research (Lindsay & Kirk, 1992, p. 370). Though considerable disagreement exists about its causes and "cure" (Epstein, 2001; Blumenfield & Epstein, 2001), the term "crisis" symbolizes the longstanding dichotomization of practice and research.

LEARNING FROM PRACTICE: THE REFLECTIVE ORGANIZATION

Over the last fifteen years, Schon's reflective practice paradigm (1983) has been applied to the study of social work practice in general (DeRoos, 1990; Goldstein, 1993; Harrison, 1987), to administrative practice (Bernstein & Epstein, 1992) and to practitioner research (Epstein, 2001; Fook, 1997).

Briefly stated for the moment (as the authors will return to the concept more fully shortly), reflective practice is a method of inquiry into the way that professionals–such as social workers–frame and conduct their everyday work. It assumes that in professional practice theorizing, thinking and action are not distinct activities, separated in time, but occur concurrently. It has been defined in the following way:

> [A] reflective approach acknowledges that, contrary to the idea that formal theorizing precedes action in a linear (from cause to effect) and deductive relationship, theory is typically implicit in a person's actions and may or may not be congruent with the theoretical assumptions the per-

son believes themself [*sic*] to be acting upon. In Argyris and Schon's terms (1974), there may be a difference between the theory implicit in action ('theory-in-use') and the theoretical assumptions a person might consciously articulate ('espoused theory'). (Fook, 1997, p. 4)

A reflective practice approach to inquiry can be said to seek to make explicit and evident both theories in use and espoused theories and examine the interaction between them and their impact on practitioner's approaches to problem solving in everyday practice situations.

More recently, Blumenfield and Epstein (2001) described efforts at Mount Sinai Medical Center to foster reflective clinical practice in a hospital social work department. Key processes and structures they highlighted included performance evaluation using ongoing feedback to build on practitioner strengths; a reward system that reinforced integration of research and practice, continuing education in clinical evaluation and access to practice-research consultation.

However, the broader construct of a "reflective organization," in which practitioners are integral to ongoing program evaluation and service design, remains relatively unexplored in social work. This article is about an attempt to do so. This collection of papers represents the product of this effort.

Admittedly, our concept of reflective organization is an *ideal* to which we aspire, rather than one we have attained. It is drawn from our own experiences in administrative practice, in clinical social work and in practice-research consultation. Its theoretical underpinnings come from the writings of several organizational theorists (Argyris & Schon, 1992; Austin, 1989; Brown & Duguid, 1991; DeRoos, 1990; Morgan, 1986) and, in particular, from Schon's (1983) seminal construct "reflection-in-action."

Although traditional rational-bureaucratic theories of organizational problem solving have been replaced with paradigms in which non-logical processes balance competing values and constraints (Simon, 1957; Patti, 1978; Morgan, 1986), practitioners' contributions to organizational development have been poorly understood and generally ignored (Weissman, Epstein, & Savage, 1983). Within social work settings, this is due in part to the theoretical dichotomization of clinical and administrative practice in social work literature and training (Meenaghan, 1995; 1998). However, Schon's concept of "reflection-in-action," which models how professionals confront challenging practice dilemmas, can be extended to understand how practitioners at every level in the agency hierarchy can participate in shaping their workplace through practice-based research.

A complex process but simply stated, reflection-in-action posits that as they routinely work, *practitioners engage simultaneously in thinking, theory-*

testing and theory-development (i.e., development of practice wisdom) *in interrelated processes that are inseparable from their actions.* Because practice problems are complex, without obvious solutions or clearly definable ends, purely bureaucratic or technical solutions rarely succeed. Instead, reflective clinical practice is an inductive process of "framing" each new practice situation in terms of a solvable problem. According to Schon (1983), all professional practitioners confront practice challenges by applying what he refers to as "theories-in-use," which are experience-based systems of thought that use analogic thinking and exemplars derived from previous situations.

Extending this concept to organizational dynamics, Argyris and Schon (1992) suggest that organizational theories-in-use are usually unstated. Rather, they are embedded in, and shape all organizational activities. And, the practices they generate are frequently extremely *valuable*, whether or not they are congruent with officially sanctioned, bureaucratic means and ends. Organizations that maximize these values may be said to be *reflective*.

WHAT IS A REFLECTIVE SOCIAL WORK ORGANIZATION?

The essence of a reflective organization lies in its ability to innovate by gathering and examining information about actual (rather than canonical) practices, learning what is valuable, adapting and changing when necessary. Morgan (1986) characterizes the challenge of organizational innovation as follows:

> [I]nnovative organizations must be designed as learning systems that place primary emphasis on being open to inquiry and self-criticism . . . The challenge to design organizations that can innovate is thus really the challenge to design organizations that can self-organize. For unless an organization is able to change itself to accommodate the ideas it produces and values, it is likely to block its own innovations. (p. 105)

Morgan (1986, p. 82) views highly "bureaucratized" organizations as poorly suited to learning because they are designed to achieve control and predictability. Consequently, during turbulent times and in uncertain conditions, they often experience "information and decision overload." More "organic," less programmed organizational styles with "flexible and *ad hoc*" approaches are better suited to adaptation.

Similarly, Brown and Duguid (1991) frame organizational learning as the bridge between everyday work and innovation. In their view, organizational change it is not a highly specialized, administrative function. Practitioners are integral to it. However, realizing this vision requires that the means and mechanisms for learning are evident at all levels of the organizational structure and culture, and that practitioners and managers have flexible, programmatically relevant role expectations.

More specifically, the authors suggest that reflective social work organizations must involve practitioners in four key activities intended to enhance *both* individual practice and program effectiveness: (1) Evaluation of services in relation to mission, consumer needs, and external environment; (2) Learning exchanges between organizational subsystems, a conception of systematic intervention in the "organization as client" that social workers may be well suited (Globerman, 1999; Globerman Davies & Walsh, 1996; Woodrow & Ginsberg, 1997); (3) Iteration of practice dilemmas and challenges within the service context; and (4) Iteration of practice competencies (in the context of the full scope of agency activities) that are the basis for individual performance appraisal.

INTERNAL PROGRAM AND POLICY CHALLENGES FACING PRACTICE SETTINGS

Because each of the aforementioned activities entails practitioner engagement in an array of reflective and evaluative activities, practitioners are challenged to expand their professional identities and orientation. Furthermore, they need to be prepared to exploit any opportunity that arises for direct involvement in shaping organizational practice. This requires a view of the practice setting as "client," i.e., as a system deserving of intervention effort. Simultaneously they are also challenged to derive and iterate the programmatic and policy lessons that can be learned from practice dilemmas (Meenaghan, 1995). If lessons are to be learned and applied to improving agency practices in general, practitioners must be able to build upon their assessment and evaluation skills by using research methodologies to examine their practice in the agency context.

In turn, managers are challenged. They must learn to facilitate vehicles that build to partnerships with direct service practitioners to improve efficiency and incorporate effects measurement into all aspects of practice. These vehicles must be flexible and non-bureaucratic if they are to bridge the management/practice divide and truly engage practitioners in the process of organizational learning. Simultaneously they must offer supports, training and rewards for practitioner engagement in ever widening professional roles, i.e., practitioner involvement in what were once considered purely *management* functions.

RESEARCH CHALLENGES FACING PRACTICE SETTINGS

The challenges described above, in turn create two highly interrelated, collective *practice-research challenges* for social work clinicians, management practitioners and educators in health and mental health services: (1) Managers, clinicians, and academic research consultants must integrate research and evaluation methodologies into all levels of organizational practice to ensure that *accountability* becomes an instrument of survival, adaptability, service enhancement and innovation; (2) Academics along with practitioners must develop new service-sensitive research and evaluation models that direct practitioners and managers to find practical, useful and beneficial in terms of the everyday challenges that they face.

IF PRACTITIONERS ARE TO ROUTINELY INCORPORATE RESEARCH, WHAT MODELS OF RESEARCH-PRACTICE INTEGRATION ARE MOST COMPATIBLE WITH PRACTICE?

For decades, research-practice models that involve partnership between academia and agency have been explicitly and implicitly advocated by proponents of Research Based Practice (RBP) and developed by academic researchers (Blythe, Tripodi, & Briar, 1994; Penka & Kirk, 1991; Fischer, 1993). However, those described in the literature (Pruett at al., 1994; Young, 1986; Subramian et al., 1994; Turnbull, Saltz, & Gwyther, 1988) fail to outline methods for addressing the differing agendas and methodologies that agency and academia each bring to the table and differentially value the contributions that each might make. Perhaps because RBP proponents tend to view agency and practice priorities as deficiencies, resulting from practitioner resistance to scientific methods or as obstacles to be overcome, they resist accommodating research strategies to practice settings.

And as guests in host settings (an unfortunate if accurate metaphor), it is reasonable to expect academic researchers to sensitively assess levels of access to patients and records, staff's willingness to fill out research forms, and the *stability* of the setting. However, an important opportunity for successful practice-research integration is missed when researchers do not fully include practitioners in the determination of the goals of inquiry based on its potential benefits to practice. It is essential that researchers not ignore practitioners' needs for understanding and instead simply provide training *to* staff in order to recruit research subjects.

For these reasons and others, Epstein (1995) is critical of the ability of university-initiated, research-driven programs to bridge the practice-research gulf. Strom and Gingerich (1993) point out that a related problem of the academic-practice partnership model is its "failure to meet current market conditions," that call for "practical evaluation . . . rather than sophisticated research designs" (p. 82). To be practice-relevant, research methodologies must accommodate the norms and ethical principles of 'best practice' in real settings and be useful in decision-making at every level of practice. In our view however, *the university-based, over-emphasis on efficacy has blinded the field to the benefits of research to practice as defined by practitioners themselves*.

Unfortunately, Blumenfield and Epstein (2001, p. 2) point out that the perception that practitioners are uninterested in research is "self-perpetuating" and real in its consequences. In the classroom and in the literature, the constancy of this message and the preoccupation with "gold-standard" experimental designs creates in practitioners a "trained incapacity to engage in research because their understanding of what research is, is overly perfectionist, incompatible with their practice values and/or their organizational role requirements."

We propose that a practice-based research approach (Epstein, 2001) is most suited to address these problems.

RESEARCH-BASED PRACTICE
VERSUS PRACTICE-BASED RESEARCH

Although many social work researchers have emphasized the importance of practice research, Epstein (2001) draws distinctions between Practice-Based Research (PBR) and Research-Based Practice (RBP). He describes RBP as "the use of research-based concepts, theories, designs and data-gathering instruments to structure practice so that hypotheses concerning cause-effect relationships between social work interventions and outcomes may be rigorously tested" (3). RBP represents the idealized academic approach to practice-research integration in social work.

By contrast, Practice-Based Research is "the use of research-inspired principles, designs, and information-gathering techniques within existing forms of practice to answer questions that emerge from practice in ways that inform practice" (4). It is naturalistic, heuristic, reflective, inductive (with key ideas derived from practice wisdom), non-experimental, or quasi-experimental, and its aim is to generate descriptive or correlational knowledge. Its uniqueness lies in the extensive involvement of practitioners in all aspects of research implementation.

While both RBP and PBR are strategies to integrate research and practice methodologies, to enhance the knowledge base and to improve the effectiveness of practitioners, each approach differs significantly in its aspirations. RBP aspires for knowledge about social work efficacy. In other words, it seeks definitive answers about what works and what does not work in practice. Implicitly, it is based on the assumption that *all* practice can and should be driven by research, and the efficacy of interventions should be demonstrated before they are selected (Bloome, Fischer, & Orme, 1995; Blythe et al., 1994; Fischer & Corcoran, 1994). The "empirical practice movement" (Fischer, 1993; Reid, 1994) and the "scientific practice movement" (Meyer, 1996) exemplify this approach.

Elsewhere, Epstein (2001) characterizes RBP as embracing the "gold standard" of academic research: it is deductive, in that it starts with a theoretically driven premise; it seeks knowledge that is causal, through research that approximates experimental, randomized control group methods as closely as possible; it is prospective; and it relies on standardized, quantitative instruments. Although RBP proponents advocate collaborative models, research priorities outweigh practice principles in the design and implementation of their studies.

Alternatively, PBR is initially inductive though it by no means ignores the research literature. However, its starting point is not social science or social work theory but practice wisdom, i.e., "currently accepted social work practice principles or organizationally embedded program theories" (Epstein, 2001, p. 4). More flexible than RBP (though some would say less rigorous), it can be retrospective or prospective, qualitative or quantitative, based on available or original information. In gathering original data, PBR emphasizes instrumentation tailored to practice needs rather than externally standardized research measures. It treats practice and research as organically related endeavors that can enhance one another by building on commonalties and parallels between them. Ultimately however, PBR is utilitarian rather than "truth" seeking, with practice principles defining its agenda. When there is conflict between the two, practice priorities outweigh research considerations. Most important, in PBR research questions are derived from practice and service delivery problems and attempt to address them.

Despite the obstacles to practitioner research that have been described earlier in this article, there is growing evidence that practitioners may not be as research averse as many academics suggest. So for example, Sidell et al. (1996) describe a successful practitioner-driven research study conducted in a health setting. In addition to generating valuable program-relevant information, the study resulted in additional resources, publications, and enhanced collegial interactions among social workers. Nonetheless, the authors warn that sustaining practitioner interest and motivation required considerable effort. "[T]he process of research takes time and it was with a dawning realization that clinicians recognized the much slower pace of research projects [as compared to] the fast paced, task-oriented practice environment (Sidell et al., 1996, p. 108)."

In a published collection PBR studies in health, Blumenfield and Epstein (2001), suggest that practitioner aversion to research is a "myth" or "half-truth" based on an overly narrow, context-insensitive conception of research that has been taught to practitioners. Two practitioner-researchers who contributed to that collection reported many "secondary" benefits of the research experience to their practice including the ability to conduct more comprehensive client assessments, more comprehensive record keeping, enhanced intra- and inter-disciplinary relationships, more positive attitudes about research and researchers, increased professional pride, and greater prestige in their organization and beyond (Hutson & Lichtiger, 2001).

In another compendium of practice-research studies, Rehr, Rosenberg, and Blumenfield (1998) demonstrate that practitioners have the research capacity and interest to make significant knowledge contributions to the field through publications in peer-review journals–calling for practitioner adoption of a PBR approach. Although university-based researchers are judged by their journal productivity, it should be clear, however, that peer-review publications are not the only vehicles for knowledge generation and dissemination.

The research-dissemination activities of practitioners at the Mount Sinai Adolescent Health Center (AHC), described elsewhere in this collection (Peake, Mirabito, Epstein, Giannone, & Hoffman, 2004), suggest that the overemphasis on published studies obscures the motivating effects of conference presentations, grand rounds and other forms of peer communication to agency-based practitioners. Equally important is the contribution that research ways of thinking contribute to daily practice. At the very least, the difficulty in engaging practitioners in research may have been grossly overestimated. More likely, it results from a very particular, academic model of practice-research integration and dissemination.

CONCLUSION

Clearly, changes in the practice environment create challenges not only for practitioners and managers but also for academics and researchers. Efforts to develop new practice approaches and to prepare new social workers for this changing world have been hampered by the dichotomization, common in the literature and in academia, between clinical practice and administrative practice, and between research/knowledge building and practice. The paradigm of the reflective organization social work organization that offers a framework for defining and bridging these divides and identifies organizational strategies that can be developed by practitioners and *designed into* practice settings. Practice-Based Research is offered as one vehicle for developing reflection and for building learning partnerships that incorporate the experiences, perspectives, and knowledge of clinical and management practitioners to improve agency practice.

However, as is evident from the literature on PBR and reflective learning in social work settings (Sidell et al., 1996; Blumenfield & Epstein, 2001; Rehr et al., 1998) and from the AHC experience, described elsewhere in this collection (Peake, Mirabito et al., 2004) the success of this approach depends on a number of factors.

First and foremost it requires a sustained effort that genuinely seeks practitioner voice and this, in turn, requires that administrators make it a core organizational strategic priority.

Second, its aim should be to become embedded in all organizational practices. As is clear from organizational learning theorists (Argyris & Schon, 1992; Morgan, 1986), organizational reflection and innovation is predicated upon the willingness of organizational leaders to integrate lessons learned and to change organizational practice.

In short, developing truly reflective organizational processes cannot be a short-term strategy or fad, or an afterthought. It requires leadership, investment of scarce resources and broad-scale practitioner involvement.

REFERENCES

Adler, G., Alfs, D., Greeman, M. Manske, J., McClellan, T., O'Brien, N., and Quam, J. (1993). Social work practitioners as researchers: Is it possible? *Social Work in Health Care* 19 (2): 115-127.
Almgren, G. (1998). Mental health practice in primary care: Some perspectives concerning the future of social work in organized delivery systems. *Smith College Studies in Social Work* 68 (2): 233-253.
Argyris, C., and Schon, D. (1974). *Theory in practice: Increasing professional effectiveness.* San Francisco: Jossey-Bass.
Argyris C., and Schon, D. (1992). *Organizational Learning: II: Theory, Method and Practice.* Reading, MA: Addison Wesley Publishing.

Austin, D. M. (1989). The human service executive. *Administration in Social Work* 13 (3/4): 13-36.

Bernstein, S., and Epstein, I. (1994). Grounded theory meets the reflective practitioner: Integrating qualitative and quantitative methods in administrative practice. In E. Sherman, and W. Reid (Eds.), *Qualitative Research in Social Work*. 435-444. New York: Columbia University Press.

Bloom, M., Fischer, J., and Orme, J. (1995). *Evaluating Practice: Guidelines for the Accountable Professional (2nd Edition)*. Englewood Cliffs, NJ: Prentice-Hall.

Blumenfield, S., and Epstein, I. (2001). Promoting and maintaining a reflective professional staff in a hospital-based social work department. *Social Work in Health Care* 33 (3/4): 1-13.

Blythe, B., Tripodi, T., and Briar, S. (1994). *Direct Practice Research in Human Service Agencies*. New York: Columbia University Press.

Borenstein, D. B. (1990). Managed care: A means of rationing psychiatric treatment. *Hospital and Community Mental Health Journal* 27: 225-229.

Brown, J. S., and Duguid, P. (1991). Organizational learning and communities-of-practice: Towards a unified view of working, learning and innovation. Special issue: Organizational learning: Papers in honor of (and by) James Marsh. *Organizational Science* 2 (1): 40-57.

Carpenter, M. C., and Platt, S. (1997). Professional identity for clinical social workers: Impact of changes in health care delivery systems. *Clinical Social Work Journal* 25 (3): 337-350.

Chernus, L. (1999). Is "humane managed care" an oxymoron? *Smith College Studies in Social Work* 69 (3): 559-572.

DeRoos, Y. S. (1990). The development of practice wisdom through human problem solving processes. *Social Service Review* 64 (2): 276-287.

Epstein, I. (1995). Promoting reflective social work practice: Research strategies and consulting principles. In E. J. Mullen, and J. L. Magnabosco (Eds.), *Practitioner-Researcher Partnerships: Building Knowledge From, In, and For Practice*. 83-102. Washington D.C.: NASW Press.

Epstein, I. (1996). In quest of a research-based model for social work practice: Or why can't a social worker be more like a researcher? *Social Work Research and Abstracts* 20 (2): 97-100.

Epstein, I. (2001). Using available clinical information in practice-based research: Mining for silver while dreaming of gold. *Social Work in Health Care*. 33 (3/4): 15-32.

Fischer, J. (1993). Empirically-based practice: The end of ideology? *Journal of Social Service Research* 18 (1/2): 19-64.

Fischer, J., and Corcoran, K. (1994). *Measures for Clinical Practice: A Sourcebook. (2nd Edition, Vols. 1 and 2)*. New York: Free Press.

Fook, J. (1997). (Ed.). *The Reflective Researcher: Social Workers' Theories of Practice Research*. New York: Allen and Unwin.

Galambos, C. (1999). Resolving ethical conflicts in a managed care environment. *Health and Social Work* 24 (3): 191-197.

Gambrill, E. (1999). Evidence-based practice. *Families in Society* 80 (4): 341-350.

Gibelman, M., and Whiting, L. (1999). Negotiating and contracting in a managed care environment: Considerations for practitioners. *Health and Social Work* 24 (3): 180-190.

Globerman, J., Davies, J., and Walsh. S. (1996). Social work in restructuring hospitals: Meeting the challenge. *Health and Social Work* 21 (3): 178-188.

Globerman, J. (1999). Hospital restructuring: Positioning social work to manage change. *Social Work in Health Care* 28 (4): 13-30.

Goldstein, H. (1986). Toward the integration of theory and practice: A humanistic approach. *Social Work* 31 (5): 352-357.

Goldstein, H. (1993). Field education for reflective practice: A reconstructive proposal. *Journal of Teaching in Social Work* 8 (1/2): 165-182.

Grasso, A., and Epstein, I. (1987). Management by measurement: Organizational dilemmas and opportunities. *Administration in Social Work* 11 (3/4): 22-34.

Hutson, C., and Lichtiger, E. (2001). Mining clinical information in the utilization of social services: Practitioners inform themselves. *Social Work in Health Care* 33 (3/4): 153-161.

Lindsay, D., and Kirk. S. (1992). The continuing crisis in social work research: Conundrum or solvable problem? An essay review. *Journal of Social Work Education* 28 (3): 370-382.

Martin, L., and Kettner, P. (1997). Performance measurement: The new accountability. *Administration in Social Work* 21 (1): 17-26.

Meenaghan, T. (1995). Social policy and clinical social work education: Clinicians as social policy practitioners. *Journal of Social Work Education* 22 (2): 38-45.

Meenaghan, T. (1998). Looking forward in social work: Challenges. Mount Sinai Medical Center, New York City. Department of Social Work Services Unpublished Paper.

Meyer, C. H. (1996). My son the scientist. *Social Work Research* 20 (2): 102-104.

Motenko, A. K., Allen, E., Angelos, P., Block, L., DeVito, J., Duffy, A., Holden, L., Lambert, K., Parker, C., Ryan, J., Schraft, D., and Swindle, J. (1995). Privatization and Cutbacks. *Social Work* 4 (4): 456-463.

Morgan, G. (1986). *Images of Organization.* Newberry Park, CA: Sage Publications.

Patti, R. (1983). *Social Welfare Administration.* Englewood Cliffs, NJ: Prentice-Hall, Inc.

Peake, K., Mirabito, D., Epstein, I., and Giannone, V. (2004). Creating and sustaining a practice-based research group in an urban adolescent mental health program. *Social Work in Mental Health,* 3(1/2): 39-54.

Penka, C., and Kirk. S. (1991). Practitioner involvement in clinical education. *Social Work* 38 (6): 513-518.

Pruett, R., Shea, T., Zimmerman, J., and Parish, G. (1991). The beginning development of a model for joint research between a hospital social work department and a school of social work. *Social Work in Health Care* 15 (3): 63-75.

Rehr, H., Rosenberg, G., and Showers, N. (1998). Social work in health care: Do practitioner's writings suggest an applied social science? *Social Work in Health Care* 28 (2): 63-81.

Reid, W. J. (1994). The empirical practice movement. *Social Service Review* 62 (2): 165-184.

Reid, W. J. (1997). Long term trends in social work. *Social Service Review* 71 (2): 200-213.

Schon, D. (1983). *The Reflective Practitioner: How Professionals Think in Action.* New York: Basic Books.

Segal, S. (1999). Social work in a managed care environment. *International Journal of Social Welfare* 8 (1): 47-55.

Sidell, N., Barnhart, L., Bowman, N,. Fitzpatrick, V., Full, M., Hillock, L., and Setoff, J. (1996). The challenge of practice based research: A group approach. *Social Work in Health Care* 23 (2): 99-111.

Siporin, M. (1992). Tough economic times require innovation and flexibility in social work practice. *Journal of Continuing Social Work Education* 5 (3): 2-9.

Strom, K., and Gingerich, W. (1993). Educating students for the new market realities. *Journal of Social Work Education* 29 (1): 78-87.

Subramian, K., Siegel, E., and Garcia, C. (1994). Case study of an agency-university research partnership between a school of social work and a medical center. *Journal of Social Service Research* 19 (3/4): 145-161.

Turnbull, J., Saltz, C., and Gwyther, L. (1988). A prescription for promoting social work research in a university hospital. *Health & Social Work* 13 (2), 97-105.

Weinbach, R. W. (1985). The agency and professional contexts of research. In R. M. Grinnel (Ed.), *Social Work Research and Evaluation.* Itasca, IL: Peacock.

Weissman, H., Epstein, I., and Savage, A. (1983). *Agency-Based Social Work: Neglected Aspects of Practice.* Temple University Press: Philadelphia.

Woodrow, R., and Ginsberg, N. (1997). Creating roles for social work in changing health care organizations: Organizational development perspective. *Social Work in Health Care* 25 (1/ 2): 243-257.

Creating and Sustaining a Practice-Based Research Group in an Urban Adolescent Mental Health Program

Ken Peake
Diane Mirabito
Irwin Epstein
Vincent Giannone

SUMMARY. This article describes the initiation, implementation, and accomplishments of a practice-based research group within a mental health program serving inner-city adolescents. Begun in 1995 and co-led by a program manager and a clinical social work practitioner, the group fosters and supports practitioner-driven re-

---

Ken Peake, DSW, is Assistant Director, Mount Sinai Adolescent Health Center. Diane Mirabito, DSW, is Assistant Professor, New York University, Ehrenkranz School of Social Work, 1 Washington Square North, New York, NY 10003. Irwin Epstein, PhD, is Helen Rehr Professor of Applied Social Work Research in Health, Hunter College School of Social Work, 129 East 79th Street, New York, NY 10021. Vincent Giannone, PsyD, is Senior Psychologist, Mount Sinai Adolescent Health Center.

[Haworth co-indexing entry note]: "Creating and Sustaining a Practice-Based Research Group in an Urban Adolescent Mental Health Program." Peake, Ken et al. Co-published simultaneously in *Social Work in Mental Health* (The Haworth Social Work Practice Press, an imprint of The Haworth Press, Inc.) Vol. 3, No. 1/2, 2004, pp. 39-54; and: *Clinical and Research Uses of an Adolescent Mental Health Intake Questionnaire: What Kids Need to Talk About* (ed: Ken Peake, Irwin Epstein, and Daniel Medeiros) The Haworth Social Work Practice Press, an imprint of The Haworth Press, Inc., 2005, pp. 39-54. Single or multiple copies of this article are available for a fee from The Haworth Document Delivery Service [1-800-HAWORTH, 9:00 a.m. - 5:00 p.m. (EST). E-mail address: docdelivery@haworthpress.com].

http://www.haworthpress.com/web/SWMH
© 2004 by The Haworth Press, Inc. All rights reserved.
Digital Object Identifier: 10.1300/J200v03n01_03

search projects as part of a "reflective" organizational development strategy. *[Article copies available for a fee from The Haworth Document Delivery Service: 1-800-HAWORTH. E-mail address: <docdelivery@haworthpress.com> Website: <http:// www.HaworthPress.com>* © *2004 by The Haworth Press, Inc. All rights reserved.]*

KEYWORDS. Practice-based research, practitioner research, practice wisdom, reflective practice, innovation, adolescent

In 1995, the Mount Sinai Adolescent Health Center (AHC), in New York City, initiated a Practice-Based Research Group (PBRG) as part of a broader effort to create and sustain a more reflective mental health program. The AHC is an outpatient center that provides comprehensive health and mental health services to inner-city adolescents, aged 10-21. This article will provide an account of the initiation, development, implementation, and accomplishments of this practice-based research group. In addition to describing the challenges and opportunities faced by the PBRG, we will provide exemplars of practice-based research, which illustrate how this group of clinicians and managers utilized their collective practice wisdom and experience to guide and develop practice-relevant research projects.

"Reflective practice" and "practice-based research" are two central concepts that were used by the PBRG. Definitions of these terms will provide a frame of reference for the following description of the origins of practice-based research within the Adolescent Health Center and the evolution of the practice-based research group. As defined by Schon (1983) the concept of "reflective practice" conveys the ways in which practitioners use their own practice wisdom and "theories in use" to confront and manage challenging practice dilemmas (Peake & Epstein, 2004). Practice-based research, as defined by Epstein (2001, p. 17), is ". . . the use of research-inspired principles, designs, and information gathering techniques within existing forms of practice to answer questions that emerge from practice in ways that inform practice."

ORIGINS OF PRACTICE-BASED RESEARCH
AT THE ADOLESCENT HEALTH CENTER

Reflecting its medical school connection, Mount Sinai's Department of Social Work Services has long embraced research as essential to practice (Rehr, Rosenberg, & Blumenfield, 1998; Blumenfield & Epstein, 2001). In the early

1990s, it was poised to expand this commitment. Alternatively, since its inception in 1968, the AHC emphasized direct services. Its structure and culture was more like that of a community-based agency than a component of an academic medical center. Within its mental health program, little or no research had been conducted by AHC social workers until 1991.

That year, five practitioners interested in understanding and preventing very early "client dropout" designed, piloted, and evaluated a time-limited treatment model. A small, quantitative, quasi-experimental design was chosen and implemented. Ultimately, the short-term treatment model that was developed by this group of practitioners did not increase client retention. However, it persuaded the participating practitioners about the value of treatment contracting and specification of treatment objectives. In addition, it provided valuable descriptive information about client characteristics previously unavailable to clinicians. More generally, it demonstrated the value of practitioner-driven research for identifying practice and service problems, for considering intervention alternatives, for evaluating their impact and for promoting practitioner dialogue and support. Moreover, presentations concerning the project's findings generated surprising enthusiasm regarding short-term and time-limited treatment approaches among staff.

In 1992, a practitioner and a manager in fulfillment of respective qualitative research doctoral coursework initiated two small-scale studies. In one study, a small sample of clinicians was interviewed about their perceptions of the reasons for client dropout from mental health treatment. In the other study, a small sample of practitioners was asked whether and how they employ theory in their practice. Despite their limited scale, modest ambitions, and lack of immediate impact of study results on practice, these exploratory studies later provided impetus and leadership to the PBRG. Because they identified the difficulties practitioners were having coping with clients' short-term utilization patterns (defined by clinicians as "premature" termination) as well as the need for more opportunities for reflection, these studies sharply highlighted the usefulness of small-scale, qualitative research projects.

In 1995, AHC service-grant acquisitions made possible program restructuring, redesign and expansion. In this climate of change, the manager and clinician who conducted the previously described qualitative research projects saw the opportunity and value of planning for research development in the mental health program at the AHC. The group they created evolved to include six practitioners and became known to them informally as the "research committee."

THE PRACTICE-BASED RESEARCH GROUP:
CHALLENGES AND OPPORTUNITIES

While the co-leaders of the PBRG had basic skills in research acquired through their concurrent doctoral studies, other group members had a strong interest in research but relatively little research experience or training. Ranging from beginning practitioners to seasoned clinicians and supervisors, the members of the PBRG had varied roles and responsibilities including direct practice, program development, supervision, and administration. As such, they brought their collective "practice wisdom" to the research process, which included: general knowledge and expertise about adolescents at risk; particular knowledge of the AHC client population and the communities where many of the adolescents lived; clinical skills in diagnostic assessment, interviewing, group and family work; program planning and organizational development skills; and finally, an awareness of the AHC's organizational structure and culture.

The organizational culture of the AHC presented significant challenges to the PBRG. Within the practice and service-oriented culture of the AHC, the PBRG anticipated that they would experience a number of challenges engaging staff in research. Most AHC practitioners, who maintained autonomous and idiosyncratic practice styles, were inexperienced with and wary about research. Members of the PBRG, who were barely more skilled in research methods themselves, worried that research-wary colleagues might view their own research activities as undermining and/or devaluing practice.

Concurrent with these challenges within the AHC, budget reductions meant that Mount Sinai's Department of Social Work Services was rationing available research consultation time. Ironically, the PBR initiative began during a time when institutional cost cutting and reorganization threatened overtly defined "research" activities as other institutionally driven factors including productivity increases and service justification gained the foreground. This resulted in a paradoxical dilemma–while research consultation and technical assistance was not available until projects were solidly conceptualized, at the same time, projects were difficult to conceptualize *without* research consultation. Finally, a significant challenge faced by all PBRG members was heavy workloads with no time explicitly allocated for research.

The PBRG responded to these challenges by conducting a strategic assessment of the opportunities and constraints it faced in developing practitioner research. Through focus groups, staff meetings and informal discussions they began to identify practice problems as defined by practitioners themselves, naturalistically, intuitively and by trial and error, developing a PBR approach. The rich themes that emerged from this form of inquiry reflected perceived disparities between client-needs and service utilization patterns. In other words, practitioners generally framed client problems in broad terms requiring long-term interventions to address them. However, because client behaviors often did not comply with clinicians' expectations regarding length or type of services, practitioners often experienced frustration and self-doubt.

In response to clinicians' frustrations, two interrelated themes emerged. Clinicians wanted to find a better fit with clients' expectations and they also wanted to change client utilization patterns by enhancing their engagement strategies. Most important from a PBR point of view, practitioners *did* believe that research could help them understand clients' motivations and definitions of help in a more rigorous manner than practice could alone. This combined information-gathering and organizational-development process encouraged practitioners to discuss common practice problems with their colleagues and fostered greater openness to research. Hence, the inquiry was also an intervention, promoting organizational change possibilities previously unlikely.

THE EVOLUTION OF A PRACTICE-BASED RESEARCH GROUP MODEL

During this period of redesign within the AHC, the newly formed PBRG framed its task as the development of practitioner-research activities. Because formal systems such as supervision and planning were still evolving, the group's structure and formal relationship to other AHC subunits was not defined and remained largely informal. Membership was open to anyone, but required a minimal commitment of weekly attendance. After almost a year, through Mount Sinai's Department of Social Work Services, the group was finally able to secure 1.5 hours per month of external research consultation with a university-based consultant who shared the group's practice-research perspective.

Still, the PBRG faced several initial choices as to its goals and approach. Should it attempt to foster practitioner participation broadly across a number of projects or work as a group on a single project? One possibility was a broad "planning study" that would focus on key service delivery issues such as the assessment of client needs and an analysis of the fit between services and users. Although this approach was considered, members felt that committing the entire group to a single study would isolate it, create barriers to wider participation, and potentially lessen its influence on practice within mental health services.

Instead, the PBRG members decided that they should undertake more modest, small-scale, methodologically "simple" projects that could be completed rapidly. These would justify additional research consultation resources without over reliance on the consultant. Ultimately, PBRG members felt that AHC staff would be more receptive to smaller-scale, practice-relevant projects that would yield findings with implications that could be directly useful for practice and program development within the clinic. Hence, less overall staff "buy-in" would be required since projects could be conducted by a few of the most motivated individuals and/or small groups, thereby maximizing the utilization of resources.

The PBRG also thought that members could serve as non-expert mentors to other interested staff to develop projects in other areas of practice. Given the limited formal research expertise in the group, this strategy was perhaps overly ambitious but reflected members' growing confidence and commitment to broad staff involvement and practice innovation.

FROM PRACTICE TO RESEARCH AND FROM RESEARCH TO PRACTICE

The focus group themes initially provided the basis for defining the mission, scale and *modus operandi* of the group. However, projects evolved incrementally and "opportunistically" based on individual practitioners' interests. All projects derived directly from perceived practice problems and new program possibilities. Weekly committee meetings provided opportunities for practitioners to share their practice wisdom to examine practice dilemmas and gaps in service delivery, identify practice needs, and consider better ways of serving at-risk adolescents.

In discussing the administrative supports necessary to engage practitioners in research, Rehr (2001, p. xxix) points out, "There needs to be institutional and administrative sanction and support for study; encouragement to pose questions; workers' articulation of needs and goals; and the means to motivate staff, and to provide resources." The PBRG helped demonstrate that management within the AHC valued this kind of inquiry and provided an avenue for staff to reflect on practice within the agency context. In keeping with the principles of PBR (Epstein, 1997; 2001) the committee process included the following components:

- *Projects were practice-driven, i.e., derived from practice concerns and dilemmas*
- *These practice concerns and dilemmas were formulated into research questions*

- *Research methodologies were chosen that were most compatible with the practice context*
- *Practitioners utilized already existing practice skills to implement projects and identified new research skills that needed to be developed*
- *Practice, program, and research innovations evolved from projects that were integrated into the mental health programs at the AHC, which resulted in enhanced and improved practice and program delivery*

Over time, PBRG members learned how to translate, refocus, reframe and utilize their clinical skills in the research process. For example, clinical interviewing skills could be modified for conducting qualitative research interviews. Practice theories could be articulated and framed in testable ways. In the process, members identified new areas for learning and skill development including the construction of indigenous practice-research instruments such as questionnaires, surveys, and interview schedules, for needs assessment, clinical intervention description, and program evaluation. Some employed "clinical data-mining" strategies (Epstein, 2001) to exploit existing information while others gathered original data and conducted focus groups with clients and practitioner groups. Members learned to conduct both quantitative and qualitative studies using SPSS (Statistical Package for the Social Sciences) or grounded theory, respectively.

The starting point for each of the projects chosen was practice. Moreover, research activities were never pursued exclusively for the purpose of "pure" research or publication. Instead, every research project chosen had direct practice implications, which were considered and discussed throughout the implementation of each project.

PRACTICE-BASED RESEARCH EXEMPLARS

In order to better convey how AHC practitioners engaged in PBR, we will describe four projects that focus on a range of issues and concerns related to at-risk adolescents and employ a range of practice-based research strategies. In the description of each, emphasis is given to the ways in which committee members utilized their "practice wisdom" to implement PBR projects and how they made use of the resources of the PBRG. Finally, dissemination and practice utilization of study processes and outcomes are discussed.

Example 1: Latino Adolescent Immigrant Experience

In a school setting, a Latina practitioner, herself an immigrant, was interested in assessing the needs of adolescents who had recently immigrated to

New York City from Latin America to plan services for them. Drawing on her personal experience as an immigrant and practice wisdom gained from five years experience with immigrants, she developed an interview guide to better understand the experiences of these adolescents. In-depth interviews conducted in Spanish were designed for the dual purposes of clinical intervention (case finding, assessment, and intake) and for qualitative data gathering. Drawing on her prior clinical interviewing skills and experience exploring personal histories, she engaged eighteen adolescents in retrospective reviews of their immigration experiences.

After translating and transcribing the interviews, she used the PBRG as a forum to learn how to use a grounded theory approach to identify themes in client narratives and systematically analyze qualitative data. Identified themes became the basis for a curriculum, which was used to conduct therapeutic support groups in local schools to new immigrants. Working from practice-to-research and then from research-to-practice, she developed and described a time-limited, narrative-therapy group that was replicated by another practitioner in a second school setting.

Example 2: Adolescent Loss Survey

In another school-based program, practitioners sought to outreach and provide clinical services to adolescents affected by HIV. A self-administered questionnaire was developed to identify youth so affected who might be interested in counseling concerning loss, fear of contagion and related issues. Though the initial impetus for the program was HIV and AIDS-related illness and death of immediate family members, questions about loss considered other diseases (e.g., cancer, drug abuse), other forms of loss (e.g., incarceration, divorce) and individuals other than immediate family members (e.g., peers, non-related adults).

Practitioners developed a questionnaire that they, along with school personnel, administered to junior-high school students in three inner-city schools. Given the complexities involved in agency/school collaborations, the project raised challenging issues regarding implementation, such as how to engage school staff in the administration of the survey and how to manage issues related to confidentiality and research implementation within a school district. AHC practitioners utilized collaborative skills in working with school staff. After much negotiation with school staff, the final version of the instrument contained an anonymous, forced-choice questionnaire and a tear-off sheet for students to confidentially self-identify if they desired counseling.

Although the tear-off sheet was not an especially effective way of recruiting clients, AHC staff recognized that aggregating the results of the returned questionnaires could provide a previously undeveloped profile of adolescent loss in the East Harlem community. To compile this profile, AHC school-based, clinical staff sought consultation and training from the PBRG regarding the use of SPSS for data analysis. In the process, they recognized some of the limitations of the original questionnaire and learned principles of question-naire construction that would become useful in future projects.

Survey findings documented the extensive and traumatic losses experienced by many adolescents in these schools as well as the high levels of distress that they experienced as sequela to these losses. For example, 96% of respondents reported having lost a family member or close friend; 73% reported that they "thought about these losses some, most, or all of the time"; and 38% reported thinking about these losses "all or much of the time." To school personnel these findings illustrated the value of mental health services within an educational setting, as students with such levels of preoccupation with loss could not be expected to be focused on learning. This, in turn, helped build visibility, legitimacy, support and referrals for new school-based counseling services the AHC was developing.

Thus, while most of the adolescents surveyed proved reluctant to request services directly because of concerns about disclosure of HIV in their lives, the project emerged as an effective program development strategy in several ways. Within the schools, the viability of the AHC's HIV program was enhanced, referrals made by individual school staff for services increased, and successful support groups for adolescents impacted by loss were developed. In addition, survey findings led practitioners within the AHC's services to a new awareness regarding the value of exploring loss during initial clinical assessment with low-income, urban adolescents.

This project resulted in national conference presentations and presentations to social work and other staff within Mount Sinai. Perhaps more significantly, the AHC's entire clinical intake/assessment process was modified to include questions about loss that were derived from this practice-based research project. In addition, clinical group services for adolescents were developed at the AHC to address loss.

Example 3: Adolescent Termination from Mental Health Services

The individual practitioner who conducted this project wondered about the process of treatment termination at the AHC because of her own practice encounters and frustrations and those of colleagues. Their collective experience suggested that in cases of both successful and unsuccessful treatment, adolescents frequently dropped out of treatment before going through any termination process. At the time a doctoral student in social work, she came to explore this practice problem more and more systematically in tandem with research courses she was taking.

In conjunction with a doctoral course in qualitative research, she conducted a pilot study based upon interviews with other clinicians that confirmed her own experience that in the vast majority of cases termination was most often unannounced and unilateral. However, in order to conduct a more systematic and comprehensive study of termination, the practitioner designed a study that combined quantitative "data-mining" and qualitative retrospective interviews, utilizing available clinical information from 100 client records and original data from interviews with 14 adolescents. The study explored both "objective" patterns of termination from mental health treatment derived from client records and client "subjective" explanations for how they terminated derived from interviews with adolescents.

Findings indicated that termination was acknowledged infrequently and was generally a brief process that occurred almost as frequently by telephone as in the context of treatment. Additionally, the study yielded several surprising and counterintuitive findings. So, for example, contrary to treatment termination theories derived from work with adults, adolescents who "dropped out" of treatment without a "clinical process" reported considerably more engagement in and satisfaction with treatment than those who acknowledged the termination of treatment.

Several practice and program innovations were derived from this study. Findings from the pilot study highlighted the importance of developing structured treatment planning teams within the mental health program to guide clinicians in reviewing and evaluating treatment. The larger study pointed out the importance of incorporating education and preparation for termination into the contracting process in the beginning of treatment as well as proactive and collaborative exploration throughout the treatment process of adolescents' perceptions of goal attainment. Other practice recommendations included support for an "open-door" approach to treatment that is consistent with adolescents' developmental needs as well as the implementation of "exit interviews" to structure termination and provide therapeutic closure.

Example 4: The Development, Implementation, Clinical, and Research Utilization of an Adolescent Intake Questionnaire (Adquest)

The most ambitious collective project to emerge from the PBRG was the development, implementation, and clinical and research utilization of an adolescent intake questionnaire (Adquest) conceived in 1997, as a practice-based clinical and research tool. The self-administered intake questionnaire (Peake, Epstein et al., 2004) was to be completed by virtually all adolescents seeking mental health services at the AHC. The only exception was HIV positive youth whose mental health assessment and counseling always began with a face-to-face interview.

The Adquest instrument includes questions about multiple domains of life, including school, work, racism, safety and violence, health, sexual issues, substance use, family, and other aspects of personal life. In 1998, a parent questionnaire was developed as a parallel to Adquest to provide family intake information and to consider the effects of parental concern and family communication on the worries of adolescents and the issues they bring to mental health counseling. The family questionnaire included parents' perceptions of how their adolescents were performing in these domains but included questions about family stressors and loss as well. Finally, they were asked how often and how well these issues were talked about.

Adquest was designed with multiple uses in mind. Clinically, it was to serve as a "bridge" in the engagement process with potential clients to keep open the therapeutic conversation about what experiences and risk factors they *wanted* to talk about. This was to be accomplished by engaging young persons requesting services in a process of self-reflection about their own lives, their accomplishments, problems, needs, worries, and reasons for seeking counseling. In addition, counselors could also consider those risk factors and possible traumatic experiences that youth didn't particularly want to talk about. In other words, what they *needed* to talk about. Thus, Adquest was intended to represent a starting point for clinical engagement with teens and their families and for comprehensive clinical assessment by a clinician.

Although initially intended as an individual clinical assessment tool, as completed Adquest forms accumulated, it became clear that it represented a *clinical* "data-base" concerning AHC adolescents with referred or self-defined mental health needs. Univariate analysis of Adquest data could be used for AHC program design and development, for identification of staff training needs and for future grant writing. Univariate, bi-variate, and multi-variate analysis of Adquest information could serve as a *research* database. This made it possible to study how factors such as age, race, gender, and other background characteristics, as well as behaviors and exposure to traumatic stress are correlated with the concerns of these young persons. Thus, Adquest became the basis for a collection of papers (Peake, Epstein, & Medeiros, 2004), each of which was written by some combination of AHC clinical and/or administrative staff, many of whom are new to the PBRG.

STABILIZING PRACTICE-BASED RESEARCH AT THE AHC

Overall, between 1995 and 1999, the PBRG completed eight relatively small-scale, low budget, but highly influential projects. The projects employed both qualitative and quantitative methods, were retrospective as well as prospective and used available as well as original data. In the process, a core group of highly motivated, increasingly skilled, practitioner-researchers was mobilized.

Themes explored in the earlier studies and increasing organizational reflectivity on the part of PBRG members led directly to the conceptualization and implementation of the more ambitious and comprehensive Adquest project. Initial consideration of this project drew attention to the need for formal integration of PBRG activities with other AHC mental health program sub-systems.

Until then, the group had developed relatively "informally" during a period when other new organizational units were still evolving, such as AHC management and treatment review teams. With the overall mental health program structure stabilized at the AHC, committee members felt that the lack of formal mechanisms for feedback and coordination between PBRG, AHC management, and Treatment Review Teams impeded implementation of PBRG generated innovations such as Adquest. As a result, the PBRG's role expanded and it undertook the task of defining professional practice competencies and empirical standards for conducting individual performance appraisal. Practitioner involvement in some form of practice-based research activities was defined as *integral* to practice and program development and as formally valued competencies. On another tack, PBRG undertook the task of planning for more formal integration of PBR activities into the practice by planning for the development of an electronic clinical information system, a current AHC project.

LESSONS LEARNED AND BENEFITS GAINED
BY INDIVIDUAL PRACTITIONERS

The success and productivity of the PBRG raises questions about the conventional "academic wisdom" regarding practitioners' antipathy toward research. And while AHC staff committed much of their energy, thought, and discretionary time to these projects, they gained a great deal professionally from them.

It should be clear, however, that practitioners who initially joined the PBRG did so largely "on faith" and experienced benefits and frustrations as a result. Lacking research experience and large blocks of dedicated research time, they pioneered clinical innovations and new research skills, in part, by trial and error. Practitioners were often frustrated by the slow speed at which projects moved forward, able to engage in research only episodically due to the demands of their direct service and administrative responsibilities. At times, their own lack of technical skills or limited organizational resources slowed them further. Though limited consultation and technical assistance was available, practitioners were sometimes unable to identify what help they needed. Over time, PBRG members learned that careful project management and forthright discussion of obstacles to progress were necessary elements in timely, practice-research problem-solving. At times the PBRG co-chairs had to pressure members for more accountability with regard to their projects, lending an increasingly formal aspect to their role and leading practitioners to want more formal acknowledgement and rewards for their participation. At other times, there were tensions regarding the allocation of resources. Questions were raised about whether projects that were favored by administration were getting more attention and resources. As a result, the program director delegated control of resource allocation to PBRG members.

Although burdened at times, individual PBRG members were enthusiastic about their development of new research skills; their increased experience of mastery, competence, and confidence about practice and research; their increased ability to engage in reflective practice and their reflective understanding of AHC as an organization; their increased practice effectiveness; their increased job gratification; their career development and enhancement; and their development of skills in professional presentation and publication.

In addition to increased job-satisfaction, staff experienced enhancement in practice effectiveness as they learned from their clients who were the subjects of their research. The opportunity to think about, talk about, and consider new ways to conceptualize their practice led to development of new ideas about their clinical practice. PBR taught them to look at their practice in new and more systematic ways. Although not emanating from "gold-standard" experiments, nor exclusively quantitative, their thinking has become more "evidence-based."

Of the six original PBRG members, the two co-founders of the group completed doctoral dissertations based upon PBRG projects, three more practitioners developed interest in doctoral education and enrolled in doctoral programs (two of them completing dissertation proposals with PBRG help), and a fourth enrolled in an MBA program focused on not-for profit agencies.

During its five-year life span, other social work practitioners became involved in the group and its membership expanded to include psychologists, psychiatrists, health educators, employment counselors, and other non-social work staff. And, now that PBRG is not solely a social work group, reflective practice is spreading to other allied health groups at the AHC. So, for example, a group of health educators recently used a PBR approach to develop a formal sexual history protocol as part of HIV counseling services and reported that their practice had become more comprehensive, thorough, and efficient.

By now, PBRG members have made several presentations at conferences nationally and internationally. These venues served as motivating occasions for completing projects, consolidating results and locating them in a wider practice-research context. However, while many PBRG members expressed interest in publishing, the realities of their schedules and inexperience with writing meant that prior to this volume (Peake, Epstein, & Medeiros, 2004) only one peer reviewed journal article has been published (Mirabito, 2001).

With this realization came a new awareness that writing and publication required considerable and specialized support, over and above what the PBRG could routinely provide. For publication, each project team needed to have at least one member with strong writing skills. Despite this new resource challenge, the opportunity to publish this volume was the turning point, which resulted in the production of significant writing about the projects.

BENEFITS TO PROGRAM

At the program level, PBRG provided an organizational space in which practitioners could reflect on their practice concerns in an organizational context, providing a vehicle for practitioners to involve themselves in programmatic decision making. It created a wider appreciation of agency challenges and constraints that might otherwise have been defined as purely administrative concerns and out of the scope of practitioners. In this way it promoted exchange between these organizational sub-systems providing a safe forum for concerns and tensions between the two to be addressed. Thus, although the central purpose of PBRG was to integrate practice and research, it was perhaps as effective in bridging the often reported, direct-service/administration dichotomy.

Admittedly, tensions between sub-systems within the AHC did arise. Examples included tensions over resource allocation (including consultant time and time practitioners needed for project work) and regarding formal recognition and rewards for research participation. Fortunately, the group was able to channel these tensions and reach agreement. Tensions between practice autonomy and accountability, common in human service organizations, led to the development of professional competency standards, a six-month project that involved two practitioners and the program director.

For the AHC, PBRG membership contributed significantly to the program overall. The loss survey resulted in new services to address previously unidentified needs. The Latino immigration study helped create and shape new services. The termination study and other studies that used data mining drew attention to the need for more comprehensive and uniform information systems and record keeping. Adquest in particular allowed the mental health program at AHC to more rigorously and thoroughly describe its clients and significantly enhanced grant writing and securing new funds.

CONCLUSION

This article described the evolution and accomplishments of a unique, practitioner-research group in an urban adolescent mental health program. Employing a practice-based research paradigm, despite limited organizational resources, the group has increased reflective clinical practice and organizational reflectivity in several new directions.

Although participation in the PBRG meant additional demands on practitioners, it gave them unique access to their director as an equal party to reflection about practice. Membership truly came to be seen as a privilege. Thus, in 1999, when expansion of membership and integration into other program sub-systems were being considered, some "charter-members" resisted this idea, concerned that the group's unique identity as a "flagship" might be compromised. This momentary lapse into elitism only showed how important PBRG membership had become to participants. As this article and others found in this volume demonstrate, the PRBR group at the AHC created a significant capacity for knowledge development with regard to adolescent mental health needs.

REFERENCES

Blumenfield, S., & Epstein, I. (2001). Introduction: Promoting and maintaining a reflective professional staff in a hospital-based social work department. *Social Work in Health Care*. 33 (3/4): 1-13.

Epstein, I. (2001). Using available clinical information in practice-based research: Mining for silver while dreaming of gold. *Social Work in Health Care*. 33 (3/4): 15-32.

Mirabito, D. (2001). Mining termination data in an adolescent mental health service: A qualitative study. *Social Work in Health Care*. 33 (3/4): 71-90.

Peake, K., & Epstein, I. (2004). Theoretical and practical imperatives for reflective social work organizations in health and mental health: The place of Practice-Based Research. *Social Work in Mental Health*. 3 (1/2): 23-37.

Peake, K., Epstein, I., & Medeiros, D. (2004). *Clinical and research uses of an adolescent mental health intake questionnaire: What Kids Need to Talk About.* New York: The Haworth Press, Inc.

Peake, K., Epstein, I., Mirabito, D., & Surko, M. (2004). Development and utilization of a practice-based Adolescent Intake Questionnaire (Adquest): Surveying which risks, worries, and concerns urban youth want to talk about. *Social Work in Mental Health,* 3(1/2), 55-82.

Rehr, H., Rosenberg G., & Blumenfield, S. (Eds.) (1998). *Creative social work in health care.* New York: Springer Publishing.

Rehr, H. (2001). Forward. *Social Work in Health Care.* 33 (3/4): xxi-xxx.

Schon, D. (1983). *The reflective practitioner: How professionals think in action.* New York: Basic Books.

Development and Utilization of a Practice-Based, Adolescent Intake Questionnaire (Adquest): Surveying Which Risks, Worries, and Concerns Urban Youth Want to Talk About

Ken Peake
Irwin Epstein
Diane Mirabito
Michael Surko

SUMMARY. This article describes an intake questionnaire (Adquest) that was designed, tested, and implemented, and later employed in clini-

Ken Peake, DSW, is Assistant Director, Mount Sinai Adolescent Health Center, 320 East 94th Street, New York, NY 10128. Irwin Epstein, PhD, is Helen Rehr Professor of Applied Social Work Research in Health, Hunter College School of Social Work, 129 East 79th Street, New York, NY 10021. Diane Mirabito, DSW, is Assistant Professor, New York University, Ehrenkranz School of Social Work, 1 Washington Square North, New York, NY 10003. Michael Surko, PhD, is Coordinator, ACT for Youth Downstate Center for Excellence, Mount Sinai Adolescent Health Center, 320 East 94th Street, New York, NY 10128.

[Haworth co-indexing entry note]: "Development and Utilization of a Practice-Based, Adolescent Intake Questionnaire (Adquest): Surveying Which Risks, Worries, and Concerns Urban Youth Want to Talk About." Peake, Ken et al. Co-published simultaneously in *Social Work in Mental Health* (The Haworth Social Work Practice Press, an imprint of The Haworth Press, Inc.) Vol. 3, No. 1/2, 2004, pp. 55-82; and: *Clinical and Research Uses of an Adolescent Mental Health Intake Questionnaire: What Kids Need to Talk About* (ed: Ken Peake, Irwin Epstein, and Daniel Medeiros) The Haworth Social Work Practice Press, an imprint of The Haworth Press, Inc., 2005, pp. 55-82. Single or multiple copies of this article are available for a fee from The Haworth Document Delivery Service [1-800-HAWORTH, 9:00 a.m. - 5:00 p.m. (EST). E-mail address: docdelivery@haworthpress.com].

http://www.haworthpress.com/web/SWMH
© 2004 by The Haworth Press, Inc. All rights reserved.
Digital Object Identifier: 10.1300/J200v03n01_04

cal data-mining studies, by practitioners in an adolescent mental health program. The instrument is primarily a practice-based, clinical information-gathering and client engagement device. Consequently, it differs in significant ways from more research-driven Rapid Assessment Instruments (RAIs). Despite these differences, when aggregated and analyzed, Adquest data provides valuable psychosocial information about hundreds of vulnerable urban youth seeking mental health services. *[Article copies available for a fee from The Haworth Document Delivery Service: 1-800-HAWORTH. E-mail address: <docdelivery@haworthpress.com> Website: <http://www.HaworthPress.com> © 2004 by The Haworth Press, Inc. All rights reserved.]*

KEYWORDS. Assessment instrument, screening tool, clinical tool, practice-based research, engagement, adolescent, risk, clinical information

Within the past decade, a variety of assessment and screening tools have been developed for clinical use with adolescents in health and mental health settings. Some assess multiple behavioral domains (Fuller & Cavanaugh, 1995; Knight, Goodman, Pulerwitz, & Durant, 2001; McPherson & Hersch, 2000; Gruenewald & Klitzner, 1990; Rahdert, 1991). Others target specific problems such as, depression and anxiety (Dierker, Alban, Clark, Heimberg, & Kendall et al., 2001; García-Lopez, Olivares, Hidalgo, Beidel, & Turner, 2001); suicide (Range & Knott, 1997); chronic and forensic mental health problems (Kroll, Woodham, Rothwell, Bailey, & Tobias et al., 1999); drug and alcohol abuse (Hallfors & Van Dorn, 2002; Chung, Colby, Barnett, Rohsenow, Spirito, & Monti, 2000; McPherson & Hersch, 2000), and delinquency (Risler, Sutphen, & Shields, 2000).

The majority of these assessment instruments have been developed for purposes of clinical screening, intervention planning and predicting future risk behaviors. Added to the list of clinical research instruments is Adquest, an adolescent self-assessment, clinical information gathering and engagement questionnaire developed at Mount Sinai Adolescent Health Center (AHC).

What distinguishes Adquest from the others, however, is that it was created *by practitioners for practitioners.* More specifically, Adquest was designed, pre-tested, piloted and implemented by members of the Practice-Based Research Group (PBRG) in AHC's mental health program (Peake, Mirabito, Epstein, & Giannone, 2004). Consequently, it is an indigenous, practice-based research tool intended to promote client, clinician, and organizational self-reflection (Epstein 2001; Peake & Epstein, 2004).

Adquest explores multiple domains of adolescent functioning and focuses on issues of particular concern to inner-city adolescents. As an engagement device, Adquest is intended to convey AHC's consumer-oriented, youth development (Pittman, Irby, & Ferber, 2000) philosophy by asking simple and direct questions about all aspects of their lives, letting them know that: (1) we care about and are interested in knowing them; (2) we are non-judgmental about their behaviors; (3) we are ready to discuss these behaviors, confidentially and openly, with them; and (4) we trust in their positive capacity to cope.

While other risk assessments are primarily self-reports and seek adolescents' concerns about themselves, Adquest is also unique in that it asks about teens' concerns about family and friends as well as their perceptions of family and friends' concerns about them. Most importantly, Adquest provides a comprehensive picture of service applicants' specific counseling requests, i.e., what they want to talk about.

Although always thought to have some research potential, Adquest's development and uses were driven by clinical priorities. Consequently, it differs in significant ways from more rigorous, research-based assessment devices conventionally referred to as Rapid Assessment Instruments (RAIs) (Springer, Abell, & Hudson, 2002). As a result, Adquest is *primarily* a clinical tool and only *secondarily* a research instrument. Even as a research instrument, its focus is on informing internal programmatic decision-making (i.e., formative evaluation) rather than generalization to other programs (i.e., summative evaluation).

Despite its limitations, when aggregated and analyzed, Adquest information can serve as a rich and valuable, exploratory research database for staff reflection and program change. This article describes Adquest and the practice-based priorities and decisions that determined its content and utilization. In so doing, the article illustrates some important differences between practice-based research (PBR) instruments such as Adquest and research-based practice (RBP) instruments such as RAIs (Epstein, 2001; Springer et al., 2002). However, treating the PBR/RBP distinction as a continuum rather than as a dichotomy, the article goes on to describe our plan for aggregating and analyzing Adquest data in subsequent articles in this collection. These articles offer *evidence-informed* insights into the risks, vulnerabilities and counseling needs of hundreds of urban youth seeking mental health services. Reminding the reader that Adquest was primarily a clinical information-gathering tool, no claim is made that it is a source of the kind of *evidence-based* knowledge that standardized research instruments might provide.

THE AGENCY PRACTICE-BASE

AHC is a comprehensive health center for inner-city adolescents providing medical and mental health services in a confidential setting, regardless of their health insurance status or ability to pay. Of AHC's yearly visits, more than 20,000 are provided by social workers and other mental health professionals who address problems ranging from substance abuse, poor school performance, depression, sexual abuse, violence, interpersonal problems with family and friends, and other difficulties that confront many urban adolescents. Individual, group and family treatment interventions represent some of the mental health services AHC offers young persons along with health education, and medical and reproductive health services.

A Practice-Based Research Group (PBRG) comprised of AHC mental health practitioners developed Adquest between 1997 and 1999 (Peake, Mirabito et al., 2004). Consistent with its practice-based research perspective, the group made use of both clinical and "research inspired principles, designs and methods to answer questions that emerge from practice in ways that inform practice" (Epstein, 2001, p. 4). The projects group members chose for themselves were intended to contribute to a reflective program development process during a period of organizational redesign and change (Peake & Epstein, 2004).

ADQUEST IN AN EVOLVING ORGANIZATIONAL CONTEXT

Four years prior to the Adquest development effort, a major program redesign and expansion took place at AHC resulting in more transparent organizational practices and new opportunities for organizational reflection. Until 1992, AHC employed a service model whose informality more closely resembled a private practice than an agency-based service. Practitioners were then providing mainly individual, insight-oriented psychotherapy to those adolescents who could benefit from this mode of intervention. By 1994, AHC offered a more comprehensive treatment array with a range of services designed to meet the needs of a more diverse client population.

In 1995, admissions and treatment decision-making, which previously had been made by individual practitioners, were delegated to four treatment-planning teams. Intake-assessment was extended from a single client interview to three face-to-face sessions. More uniform admission and treatment planning criteria were established and forms were redesigned to improve short-term treatment planning and increase worker accountability. The team structure became the foundation for program administration, with team leaders actively participating in operational management and program development. During this period, new funding resulted in new services, greater levels of community involvement, a doubling of staff, and the establishment of group and family therapy programs. Although intake and assessment practices were more uniform and centralized, flexibility, diversification, and experimentation were encouraged in all program areas.

Not all staff members were pleased about these changes. However, staff turnover, new hires and team development created opportunities for the remaining direct service staff to serve as team leaders, supervisors, and mentors, and to participate more in programmatic decision-making. Practitioners became more cognizant of what each was doing and why they were doing it. Those who remained became informally "accountable" to each other as decisions regarding intervention were discussed and debated. This new emphasis on accountability to one's peers raised the climate of professionalism significantly at AHC (Billingsley, 1964; Etzioni, 1969; Reeser & Epstein, 1990).

ADQUEST'S OBJECTIVES

Adquest emerged out of widely shared clinical concerns about problems of initial client engagement and premature disengagement at AHC. These issues were discussed frequently and researched in various ways by PBRG members (Mirabito, 2001; Peake, Mirabito et al., 2004). Comparable patterns of disengagement were described in the adolescent mental health literature (Mirabito, 2001). In response, Adquest was intended to inform decisions about the first contact between client and clinician and to promote better rapport and clinical engagement.

The theory behind Adquest was quite simple. Applying a combined *consumer research* and youth development (Pittman et al., 2000) approach to adolescent help-seeking, PBRG members assumed that by comprehensively querying service applicants about their lives, problems, needs, worries, coping, and reasons for seeking counseling, and by having intake practitioners review and attend to client responses, initial engagement in psychotherapy would be enhanced. In other words, clinicians would be better attuned to what their prospective clients wanted to talk about. And, clients would feel that their "voices were heard."

Practice-wisdom and subsequent analysis of Adquest data has taught us that our original theory was overly simplistic and that a direct, purely client-oriented approach to initial assessment was inadequate. Simply stated, what adolescents say they *want* to talk about is not necessarily what they *need* to talk about. The clinical, programmatic, and research implications of this evidence-informed reflection are amply illustrated in this and subsequent articles in this volume.

Additionally, organizational self-reflection has taught us that it is also simplistic to assume that having clients complete a self-assessment instrument will result in practitioners' actually reviewing and clinically utilizing the information it provides. Instead, promoting Adquest utilization has represented a continuous challenge for AHC organizational development, supervision and training. Nonetheless, several AHC clinicians have invented varied and creative ways to integrate Adquest into their practice (Elliott, Nembhard, Giannone, Surko, Medeiros, & Peake, 2004; Ciro & Nembhard, 2005).

ADQUEST'S CONTENTS AND IMPLEMENTATION

Adquest is an 80-item, adolescent self-report questionnaire that asks about demographic factors, traumatic experiences, risk behaviors and exposures, school performance and work, health and safety concerns, experience of racism, concerns of and about family and friends, worries, coping, and the desire to talk about each of these areas in counseling (a full version of Adquest appears in the Appendix to this article). Questions are grouped across a number of psychosocial parameters–education, work, safety, health, sexuality, substance abuse, and personal/family life, etc.

Adquest is routinely administered to all adolescents seeking mental health service prior to their first meeting with a counselor. The only exception to this practice applies to emergency psychiatric cases and AHC health service patients who have been referred for mental health services because they are HIV-positive. For obvious reasons both groups see counselors immediately.

With remarkable levels of acceptance, all other mental health program applicants complete the questionnaire before seeing a counselor. Completion time rarely exceeds twenty minutes. For those few who seem to have problems understanding the simple and colloquial Adquest language and instructions, help is available.

Counselors conducting intake assessments are strongly encouraged to review each adolescent's responses to Adquest prior to the first face-to-face meeting. This review allows the practitioner to identify specific areas of concern in order to begin the assessment and engagement processes and to plan future interventions. Where there are differences of opinion between client and clinician, these can be noted and kept on the clinical agenda for future discussion (Elliott et al., 2004).

On those occasions when adolescents come accompanied by a parent or guardian and it is clinically appropriate, Adquest intake information is supplemented by a shorter questionnaire completed by parents or guardians. The latter focuses on parental observations and concerns about the youth and her/his friends. In addition, it attempts to assess the climate of communication in the home. Although that instrument was developed by PBRG as well and was based on the same principles as Adquest, the articles in this collection focus on data generated by Adquest alone.

ADQUEST AS A CLINICAL DATA-MINING RESOURCE

While Adquest was primarily intended for clinical use with individual clients, by aggregating and *mining* (Epstein, 2001) client responses as a research database, Adquest has the potential for providing rich information about AHC's client population. More specifically, it can be used for describing the risks, vulnerabilities, concerns and counseling desires of a large clinical population of urban youth. By cross-tabulating demographic characteristics with counseling requests, the data-base offers the possibility of studying how factors such as age, race, and gender are related to risk exposure, risk behaviors, and counseling needs.

Ultimately, Adquest represents the first element of a future AHC clinical information system to which will be added information about practitioner interventions and client outcomes. All of the above will enhance AHC's capacity for evidence-informed, clinical, and programmatic reflection (Peake & Epstein, 2004).

PRACTICE-BASED CONTRIBUTIONS
TO THE DEVELOPMENT OF ADQUEST

Unlike research-based protocols for constructing and validating RAIs (Springer et al., 2002), the development of Adquest was neither a linear nor tightly organized process. Paralleling life in a practice agency, the process was organic, incremental and somewhat messy. Over the course of many PBRG meetings, sample practice questions in each life sector were drawn from clinical experience and gradually distilled into this single but far-reaching PBR innovation. In the process, practice considerations were generally given precedence over research priorities. However, basic research principles were used to systematize information-gathering and make it more rigorous.

At first, the Adquest development effort was referred to as the "risk project" and its focus was entirely individual. Over time, however, programmatic implications were recognized which led to wider aims which included: (1) providing aggregate information on client risks and client expectations of services; (2) improving clinical assessment practices by developing uniform methods for identifying client risk factors and vulnerabilities; and (3) creating a data- base that could be used to enhance program development, contribute to knowledge, and assist in grant development and retention.

RESEARCH-BASED CONTRIBUTIONS
TO THE DEVELOPMENT OF ADQUEST

In thinking through how to strengthen risk assessment and create a "risk data-base," PBRG members gave consideration to existing standardized re-search instruments as well as to available RAIs. In so doing, however, the im-plications of importing existing instruments into the practice brought the project's true goal–to enhance intake processes through PBR methodologies–into sharper focus.

For example, consideration was given to incorporating the Youth Risk Be-havior Survey (YRBS) (Commonwealth of Massachusetts Department of Ed-ucation, 1993; Centers for Disease Control, 2003) into intake procedures but this approach was determined to be unsuitable for the setting. YRBS was rec-ognized as valuable from a research perspective in that it would make possible comparison of the AHC client population with national norms. However, members felt that it would generate *universal* information that was "too broad" for clinical decision-making purposes and that "the price" of client time in com-pleting the instrument might be disengagement.

Instead, practitioners favored more *local* information-gathering tools that were briefer and contributed more directly and specifically to initial assessment of AHC applicants. However, reviewing standardized risk assessment instru-ments helped practitioners think holistically about risk factors that were relevant to their own practice context. Existing instruments were used as a yardstick to measure rigor against relevance, to think comprehensively about risk factors based on national norms and to decide what dimensions of client risk and vul-nerability were most pertinent to AHC practice.

Creating a first draft of Adquest as a risk inventory brought the realization that such an instrument could do far more than identify risk behaviors. Practice considerations suggested that inventorying client behaviors, without eliciting their *meanings to clients* was, from a clinical standpoint, a meaningless exer-cise. From a PBR standpoint, having AHC clients efficiently assess their own risks, worries, and counseling wants on an original instrument was far prefera-ble. In this reflective process, while review of existing research instruments in-formed the process, practice priorities shaped the final product.

For example, the YRBS, the Child Behavior Checklist (CBCL) (Achenbach, Howell, Quay, & Conners, 1991), the Beck Depression Inventory (Beck, 1967), Offer's (1967; 1972) Adolescent Self-Esteem Questionnaire, and the Coopersmith Self-Esteem Inventory (Coopersmith, 1959; 1967) were reviewed and rejected because of their length and/or narrowness of focus.

Thought was given as well to the creation of indigenous RAIs. Discussion of this approach–from both a research and practice point of view–led to further clarification of the group's aims. Practitioners reasoned that RAIs might well improve diagnosis or screen for particular problems but would not generate broader information about risk exposure, risk behaviors, and help seeking which by then were emerging as PBRG's central interest.

Rightly or wrongly, clinicians perceived RAIs as *impersonal*, limited in scope and potentially alienating to teens. While they might be more effective for diagnostic purposes they would not contribute directly to the client-therapist relationship. Consequently, the RAI option was rejected.

ADQUEST VALIDITY AND RELIABILITY

In contrast to RAIs, a unique aspect of Adquest is that it seeks adolescents' perspectives on their total lives in a broad, holistic but relatively cursory manner rather than having them respond to disjointed, in-depth, multiple-item batteries of questions about single dimensions such as depression or self-esteem. Protocols for constructing RAIs, on the other hand, reflect researchers' predominant concern for instrument reliability and validity (Springer et al., 2002).

RAI developers seek to achieve these ends through extensive data collection and lengthy and complex statistical analysis, which greatly exceed the skill repertoires and resource capacities of most clinicians and practice settings (Epstein, 2001). Moreover, although "widely-available" (Springer et al., p. 409) and intended as a strategy for integrating research into social work practice, practitioners have not taken up RAIs with great enthusiasm.

Because PBRG members were more concerned about clinical rather than research priorities their approach to establishing reliability was practice-based rather than statistical. Nonetheless, understanding the importance of having reliable information for clinical decision-making, PBRG's initial approach to instrument reliability meant asking questions in such a way as to promote response consistency and assessing response consistency thematically across and within behavioral risk dimensions. The former involved using clear and simple question formats whenever possible. The latter involved clinically assessing the consistency of questionnaire responses across Adquest dimensions for individual clients and assessment of the consistency of questionnaire responses with client interview data. This latter approach allowed clinicians to explore those responses that seemed unreliable (i.e., inconsistent) within the context of a clinical interview. In this way, practitioners were also incorporating the basic principle of reliability into their clinical practice. In subsequent studies based upon Adquest data, however, conventional statistical procedures were introduced to establish the inter-item reliability of Adquest-generated scales.

With regard to validity (and in contrast to RAI developmental criteria), instrument validation efforts were limited to what researchers refer to as establishing *face validity* or *content validity*. In this approach to instrument validation, expert clinical judgments are made concerning the extent to which item responses reflect underlying dimensions. Springer et al. (2002) reject reliance on expert judgment as "too casual to be given much credence" (p. 428).

For PBRG members (who were such experts), however, collective judgments about face and construct validity were anything but casual. Instead, they derived from many hours of discussion and consensus-building as well as piloting Adquest with former clients. For AHC practitioners and for PBR purposes it was decided that these judgments were "good enough." After all, the clinical judgments for which clinicians are paid rely on precisely the same principle of *goodness of fit* between theoretical concept and practical application.

Admittedly, AHC staff did not have the luxury of time, statistical skills, nor the inclination to follow the validation procedures recommended by Springer et al. (2002) in developing Adquest. Nonetheless, PBRG took the reliability and validity very seriously, *conceptually* though not statistically. As concepts, they provided useful practice analogs (Epstein, 2001). In addition, consensus building about questionnaire items and the meaning of their response categories legitimated the use of Adquest among AHC clinicians. Finally, and perhaps most interesting, was the realization that emerged from the process that researchers regard questions that generate "unreliable" or "untrue" responses as useless and they routinely discard them. For clinicians, however, the recognition of and therapeutic reflection upon inconsistent and/or possibly "untrue" responses can have enormous clinical utility.

So, while Adquest may not measure up to idealized RAI statistical standards, it does offer an efficient initial picture of how young persons experience how they are managing multiple sectors of their lives. Most importantly, it represents a starting point for clinical engagement with young persons and their families and for in-depth clinical assessment by mental health counselors (Elliott et al., 2004).

PRACTICE-BASED RESEARCH
AND RESEARCH-BASED PRACTICE
AS A DIALECTICAL CONTINUUM

Although Adquest was generally considered to be a practice tool by PBRG members, at times it was viewed more from a research perspective. For example, research considerations shaped the decision to introduce it into the treatment process before a client's first encounter with a practitioner. Doing so would ensure collection of data on the largest number of adolescents seeking services and would include any who might drop out during the intake process. This would allow study of the differences between those who left during the assessment process and those stayed in treatment.

When conceptualized as a *research protocol*, Adquest did, however, raise concerns for PBRG practitioners. Would the desire for more systematic client information interfere with practice priorities? Staff worried that if the experience of responding to Adquest was our clients' first encounter with the mental health program, they might experience the service as impersonal and off-putting. Moreover, PBRG members wondered how clients would be informed about confidentiality limits; should client consent to research be obtained upon administering Adquest and, even if not, should clients be given the choice of refusal?

Prior to pre-testing the instrument, concerns about Adquest's potential to "turn clients off" were temporarily suspended, outweighed by considerations that its implementation might better prepare clients for therapy and indirectly educate them about services. All of these concerns were greatly allayed, however, when Adquest was piloted with long-term clients. In fact, the feedback they gave staff was that the questions "did not go far enough."

Despite client reassurance, PBRG members frequently expressed lingering fears that Adquest was too "research-driven" and a threat to the clinical principle of confidentiality and the research principle of informed consent. Reframing these issues as practice dilemmas was helpful. For example, clarification that Adquest was only part of an intake process and a component of the service record brought the realization that there were current inconsistencies in the way confidentiality and consent were being handled with clients. The service record was rarely discussed with clients and they were rarely informed that under certain circumstances, the written record could be made public in legal proceedings. As a result of these discussions, new protocols were created to address this issue uniformly within the clinic.

In a parallel process, practitioner concerns about research ethics led staff to the question of whether adolescents would have to consent to research participation before completing Adquest. The group's reminding itself that Adquest's primary purpose was not research helped refocus on how client consent to treatment was handled in the broader practice. Subsequently, however, when a decision was made to have Adquest information analyzed for PBR purposes, Institutional Review Board approval was secured.

The research-practice dialectic also shaped and limited Adquest content. Questions regarding gang membership, perpetration of violence, and weapon possession were eliminated because answers might implicate clients as criminally liable. In the context of a study of juvenile delinquency in which individual subjects cannot be identified even such questions might be explored. These questions, however, would be inappropriate in this clinical context and might truly "turn off" potential AHC service recipients.

What became clear as a result of many of these discussions was that although treating RBP and PBR as a dichotomy is useful for pedagogical and rhetorical purposes (Epstein, 2001), for practice utilization purposes, they are best viewed as ends of a *dialectical continuum.*

ADQUEST AS AN INTERVENTION

To make Adquest more palatable to respondents, the questionnaire itself was entitled "All About You." With engagement as well as information gathering in mind, the sequencing and grouping of its questions are arranged to mirror the flow of a typical clinical interview, moving from the least "personal" to the most. Its content and organization are intended to inform AHC applicants about its service philosophy, services and available clinical expertise. For example, the question "Have you ever experienced racism?" conveys that this is a legitimate issue for discussion and that counselors are equipped to handle such experiences. As one clinician remarked, "It lets minority clients know that this place is prepared to help them."

Content groupings reflect adolescent experiences within psychosocial domains such as "school and work," "safety," "health," "sex and sexuality," "cigarettes, alcohol, and drugs," and "personal life." Carefully worded introduction precedes each new set of questions. Following is an example for the health section.

> YOUR HEALTH–Many things can affect your health, including how you feel about yourself, your sexuality, your family, your friends, your community, and seeing drug and alcohol use. Here at the Adolescent Health Center we can help you understand yourself, your health, and your body. We can help you with any concerns or questions. Please answer as many of the following questions as you can.

A "safety" domain was created to signal that a young person's "right to safety" is highly important to AHC practitioners and that they will devote their attention to protecting clients. Locating questions about sexual abuse and rape within the domain of "safety" was intended to help begin to reframe cognitive distortions common among abuse victims that these experiences are more related to sexuality than they are to violence and exploitation.

Interest in intervention with parents influenced the design of Adquest in other ways. Believing that parents who minimized their child's concerns increased her/his overall risk, and wanting to be able to consider adolescents' views of their problems in comparison with the views of their parents, PBRG members developed questions to elicit client perceptions of parents' levels of worry about them, their friends' worries about them, and about client willingness to discuss these various issues in treatment. Such questions complete each substantive section of the questionnaire.

For illustrative purposes, Figure 1 illustrates a series of questions as they appear in the "sexuality" section of Adquest. PBRG members considered these particular questions as the clinically most valuable, direct, and inoffensive approach to information gathering and engagement in this sensitive area.

FIGURE 1. Sample Adquest Items Concerning Adolescent Perceptions of Coping Skills and Worries Regarding Sexuality

52. Do you ever worry about anything to do with sex, your body or birth control?
    Yes____ No____

53. Do you have any questions or concerns about sex, your body, or birth control?
    Yes____ No____ Don't Know____

54. Do your friends or family members ever worry about your sexual behavior?
    Yes____ No____ Don't Know____

55. When it comes to sex, your body and birth control how would you say you are doing?

1	2	3	4	5
Very Poor	Poor	Average	Well	Very well

56. How much do you want to talk to your counselor here about anything to do with sex, your body or birth control?

1	2	3	
Not At All	Somewhat	Very Much	Don't Know

PILOTING ADQUEST

Practice-research dialectics within PBRG continued to shape the development and implementation of Adquest. Out of these discussions a three-stage piloting process emerged. Stage One involved client focus groups, Stage Two involved administering Adquest to long-term clients, and Stage Three involved a time-limited implementation of Adquest as an intake and engagement tool in one treatment team.

All Adquest piloting efforts followed youth development and participatory action research principles. By involving adolescent consumers in the shaping of the project, further refinements were made in the instrument itself and in the implementation process. Piloting also served to allay practitioner fears and concerns about integrating research methodology into the mental health practice. The following discussion describes the piloting process in greater detail.

Stage One: Focus groups were constituted from adolescent health educators in AHC's peer-education program. Recommendations emerged regarding the wording of Adquest, content areas for exploration and its "look." As with individual pre-test respondents described earlier, teen focus-group participants thought questions should be posed more pointedly and would be welcomed as evidence of caring. However, the overriding concern expressed within focus groups and again in interviews with long-term clients was that they not be "blamed" for revealing parental and family problems. They worried that such disclosures might make them "lightning rods" for parental anger. This widespread concern was important for clinicians to know about and take into account in their clinical interviews with Adquest respondents.

Stage Two: PBRG members then piloted Adquest with long-term clients in their own caseloads. These clients indicated that Adquest was helpful to them in focusing previously unaddressed concerns and experiences with their therapists. In virtually every case, therapists were surprised at the discoveries they made. One dramatic example involved uncovering a history of incest in the case of a fourteen-year-old girl nine months after her therapy had begun. This was particularly striking because the therapist–an expert on child sexual abuse –had explored this issue during an earlier clinical interview. One possible explanation is that in a later stage of treatment the client was more willing to disclose. Another is that the client felt more comfortable disclosing in a questionnaire than a face-to-face interview. Irrespective of the explanation, it is particularly ironic that the piloting strategy had been undertaken to allay clinician concern about Adquest's intrusiveness. Instead, in several piloting instances it provided invaluable information never before revealed over the course of months of therapy.

Stage Three: As a result of stages one and two, Adquest was revised for the last time and implemented in one treatment planning team for a five-month period. During that time, no formal protocols were created as to how Adquest would be integrated by practitioners into their work. Rather, PBRG viewed this trial implementation as another aspect of an exploratory PBR development and utilization process. Once trial implementation had begun, planning for full implementation with new clients could commence.

Most importantly, the practice discoveries made in piloting Adquest helped PBRG members relieve other AHC practitioners of the fear that Adquest was essentially a research tool. Adquest was ready for full implementation in November 1999.

THE DISTINCTION BETWEEN CLIENT "WANT" AND "NEED" OF COUNSELING

In the piloting, an unanticipated but highly significant discovery was made concerning the use of forced-choice ("yes" or "no") questions in Adquest. Clients and peer educators alike suggested that in some contexts an adolescent might be confused about what is normative and, therefore, unable to respond categorically. This was of particular concern regarding exposure to traumatic events. Wisely, they suggested that in some domains a "don't know" option should be added.

For example, a "don't know" answer in response to the question, "Have you ever had forced sex?" might reflect an adolescent's "acceptance" of abuse, lack of clarity about what is normative in relationships, or other misconceptions that require intervention. Similarly, in questions regarding sexual orientation, response categories should make it possible for clients to indicate a lack of certainty. As a result, the "don't know" category was added to seven items on Adquest where such considerations are developmentally relevant, empirically valid, and clinically significant.

Empirical validation of this insight appears in Table 1. These findings indicate that young persons who say they "don't know" whether they have been raped, abused or experienced other safety violations are about as likely, or even more likely, to want to speak to a counselor about safety as those clients who simply respond "yes" to the item. A parallel practice-based decision was made concerning how to treat "don't know" responses to questions about their desire to speak to a counselor. Here again, a "don't know" response was treated as a "yes" for the purposes of case finding and treatment planning.

Taken together, these two sets of items and their response patterns changed the practice-research focus of our analysis in a fundamental way. It shifted from a simplistic consumer-oriented interpretation of Adquest-generated information to a more clinically and empirically refined conception. This transition is reflected in the difference between a clinical decision based entirely upon the client's direct expression of "wanting" to speak to a counselor and a more collaborative, clinically sophisticated judgment about a client's "needing" service.

This distinction is illustrated as a typology in Table 2. In the typology, client exposure to significant risk or trauma is cross-classified with client desire to speak with a counselor about this problem. Affirmation of exposure to risk or trauma and "not knowing" are combined into one category as opposed to a definitive "no" exposure response. Likewise, client affirmation of or "not knowing" whether she/he wants to speak with a counselor about a given problem dimension are combined. A clear "no" response to wanting to speak with a counselor is, by itself, taken at face value.

These distinctions and combinations are illustrated as a typology in Figure 2. In the typology, client exposure to significant risk or trauma is cross-classified with client desire to speak with a counselor about this experience. Four dis-

TABLE 1. Proportions of Adolescents Expressing Desire to Talk About Safety, by Reported Experience of Safety Risks

Type of safety risk	Safety risk present?			χ^2
	Don't Know	Yes	No	
	% (n)	% (n)	% (n)	
Victim of violence	90.4 (47)	71.2 (195)	66.0 (278)	13.470**
Touched uncomfortably	81.3 (13)	84.6 (154)	64.4 (355)	27.430***
Forced sex	100.0 (10)	81.9 (59)	68.6 (452)	9.827**

*$p < .05$, **$p < .01$, ***$p < .001$

TABLE 2. Typology of Client Need for Counseling

Wants to Talk to Counselor	Exposure to Risk	
	No	Yes/DK
No	Type I	Type IV
Yes/DK	Type II	Type III

tinct and clinically relevant typological categories result from this cross-clas-sification:

> Type I–are those clients who say that they have *not* been exposed to risk or trauma and *do not* wish to speak to a counselor about this area of concern. These clients would have *no immediate need* for further clinical exploration in this area.
>
> Type II–are those clients who say they have *not* been exposed to risk or trauma but indicate that they *do* want to speak to a counselor about it or indicate that they *don't know* whether they want to or not. These clients would be identified as having a *need* for intervention.
>
> Type III–are those clients who say they *were* exposed to risk or trauma or indicate that they *don't know* whether they were but either *do* want to speak to a counselor about it or *don't know* whether they want to or not. These clients would be identified as having a *need* for intervention.
>
> Type IV– are those clients who say they *were* exposed to risk or trauma or indicate that they don't know whether they have but *do not* want to speak to a counselor about it. These clients would be identified as having a *need* for intervention.

Based on client feedback, practice wisdom and preliminary Adquest findings, Types II, III, and IV each have a *need* for further exploration and possibly clinical or programmatic intervention. Differential use of this typology in case finding, treatment planning and program development is just beginning to be discussed in the PBRG. So for example, Type II clients might be seen having the least urgent need for intervention as compared to Type IV who might be most in need, i.e., having been traumatized but not wanting to talk about it. This typological paradigm for establishing client need for service will be tested throughout our subsequent empirical analyses of Adquest data.

Clearly, Adquest remains a work in progress, and its practice, program, and research applications are still evolving.

SAMPLE

The sample on which the subsequent studies are based included 759 adolescents presenting for mental health intake at AHC between 4/27/99 and 4/9/02. Thirty-six percent were male and 64.0% were female; 33.7% were ages 11-14, 39.9% were ages 15-16, and 26.4% were ages 17-21. When asked about race/ethnicity 1.4% did not respond. Of those responding, 44.7% identified as Hispanic/Latino, 29.8% African-American, 4.5% West Indian/Caribbean, 1.6% Asian/Pacific Islander, 6.0% White (non-Hispanic) and 13.4% checked more than one race/ethnicity category, "other" race/ethnicity, or "don't know."

USING ADQUEST FOR EXPLORATORY RESEARCH PURPOSES

In addition to its clinical and programmatic contributions, Adquest findings are already being used to augment organizational reflection within AHC and to add to PBR knowledge for consumers beyond AHC. One example of this extramural research contribution is the publication of this volume. In planning this collection of articles the PBRG committed itself to describing the clinical uses of Adquest (Elliott et al., 2004) but also more fully exploiting its research potential as a database.

To accomplish the latter objective, PBRG conceived a simple initial approach to data analysis and interpretation aimed at providing practice- and program-relevant information for reflection by AHC clinicians and managers. This involved separate groups of AHC practitioners looking within each of Adquest's psychosocial domains, e.g., work and school, safety, health, sex and sexuality, alcohol and drugs, race and racism, etc. Each group would produce an article on their chosen topic. A final group made up of representatives from each of the workgroups would analyze and integrate data across all domains in a "multiple risks/multiple worries" article.

Throughout this analysis, the "need to talk to a counselor" constitutes the central *dependent variable* or ultimate focus of the analysis. However, as indicated earlier, "need to talk" was operationalized by creating four empirically derived, clinically relevant groupings as follows: (1) Adolescents with no risk exposure and no desire to talk; (2) Adolescents with no risk exposure who want to talk; (3) Adolescents with risk exposure who want to talk; and (4) Adolescents with risk exposure and no desire to talk. In addition, to aid analysis, risk exposure was re-conceptualized by PBRG into four categories: environmental risk or vulnerability, behavioral risk, worries, and self-perceived coping.

In planning for subsequent data analysis, PBRG members decided that for each problem domain, analysis should take place on several different *levels*. The first level is intended to provide a univariate "snapshot" of the prevalence of exposure to risk within a particular domain for our sample. The second level involves bivariate analyses concerning age and gender determinants of exposure to risk and desire for counseling within a given area of concern. A third level is multivariate and looks at age and gender combinations with different configurations of need for service. A fourth level of analysis was left unspecified by

PBRG members and allows members of each study group to explore empirically practice- and program-relevant questions that emerge from the prior levels of analysis or from their own practice interests. The products of these individual study groups and a final chapter linking all of the risk domains form the empirical research core of this collection of articles.

CONCLUSION

This article has described the development of Adquest and the PBR considerations effecting its construction. In addition, it enumerated the contributions that AHC service recipients made to its development. We believe that as a research instrument as well as a process of practice-based instrument design and development, Adquest development and utilization represents a legitimate option for social workers wanting to integrate practice and research. It is offered here as an exemplar of a practitioner designed, context-specific tool to enhance assessment, client engagement, program development, *and* knowledge about urban adolescent vulnerability and need for counseling.

Adquest took almost five years from its initial development to its being used for both practice and research. This might seem like a lifetime to clinicians working in a "fast paced, task-oriented practice environment" (Sidell, Barnhart, Bowman, Fitzpatrick, Fulk, Hallock, & Metoff, 1996, p. 108). Sustaining this effort within a busy practice setting such as AHC has required not only a major commitment on behalf of practitioners and administrators, but also a theoretical and conceptual framework that was consistent with the everyday challenges and resources of the practice setting. However costly this effort has been, it has paid off with benefits to clinical practice and organizational reflection from the very start and continues today. These benefits and costs to clinicians as well as to program managers and administrators are discussed more fully in the final two articles in this collection.

Put more succinctly, however, as practice-research dialectics drove Adquest development, AHC staff became more mindful of client needs, more aware of inconsistent and uneven clinical practices, more cognizant of program inadequacies and more willing to respond to these problems individually and organizationally. Had Adquest not come to fruition, the development process alone would have contributed to practice *conceptually*. Now that we have completed the first phase of development and begun to exploit its research potential, however, Adquest is also informing us *empirically* about what our clients need to be talking about, what our clinicians need to be asking about and what our program managers and planners need to know.

REFERENCES

Achenbach, T. M., Howell, C. T., Quay, H. C., and Conners, C. K. (1991). National survey of problems and competencies among four-to-sixteen-year-olds. *Monographs of the Society for Research in Child Development.*

Beck, A. T. (1967). *Depression: Clinical experimental and theoretical aspects.* New York: Harper & Row.

Billingsley, A. (1964). Bureaucratic and professional orientation patterns in social casework. *Social Service Review, 4,* 400-407.

Centers for Disease Control, (2003). Youth Risk Behaviors Surveillance System (YRBSS) retrieved November 22, 2003. from *http://www.cdc.gov/nccdphp/dash/yrbs/about_yrbss.htm*

Chung, T., Colby, S., Barnett, N., Rohsenow, D., Spirito, A., and Monti, P. 2000. Screening Adolescents for Problem Drinking: Performance of Brief Screens Against DSM-IV Alcohol Diagnoses. *Journal of Studies on Alcohol,* 579-587.

Ciro, D., and Nembhard, M. (2005). Collaborative data-mining in an adolescent mental health service: Clinicians speak of their experience. *Social Work in Mental Health, 3*(3), 305-317.

Commonwealth of Massachusetts Department of Education. (1993). Youth Risk Behavior Survey. 1385 Hancock Street, Quincy, MA, 02169-5183.

Coopersmith, S. (1959). A method for determining types of self-esteem. *Journal of Abnormal & Social Psychology, 59,* 87-94.

Coopersmith, S. (1962). Clinical explorations of self-esteem. In G. Nielsen (Ed.), *Proceedings of the XIV International Congress of Applied Psychology. Vol. #. Child and Education* (p. 61-78). Oxford, UK: Munksgaard.

Deas, D., and Thomas, S. E. (2001). An overview of controlled studies of adolescent substance abuse treatment. *The American Journal on Addictions, 10,* 178-189.

Dierker, L. C., C., Albano, A., Clarke, G. N., Heimberg, R. G., Kendall, P. C., Merikangas, K. R., Lewinsohn, P. M., Offord, D. R., Kessler, R., and Kupfer, D. (2001). Screening for Anxiety and Depression in Early Adolescence. *Journal of the American Academy of Child Adolescent Psychiatry, 40* (8), 929-936.

Elliott, J., Nembhard, M., Giannone, V., Surko, M., Medeiros, D., and Peake, K. (2004). Clinical uses of an adolescent intake questionnaire: Adquest as a bridge to engagement. *Social Work in Mental Health, 3*(1/2), 83-102.

Etzioni, A. (1969). *The Semi-Professions and Their Organization.* New York: Free Press.

Fuller, P. G., and Cavanaugh, R. M. (1995). Basic assessment and screening for substance abuse in the pediatrician's office. *Pediatric Clinics of North America, 42,* 295-307.

García-Lopez, L. J., Olivares, J., Hidalgo, M., Beidel, D., and Turner, S. (2001). Psychometric properties of the social phobia and anxiety inventory, the social anxiety Scale for Adolescents, the Fear of Negative Evaluation Scale, and the Social Avoidance and Distress Scale in an Adolescent Spanish-Speaking Sample. *Journal of Psychopathology & Behavioral Assessment, 23* (1), 51-59.

Gruenewald, P. J., and Klitzner, M. (1990). *Results of Preliminary POSIT Analyses.* Pacific Institute for Research and Evaluation, Inc. Unpublished report to the National Institute on Drug Abuse.

Hallfors, D., and Van Dorn, R. A. (2002). Strengthening the Role of Two Key Institutions in the Prevention of Adolescent Substance Abuse. *Journal of Adolescent Health, 30,* 17-28.

Hastings, R. P., Brown, T., Mount, R. H., and Cormack, K. F. M. (2001). Exploration of Psychometric Properties of the Developmental Behavior Checklist. *Journal of Autism & Developmental Disorders, 31* (4), 423-431.

Knight, J. R., Goodman, E., Pulerwitz, T., and Durant, R. H. (2001). Reliability of the problem oriented screening instrument for teenagers (POSIT) in adolescent medical practice. *Journal of Adolescent Health, 29,* 125-130.

Kroll, L., Woodham, A., Rothwell, J., Bailey, S., Tobias, C., Harrington, R., and Marshall, M. (1999). Reliability of the salford needs assessment schedule for adolescents. *Psychological Medicine, 29* (4), 891-902.

McPherson, T. L., and Hersch, R. K. (2000). Brief substance use screening instruments for primary care settings: A review. *Journal of Substance Abuse Treatment, 18,* 193-202.

Mirabito, D. M. (2001). Mining treatment termination data in an adolescent mental health service: A quantitative study. *Social Work in Health Care, 33* (3/4), 71-90.

Offer, D. (1969). *The Psychological World of the Teenager.* New York: Basic Books.

Offer, D., and Howard, K. I. (1972). An empirical analysis of the self-image questionnaire. *Archives of General Psychiatry, 27* (4), 529-533.

Peake, K., and Epstein, I. (2004). Theoretical and practical imperatives for reflective social work organizations in health and mental health: The place of practice-based research. *Social Work in Mental Health, 3*(1/2), 23-37.

Peake, K., Mirabito, D., Epstein, I., and Giannone, V. (2004). Creating and sustaining a practice-based research group in an urban adolescent mental health program. *Social Work in Mental Health, 3*(1/2), 39-54.

Pittman, K., Irby, M., & Ferber, T. (2000). Unfinished business: Further reflections on a decade of promoting youth development. In *Youth Development: Issues, Challenges, and Directions.* Philadelphia, PA: Public/Private Ventures.

Rahdert, E. R. (1991). The Problem Oriented Screening Instrument for Teenagers (POSIT). In E. R. Rahdert (Ed.), *The Adolescent Assessment/Referral System Manual.* Rockville, MD: U.S. Department of Health and Human Services, *DHHS Publication No. (ADM)* 91-1735.

Range, L. M., and Knott, E. C. (1997). Twenty suicide assessment instruments: Evaluation and recommendations. *Death Studies, 21,* 25-58.

Reeser, L., and Epstein, I. (1990). *Professionalization and Activism in Social Work: The Sixties, the Eighties, and the Future.* New York: Columbia University Press.

Risler, E. A., Sutphen, R., and Shields, J. (2000). Preliminary Validation of the Juvenile First Offender Risk Assessment Index. *Research on Social Work Practice, 10* (1), 111-126.

Sidell, N., Barnhart, L., Bowman, N., Fitzpatrick, V., Full, M., Hillock, L., and Setoff, J. (1996). The challenge of practice based research: A group approach. *Social Work in Health Care, 23* (2), 99-111.

Springer, D. W. (1998). Validation of the adolescent concerns evaluation (ACE): Detecting indicators of runaway behavior in adolescents. *Social Work Research, 22* (4), 241-250.

Springer, D. W., Abell, N., and Hudson, W. W. (2002). Creating and validating rapid assessment instruments for practice and research: Part I. *Research on Social Work Practice, 12* (3), 408-439.

APPENDIX

ALL ABOUT YOU!

The following questions are about you, your opinions, and issues that affect teenagers and young adults.

Your answers will be reviewed privately, between you and your counselor today.

Please answer as many questions as you can so that we can be sure we understand you and how to best help you. Your answers will help us to provide the best possible services to you and other young people.

If you have any questions about anything below, your counselor will be glad to talk with you.

If you need help or don't understand any of the questions please ask us.

Intake Worker: Team: Date: #

ALL ABOUT YOU

The first questions ask you some personal information to help us understand you better.

1. Your Name: _____

2. Your Date of Birth:_____

3. How old are you? (Please circle one)

    10   11   12   13   14   15   16   17   18   19   20   21

4. What sex are you? Male ____ Female ____

5. What is your race or ethnicity?

_____African American   _____West Indian/Caribbean

_____Asian of Pacific Islander   _____White (non-Hispanic)

_____Hispanic/Latino   _____Don't know

_____Other (Please write in)_____

6. Are you proud of your race and ethnicity?   Yes_____ No_____ Don't Know____

7. Have you ever experienced racism?   Yes____ No____

8. What Religion are you? (Please write in) _____

9. How much do you want to talk to your counselor here about any issue with your race or ethnicity?

1	2	3	
Not At All	Somewhat	Very Much	Don't Know _____

SCHOOL AND WORK
The next questions ask about school and work. Education and work are important parts of every young person's life. We are interested in your needs, opinions, and experiences.

10. Are you in school?   Yes ____ No____

   If NO, please skip to question 15

   11. If you are in school or college, what grade are you in?   ____ Don't Know____

   12. Are you failing any classes?   Yes____ No____ Don't Know____

   13. How do you rate the school you attend?

1	2	3	4	5
Very Bad	Bad	Average	Good	Very Good

   14. Which of the following describes your school attendance best?

1	2	3
I often miss classes	I sometimes miss classes	I almost never miss classes

15. Do friends or family members worry about how you are doing in school or with your education?   Yes____ No____ Don't Know____

APPENDIX (continued)

16. In general how are you doing with your education?

1	2	3	4	5
Very Poor	Poor	Average	Well	Very well

17. How much do you want to talk to your counselor here about any school or education issues?

1	2	3	
Not At All	Somewhat	Very Much	Don't Know _____

18. Are you currently working?   Yes____ No____

   If No, please skip to question 21

   19. Do you have any problems on the job?   Yes ____ No____

   20. Do you have any problems balancing
       work and other responsibilities?   Yes ____ No____

21. If you are not working, do you want to work?   Yes ____ No____ Don't Know____

22. How much do you want to talk to your counselor here about any work or employment issues?

1	2	3	
Not At All	Somewhat	Very Much	Don't Know _____

YOUR SAFETY
**Many young people have concerns about their own personal safety.
The following questions are about your experiences.**

23. Have you ever witnessed violence?   Yes___ No ___

24. Do you ever feel unsafe?   Yes___ No ___

25. Have you ever been threatened with a weapon?   Yes___ No___

26. Have you ever been a victim of violence?   Yes ___ No___ Don't Know____

27. Has anyone ever touched your body in a way that made you feel uncomfortable?
                                                                Yes___ No___ Don't Know____

28. Do you and your boyfriend/girlfriend ever physically fight?
                                                                Yes___ No___ Don't Know____

29. Have you ever been forced to have sex when you didn't want to?
                                                              Yes ___ No___ Don't Know____

30. Have you ever worried about hurting yourself or someone else in any way?
                                                                Yes___ No___ Don't Know____

31. Do you ever worry about the friends or associates that you hang out with?
                                                                Yes___ No___

32. Do you ever worry that things you do are dangerous? Yes___ No___

33. Do your friends or family members ever worry that things you do are dangerous?
Yes___ No___ Don't Know___

34. Could you get a gun if you wanted to? Yes____ No___

35. Do your friends or family members ever worry about your safety?
Yes ___ No___ Don't Know___

36. In general, when it comes to your own safety, how often do you feel unsafe?

1	2	3	4	5
Always	Often	Sometimes	Rarely	Never

37. How much do you want to talk to your counselor here about your safety?

1	2	3	
Not At All	Somewhat	Very Much	Don't Know _____

YOUR HEALTH
Many things can affect your health, including how you feel about yourself, your sexuality, your family, your friends, your community, and seeing drug and alcohol use. Here at the Adolescent Health Center we can help you understand yourself, your health and your body. We can help you with any concerns or questions.
Please answer as many of the following questions as you can.

38. Do you have any health problems or worries? Yes___ No___ Don't Know___

39. Do you worry that you are overweight or underweight? Yes____ No ___

40. Do you throw up to lose weight or binge (really over eat)? Yes____ No ___

41. Do you ever try to go a whole day or days without eating? Yes____ No ___

42. Do you worry that you sleep too much or too little? Yes____ No ___

43. Do you have frequent headaches or stomachaches? Yes____ No ___

44. In general, when it comes to your own health how would you say you are doing?

1	2	3	4	5	
Very Poor	Poor	Average	Well	Very well	Don't Know___

45. How much do you want to talk to your counselor here about any health issues?

1	2	3	
Not At All	Somewhat	Very Much	Don't Know _____

APPENDIX (continued)

YOUR HEALTH: SEX AND SEXUALITY

46. How would you describe yourself? (Check any below)

Straight (Heterosexual)_____   Bisexual_____

Gay_____   Transgender_____

Lesbian_____   Not sure_____

47. Have you been taught about your body and sexuality? Yes___ No___ Don't Know___
48. Have you ever had sex? Yes___ No___
49. Have you ever been pregnant or gotten someone pregnant?   Yes___ No___
50. Have you ever thought about testing for HIV/AIDS?   Yes___ No___
51. Have you ever used drugs or alcohol to make sex easier, longer, or more fun? Yes___ No___ Don't Know___
52. Do you ever worry about anything to do with sex, your body, or birth control? Yes___ No___
53. Do you have any questions or concerns about sex, your body, or birth control? Yes___ No___ Don't Know___
54. Do your friends or family members ever worry about your sexual behavior? Yes___ No___ Don't Know___
55. When it comes to sex, your body, and birth control how would you say you are doing?

1	2	3	4	5
Very Poor	Poor	Average	Well	Very well

56. How much do you want to talk to your counselor here about anything to do with sex, your body, or birth control?

1	2	3

YOUR HEALTH: CIGARETTES, ALCOHOL AND DRUGS

Not At All	Somewhat	Very Much	Don't Know ____

57. Has anyone ever offered you any drugs?   Yes___ No___
58. Do you spend time with anyone who uses drugs or alcohol?   Yes___ No___
59. Check any of the following that you have tried.
    ___ Tobacco (cigarettes, snuff, chew)
    ___ Alcohol (beer, wine, wine coolers, hard liquor)

____ Marijuana (pot, weed, reefer, boom, chronic, blunts, joints)

____ Other drugs (e.g., crack, cocaine, ecstasy, special K, LSD, acid, glues, heroin, uppers, downers, steroids)

60. In the last month have you used alcohol, marijuana or any other drugs? Yes___ No ___

61. Have you ever worried about your use of alcohol or drugs, or tried to cut down?
                                                                    Yes___ No ___

62. Do you know someone whose drug or alcohol use worries you?   Yes___No ___

63. Do your friends or family members ever worry about your alcohol or drug use?
                                                        Yes ___No___ Don't Know___

64. In general, when it comes to alcohol and drugs how would you say you are doing?

1	2	3	4	5
Very Poor	Poor	Average	Well	Very well

65. How much do you want to talk to your counselor here about anything to do with alcohol or drugs?

YOUR PERSONAL LIFE

1	2	3	
Not At All	Somewhat	Very Much	Don't Know ____

66. Do you have any worries about your friends or associates?
                                                        Yes ___ No ___

67. Do your family members ever worry about your friendships?   Yes ___ No ___
                                                        Don't know___

68. In general, when it comes to friendships how would you say you are doing?

1	2	3	4	5
Very Poor	Poor	Average	Well	Very well

69. How much do you want to talk to your counselor here about friends or associates?

1	2	3	
Not At All	Somewhat	Very Much	Don't Know ____

70. Has anyone close to you died in the last year?   Yes___ No ___

71. Do you have any worries about your family or home life?   Yes___ No ___

72. In general, when it comes to your family or home life how would you say you are doing?

APPENDIX (continued)

1	2	3	4	5
Very Poor	Poor	Average	Well	Very well

73. How much do you want to talk to your counselor here about your family or home life?

1	2	3	
Not At All	Somewhat	Very Much	Don't Know _____

74. Do you ever worry about any other personal things that we have not asked you about today?   Yes___ No ___

75. In general, when it comes to your personal life how would you say you are doing?

1	2	3	4	5
Very Poor	Poor	Average	Well	Very well

76. How much do you want to talk to your counselor here about your personal life?

1	2	3	4
Not at all	Somewhat	Very Much	Don't Know

77. Do you consider yourself a spiritual person?   Yes ___   No___ Don't Know___

78. How often do you attend religious services (Church, Synagogue, Mosque, Temple, Other)?

> **THANK YOU FOR ANSWERING THESE QUESTIONS. IS THERE ANYTHING WE FORGOT TO ASK ABOUT?**
>
> **IF THERE IS FEEL FREE TO WRITE IT DOWN BELOW**
>
> **OR TO TELL YOUR COUNSELOR ABOUT IT**

1	2	3	4
Never	Rarely	Sometimes	Often

79. Please write down any personal views or concerns that we forgot to ask you about.

_____
_____
_____
_____

80. If you have any questions or comments please write anything you want to in the space below:

_____
_____
_____
_____

Clinical Uses of an Adolescent Intake Questionnaire: Adquest as a Bridge to Engagement

Jennifer Elliott
Michael Nembhard
Vincent Giannone
Michael Surko
Daniel Medeiros
Ken Peake

SUMMARY. Open dialogue concerning behavioral and environmental risks is key to effective, holistic intervention with urban adolescents. Topics for discussion must include substance use, sexual behaviors and abuse, health concerns, exposure to violence and racism, school performance, and relationships with family and peers. Clinical engagement of adolescents requires focusing the therapeutic relationship on issues of their own choice, at their own pace. This article describes the clinical

Jennifer Elliott, MSW, and Michael Nembhard, MSW, are Clinical Social Workers, Mount Sinai Adolescent Health Center (AHC). Vincent Giannone, PsyD, is Senior Psychologist, AHC. Michael Surko, PhD, is Coordinator, ACT for Youth Downstate Center for Excellence, AHC. Daniel M. Medeiros, MD, is Director of Mental Health Services, AHC, and Assistant Professor in Pediatrics and Psychiatry, Mount Sinai School of Medicine, Mount Sinai. Ken Peake, DSW, is Assistant Director, AHC, 320 East 94th Street, New York, NY 10128.

[Haworth co-indexing entry note]: "Clinical Uses of an Adolescent Intake Questionnaire: Adquest as a Bridge to Engagement." Elliott, Jennifer et al. Co-published simultaneously in *Social Work in Mental Health* (The Haworth Social Work Practice Press, an imprint of The Haworth Press, Inc.) Vol. 3, No. 1/2, 2004, pp. 83-102; and: *Clinical and Research Uses of an Adolescent Mental Health Intake Questionnaire: What Kids Need to Talk About* (ed: Ken Peake, Irwin Epstein, and Daniel Medeiros) The Haworth Social Work Practice Press, an imprint of The Haworth Press, Inc., 2005, pp. 83-102. Single or multiple copies of this article areavailable for a fee from The Haworth Document Delivery Service [1-800-HAWORTH, 9:00 a.m. - 5:00 p.m. (EST). E-mail address: docdelivery@haworthpress.com].

http://www.haworthpress.com/web/SWMH
© 2004 by The Haworth Press, Inc. All rights reserved.
Digital Object Identifier: 10.1300/J200v03n01_05

83

uses and practice impacts of a comprehensive adolescent self-assessment questionnaire (Adquest). By normalizing sensitive topics and allowing clients to exercise control over the therapeutic agenda and pace, Adquest serves as a "bridge to engagement," a device for keeping the clinical dialogue open and a mode of induction to the client role. For staff, it represents a way of standardizing and broadening clinical assessment, identifying treatment objectives, and framing psycho-educational interventions. *[Article copies available for a fee from The Haworth Document Delivery Service: 1-800-HAWORTH. E-mail address: <docdelivery@haworthpress.com> Website: <http://www.HaworthPress.com> © 2004 by The Haworth Press, Inc. All rights reserved.]*

KEYWORDS. Instruments, assessment, adolescents, engagement, risk, practice-based research

INTRODUCTION

Clinical practice in an agency setting with urban adolescents offers many challenges and places many constraints on practitioners. Uppermost is the need to engage the client in treatment. This involves accomplishing a number of highly complex tasks in a limited amount of time. The tasks include establishing trust with the young person while gathering sufficient information to make a sound diagnosis and developing a viable treatment plan.

Adquest is a self-assessment questionnaire designed by practitioners at Mount Sinai's Adolescent Health Center (AHC), with the aim of enhancing the effectiveness of psychotherapy with urban adolescents (Peake, Epstein, Mirabito, & Surko, 2004). It asks adolescents to reflect on their own experiences, concerns, behaviors, needs, and preferences regarding what they would like to talk to a counselor about. Introduced under the title "All About You," Adquest is given to prospective clients to be completed immediately before their first intake interview. Adquest is organized into seven sections of questions that are designed to mirror the flow of a clinical interview. It ends with a final, open-ended section intended to generate qualitative information concerning anything that the prospective client thinks might have been left out of the forced-choice questions. Completion usually takes about twenty minutes.

When a parent or guardian is present, he or she is asked to complete a parallel, but briefer, questionnaire about the adolescent and the family environment. Together, this information provides a comprehensive overview of how the adolescents and their families perceive multiple sectors of their lives. As such, it represents a starting point for clinical engagement with young persons and their families and for a comprehensive clinical assessment by a mental health professional.

This article describes how AHC clinicians use Adquest in planned and unplanned ways. Part of its unique contribution is that it describes a practitioner-led inquiry into the impact of a formal assessment instrument on their own practice and that of colleagues–an area of inquiry currently missing in the literature. To accomplish this line of inquiry a practice-based research approach was developed and utilized by AHC practitioners, borrowing from Epstein's (1995) exemplar of how a reflective method might be applied using a single case methodology. Epstein proposes that a practitioner can examine his or her own premises and practices by focusing on identifying central assumptions, constraints, challenges, and identifying guiding metaphors. Central questions in this reflective inquiry are: What metaphors arise? How do these metaphors arise? And what is their function?

ASSESSMENT INSTRUMENTS IN SOCIAL WORK PRACTICE

Accountability for service outcomes and the introduction of research methodologies into organizational practice has led to increasing interest in the development and use of formal instruments in direct practice situations (Blumenfield & Epstein, 2001; Peake & Epstein, 2004). There is evidence that indigenous tools–designed to supplement rather than replace interpersonal assessment methods–can enhance practice. Screening tools have long been used in health care to identify high-risk clients where not all patients are seen by social workers (Becker & Becker, 1986; Berkman, Rehr, & Rosenberg, 1980; Wolock & Schlesinger, 1986). Similarly, indigenous self-report questionnaires that screen for family violence have been effective in identifying candidates for psychotherapy in community settings (Guterman & Cameron, 1997). Recently, Springer and Abell (2002) called for increased development and implementation of context-sensitive instruments derived from standardized, research-derived tools so that practitioners can define and measure practice parameters. Researchers, academics, and managers see many potential benefits of introducing research-derived instruments into practice settings (Peake & Epstein, 2004).

Despite this, social work practitioners–especially those trained in psychodynamically derived and interpersonal practice models–have not widely embraced the use of research methods in direct practice, nor have they integrated the use of formal assessment instruments into their clinical work (Balassone, 1991; Bloom, Fischer, & Orme, 1995; Chapman & Richman, 1998; Savaya,

1998; Savaya & Spiro, 1997). While the reasons for this are numerous and complex, and have not been fully understood, some have been identified in the literature.

Chief among the organizational factors that make practitioners aversive to assessment instruments is the failure of managers and researchers to create an atmosphere conducive to such innovations, resulting in clinicians rarely being given adequate time, training, support, and preparation for these "new" methodologies (Savaya, 1996). Perhaps because–in the minds of many practitioners–*standardization* in intervention is associated with monitoring practitioner performance, practitioners often resist such approaches for fear that they will expose practitioner weaknesses and practice problems in agency practice (Bloom et al., 1995). Such fears have been reinforced by the fact that many who call for research integration into practice are blind to the real challenges of practice and are critical of practitioners' effectiveness (Epstein, 2001). Perhaps the most important factor has been a failure among researchers and administrators to include clinicians as leading partners in efforts to integrate research into practice in ways that improve practice (Blumenfield & Epstein, 2001; Peake & Epstein, 2004).

Practitioners are generally unfamiliar with instruments and view them as "blunt and irrelevant" (Pasahow, 1989, p. 41) and as antithetical to the human qualities of direct practice. Rubin and Babbie (1989) note that social workers see formal measurement of problems as cold and in conflict with the warm, intuitive, spontaneous aspects of interpersonal practice. This view may be reinforced by the fact that standardized instruments are developed on the basis of shared characteristics of broad populations (Epstein, 2001) and much of practice is geared toward understanding the unique individuality of the client.

Adquest was developed *by practitioners* as a Practice-Based Research tool, a process of development in which clinical priorities superseded research requirements (Peake, Epstein et al., 2004). As a result, Adquest is locally based and may fall short of ideal research standards of reliability and external validity. On the other hand, Adquest allows AHC clinicians to collect important client information in an efficient manner, while maintaining an approach that is consistent with the overall agency philosophy. One of the major driving forces behind the development of Adquest was the aim of trying to capture the experiences and perceptions of adolescents and to enhance their involvement in therapy.

An initially informal line of inquiry–practitioner to practitioner–followed by a focus group was conducted with AHC practitioners who volunteered to discuss how they apply Adquest routinely to the assessment and treatment process. Practitioners self-selected for the focus group after being told that it was intended to explore how Adquest fit with practice so as to improve its practice utilization. The focus group supplies the metaphors, descriptions, and anecdotes used in this article.

THE PRACTICE SETTING

AHC is a comprehensive, adolescent-specific health center that serves highly vulnerable, high-risk, poor, minority, urban adolescents, ages 10 through 21 (Diaz, Peake, Surko, & Bhandarkar, 2004). AHC provides confidential health, mental health, and reproductive health services without parental notification or consent. More than 20,000 of AHC's yearly visits are for mental health services.

AHC's mental health staff includes clinical social workers, clinical psychologists, and psychiatrists who provide short- and long-term individual, group, and family treatment. Typical presenting problems include sexual assault, abuse and other exposure to violence, family conflicts, sequelae to HIV/AIDS, depression, school failure, and substance abuse. Youth are referred from schools, families, friends, and community-based organizations. Many are self-referred as a result of AHC's reputation for nonjudgmental quality services, easy access and commitment to confidentiality.

As a clinical tool, Adquest is a component of every client's service record and is presented to clients as such, not as a research project. Confidentiality, and its scope and limitations, is discussed with clients prior to intake and completion of Adquest, including how concerns over client safety might result in a practitioner breaching confidentiality.

Although it was not primarily intended as a research instrument, Adquest does offer unique opportunities for data mining (Peake & Epstein, 2004). Research projects resulting from Adquest, like studies that utilize any other component of the service record, require approval through Mount Sinai's Institutional Review Board, as does all research. All data from Adquest have been de-identified and aggregated so that client confidentiality and anonymity cannot be compromised. (A more detailed discussion of confidentiality and research is included in Peake, Epstein et al., 2004).

IMPLEMENTING ADQUEST

Perhaps because Adquest was developed by a group of practitioners and supervisors, its initial implementation, begun in 1999, was intentionally incremental, highly informal and non-prescriptive. This approach was chosen in recognition that Adquest might represent a potential threat to many of the practitioners being asked to integrate it into their practice (Peake, Epstein et al., 2004). *Except for the expectation that the completed Adquest form would be reviewed with each client at some time during the intake process, clinicians received no initial instruction about exactly how it should be used.*

At first, many clinicians found it difficult to incorporate Adquest into their routine assessment practices, oftentimes considering it a threat to their autonomy and an obstacle to building a therapeutic relationship. In response, over a one-year period several staff and team meetings were devoted to giving clinicians a chance to offer their negative feedback about this new tool, and explore ways in which it might be used to complement their practice. Practitioners were encouraged to recognize the potential value of having access to the information it provided.

Although Adquest was designed by practitioners and intended for use within the first interview, the initial experience of implementation showed that few clinicians used it routinely. Those who did use Adquest used it inconsistently and in idiosyncratic ways depending on the unique circumstances of each case. Chief among practitioners' concerns about Adquest were time constraints, particularly when other tasks were deemed more important in getting an intake completed. In addition to completing extensive paperwork, they also had to complete a number of rapid assessment instruments (RAIs). These RAIs, such as the Child Behavior Checklist [CBCL] (Achenbach, 1991) and the Global Assessment of Functioning scale [GAF] (American Psychiatric Association, 2000, p. 34), were required by AHC psychiatrists prior to their scheduling a psychiatric evaluation. Practitioners valued these RAIs far less than Adquest, but saw them as essential to satisfying the demands of others and, therefore, to managing the intake process, or as they called it, "getting past the gate."

Faced with time constraints and the need to ensure the completion of intake paperwork such as a full psychosocial assessment, practitioners often decided that they could adequately assess adolescents' concerns solely by interviewing. This was further reinforced by practitioners' perceptions that key organizational players, such as psychiatrists, supervisors, and treatment planning team leaders, did not view Adquest as an essential component of intake. On balance, practitioners appeared to conduct an implicit cost-benefit analysis that other tasks were of more instrumental value in managing intake processes, though they might be viewed as of less direct clinical value. As a result, Adquest was mainly used when practitioners were faced with problematic cases.

A number of organizational strategies were initiated to more fully integrate Adquest into intake practice. Intake forms were revised and streamlined, wherever possible, to reduce the time required for completion. Team leaders and psychiatrists were asked to ensure that practitioners presented their discussions with clients regarding Adquest as part of treatment planning. Staff meetings were used to explore ways that more use could be made of Adquest. The expectation was clarified that during the three-session face-to-face intake process the clinician would review the adolescent's responses on Adquest and use them clinically.

Over time, clinicians began to find it easier to integrate Adquest into the assessment process. Now, many report that it has become integral to the engagement process, provides a wide range of important information, offers an additional reliability check on face-to-face information gathering, and is a basis for treatment goal-setting and ultimately for treatment evaluation.

A PRACTITIONER-LED REFLECTIVE PRACTICE INQUIRY INTO CLINICAL USES OF ADQUEST

To further enhance integration of Adquest into practice, a best practices approach was used to identify *how* practitioners used Adquest through a peer-led practitioner focus group. Group members were asked to reflect on when and how they used Adquest, and how it impacted on and changed practice, both in helpful and unhelpful ways. The *methodology for analysis* utilized Epstein's (1995) application of Schon's (1983) *reflective practice* concept to case study. This methodology focuses on having practitioners reflect on their practice to identify the central theoretical assumptions and *guiding metaphors* that are in play, what functions they play, and how these metaphors interact with one another. This article reports the results of that inquiry.

Practitioners overwhelmingly identified Adquest as *helpful* and reported no negative experiences with clients, whom they viewed as well able to regulate how much they shared in completing the questionnaire. However, obstacles to integrating Adquest into practice were identified. Practitioners still felt limited by time constraints, the primary limitation being the need to ensure that sufficient information was gathered by interview to allow completion of the assessment forms required at intake. Practitioners also reported that discussing Adquest in the first session was often not possible when there was a concern about client safety, and all felt that it was essential to thoroughly assess for safety in the initial interview. Additionally, some ambivalence remained that Adquest might be used for *monitoring* how practitioners performed their assessments or might leave practitioners exposed to criticism from colleagues. This concern is reflected in the discussion of the metaphors that arose in the focus group.

A BRIDGE TO ENGAGEMENT

After initial struggles with integrating the Adquest into practice, clinicians overall have reported that using the questionnaire has served as a "bridge to engagement" with adolescents. By allowing easy identification of which issues adolescents want to talk about (along with some idea of which issues adolescents *need* to talk about), clinicians can begin to engage clients in areas where they are ready to begin and return later to those issues adolescents are reluctant to discuss. Many of the metaphors that follow describe how Adquest serves as a bridge in the therapeutic process.

GIVING KIDS PERMISSION TO TALK

In addition to providing clinicians with an immediate wealth of personal information, clinicians have observed that *Adquest signals to adolescents that under the right circumstances it is appropriate to relinquish the social expectation that one must first get to know someone before disclosing personal information.*

Nevertheless, clinicians report that some clients will admit during later stages of treatment (when trust is firmly established) that they omitted some information from their Adquest because they "just couldn't imagine walking in here and saying, yeah, that happened to me, and yeah, that, too." Just knowing that they can talk about these subjects, when they are ready, can be very valuable to the engagement process and the development of a relationship with the counselor.

On the other hand, practitioners report that most clients feel an immediate need to discuss highly sensitive issues. They are relieved to find that they have been given the chance to begin talking about such painful subjects as incest and rape, which perhaps they have never yet had the opportunity to discuss with anyone. On the whole, practitioners are struck by how open and forthcoming youth are in their responses to Adquest, and how helpful it can be in starting that first conversation. As one practitioner put it: "I think it does bridge the gap, if you will, between total strangers . . . and by the end of that session, I think you both move a little closer, by just being able to talk about a lot of different things because of what's in the Adquest."

Whether or not a client is initially hesitant to reveal him or herself, it also offers some preparation for what topics might be discussed in treatment. And, as it covers such a wide range of adolescent experience, it provides young persons with *permission* to talk about virtually anything that is troubling to them.

As a consequence, adolescents have time and privacy to decide how much they feel ready to reveal about themselves initially.

GIVING CLINICIANS PERMISSION TO ASK

From the standpoint of the clinician, Adquest gives the practitioner "permission" to ask prospective clients questions that both can find difficult to discuss. And by communicating that *all* new clients are asked the very same questions, Adquest normalizes the discussion of these topics. One clinician comments: " I think . . . it also normalizes things, because you're getting something that you know everyone is getting asked, so it's pretty normal to be asked if you're having sex or if you've been exposed to violence or what drugs you're doing. So, it's not like 'I'm the only one coming in here who may have these issues.'"

Even for seasoned clinicians, approaching some personal domains can be difficult and requires sensitivity to adolescents' verbal and nonverbal reactions. Overall, as a consequence of the routine implementation of Adquest, clinicians cited an increased comfort level for both the client and counselors. They observed that as clients got to know what to expect when meeting for the intake, workers became less worried about shocking adolescents with direct, personal questions so early in the therapeutic relationship. As one such practitioner put it, "One of the things I find that the Adquest helps with is I have to spend less time *setting up* a question around drug abuse or around sexual abuse." Another clinician comments:

> I think it makes the dialogue significantly easier, because you don't have to think too much about how to ask this question so this kid doesn't feel uncomfortable, and so that you also feel comfortable asking the question. It's already there and you can go right into it . . . without giving it too much thought. And they're expecting to be asked about these things.

Utilizing the adolescent's responses to Adquest can help both client and clinician negotiate where it feels safe to begin a therapeutic dialogue. Regardless of the rest of the client's profile, beginning with what he or she worries about is often the best place to start. At times, however, the young person may be more comfortable reporting that other people worry about him or her, or that he or she worries about other people, which allows the clinician to begin by asking about these particular worries. When this occurs, clients may be indirectly exposing concerns about their own behaviors. For example, a clinician observes:

[I]t's interesting though, they'll say that they've been a victim of crime, that they've been forced to have sex, that they're using a lot of substances and they don't want to talk about that. But then you go to the "family" [section on Adquest] and [their response is] "very much, I want to talk about my family" . . . because they perceive that to be the problem that explains the other stuff.

Adquest's format is especially useful in the early stage of clinical engagement because it allows the therapist to simultaneously monitor risk indicators as well as the young person's willingness to talk about them.

THE SILENT DIALOGUE

Adquest also provides young people with an *internal* forum for self-reflection in addition to their face-to-face encounters with clinicians. Without yet having to verbalize any of their feelings, experiences, or concerns, Adquest invites adolescents to take stock of their own lives in a way they have never before done. Although this may seem to some an unrealistic expectation, clinicians agree that adolescents as a rule take great care when filling out the Adquest, and seem to find it meaningful and engaging.

While the adolescent's responses to Adquest begin to tell his or her story, its format and headings initiate the clinician's contribution to this silent dialogue. Section titles and the carefully worded introductions that accompany each of them are meant to indicate AHC's philosophy about many issues (Diaz et al., 2004; Peake, Epstein et al., 2004). It is intended that the questions and their location within Adquest are both information-gathering devices and clinical interventions, helping adolescents to better understand how clinicians might perceive their clients' experiences and behaviors.

Despite predictable feelings of resistance, fear, shyness or resentment, adolescents seen at AHC want to be understood and appreciated by a caring adult. When they take responsibility for their side of the conversation, it gives the clinician a welcome opportunity to further explore and try to better understand the individual. Though Adquest starts with forced-choice questions, together the practitioner and client will work to ultimately put an adolescent's story into his or her own words.

A SECOND VOICE

Some practitioners went so far as to describe Adquest as a "second voice" for adolescents. One said, "They want to be heard. They want their side of the story to be told. And this is a way of telling their side of the story." When accompanied by a parent who is upset and angry, an adolescent often limits what he or she has to say in the initial session–even when seen alone. As a second voice for the adolescent, *Adquest provides adolescents with an opportunity to balance the power between themselves and their parents.* One clinician describes it as a "safe place" for adolescents to develop their story about themselves, because each account is shared with only the clinician, making it less likely they will be contradicted. Clinicians overall agree that adolescents seem to be reassured that by completing Adquest they have begun to silently share their side, and that this story will be heard at some point by the counselor.

Some practitioners report that they consult this "second voice" more directly with some clients, particularly those who do not spontaneously talk about their problems and concerns. In such instances, Adquest responses provide insight into the adolescent's silence. For example:

> I always find it interesting when they act like they don't want to talk about anything and they seem really resistant, and I go back over the . . . questions that ask "how much do you want to talk to your counselor about whatever issue?" And they say "a lot." So, that's always helpful when I [originally thought] . . . "oh, they're not interested."

When confronted by a silent adolescent, clinicians find that rather than explore the reasons why someone else may have referred the youth for treatment, they can ask about worries and concerns that the adolescent has indicated on Adquest. And there are almost always concerns. For instance, a youth may be referred by a parent due to school failure or drug use, but when reviewing Adquest responses what stands out might be the adolescent's worries about family and home life. From here this adolescent–who might not be open to discussing drug use–can be engaged around these domestic issues, and the other problems can be reframed in relation to these concerns as engagement progresses.

Likewise, AHC counselors report that often clients appear to want to be asked about personal or sensitive topics, but aren't prepared to broach the topics themselves. The result can be a "mismatch" between clients' responses to Adquest and what they volunteer in the first assessment interview. Clinicians describe several ways this mismatch is identified and monitored in order to capitalize on opportunities for dialogue about key issues. Although many adolescents might appear to be oppositional, guarded or withdrawn in their first session, they may check forced-choice items or write in responses to open-ended questions that are revealing about what they want and need to talk about. Mismatches are most commonly identified when adolescents acknowledge risky behaviors but minimize their worries about these behaviors or their desire to talk about them.

Of course, the most direct expression of an adolescent's desire to talk about an issue in counseling comes in response to the summary question at the end of each Adquest section, about how much they want to talk to a counselor about the particular issues the section explores. Even with adolescents who are not particularly verbal initially, clinicians report that their paying careful attention to client responses about wanting to talk leads adolescents eventually to talk.

BUILDING TRUST

For the majority of clients, the array of issues that they face can feel overwhelming and frightening when first broached in counseling. This may prevent an adolescent from feeling safe enough to begin the conversation. Because Adquest's structure allows adolescents to see the conceptual framework of the intake in advance, they can plan ahead of time about how and what they will disclose. This augments feelings of control over the process of beginning treatment, which is an important aspect of developing trust between the client and the clinician: "I think it's reassuring [that Adquest helps] not to flood them–they're [responding to] . . . questions that they've seen before. The Adquest provides a little structure to the interview, so that is a little reassuring, too. Not that they have to come in here and start spilling everything."

Clinicians cite many examples in which the structure potentially provided to the intake process by Adquest–for they can use it to structure the intake or not, as suits the situation–has accompanied increased rapport between therapist and client. Although the fact that the clinician knows that sensitive information doesn't automatically create closeness, the way that clinicians respect and protect privileged information quickly gives them opportunities to earn trust.

In other cases, adolescents can test the therapist by not fully revealing information. Though many Adquest questions force a choice between a "yes" or "no" response, a "don't know" option is available in most of Adquest's more sensitive questions such as: "Have you ever been forced to have sex?" This option provides adolescents the freedom to develop trust with the counselor before acknowledging rape or abuse, the revelation of which might precipitate a clinician taking legal action or have other unforeseen consequences. Adolescents with a history of being sexually abused are rarely ready to take action against the perpetrator at intake. They must first organize their thoughts and feelings about what has happened to them. Adquest may be the first chance they have to safely disclose this painful experience and to manage the extent of disclosure at a pace within their own comfort level.

And because Adquest asks about a range of behaviors and experiences in a nonjudgmental way, it conveys AHC's stance that young people will experiment and that adults can be of most use helping them weigh options, understand themselves and their choices better, and provide a safe and supportive place to talk. Clinicians will of course challenge clients about their risky behaviors when appropriate, but the content of Adquest tells adolescents from the start that their behaviors and experiences will not shock or dismay clinicians and implies that practitioners will respond with empathy, concern, and understanding.

KEEPING THE CONVERSATION OPEN

Clinicians report that by reviewing a client's responses on the Adquest, respecting their "don't know" answers or not wanting to talk about certain issues that may be of concern to the practitioner, they still can return to issues at a later time. Often in such cases, there is an "unspoken agreement" between client and worker that the topic is off limits for the moment, but that the clinician will respectfully return to it in the future without being too intrusive. As one practitioner indicates:

> [I]t sort of depends on how you feel as far as the engagement is going. If it's something that they don't really want to talk about, but they have indicated on the list that they have a lot that needs to be talked about . . . I don't want to overwhelm them the first or second time I've met them so they don't come back. So, it's sort of like a mental note or . . . you include it in the treatment plan.

Clinicians also give central importance to allowing adolescents to set the pace for exploring sensitive issues. They sometimes share their desire and intention to explore issues they have concerns about when the adolescent becomes ready. This approach requires patience as well as openness: "I'll acknowledge that it's their right not to talk about these things . . . but I think it's important and I'll bring it up when it's necessary and their responsibility is just to tell me they don't want to talk about it. A lot of the kids kind of accept that and I think it's good that we earmark for them that we do consider it important."

The range of information that Adquest provides about an adolescent's risks and willingness to talk about them allows clinicians to plan for future engagement of problems that the client will not discuss at the moment. For example, when a female adolescent is in a sexual relationship with a much older partner (a common AHC experience) where there are dramatic power dynamics and coercive manipulation, the adolescent rarely defines this as abusive. The clinician must help the adolescent begin to understand ways in which the relationship is abusive, and what kind of an effect it can have on her future emotional and physical health.

Another frequent "mismatch" is between self-reported drug use and young people's desire to talk about it. This is one of the most difficult topics to engage youth around, since they are accustomed to conflicts with their parents over their substance use, or to hiding it, or to viewing substance use as normative in their reference group.

Here again, Adquest prepares adolescents for the clinician's perspective that tobacco, alcohol, and drug use are all health issues, and are a matter of concern. At the same time, the reality of the prevalence of substance use in urban communities requires asking about the youth's experience in a straightforward, accepting way. Clinicians agree, however, that respecting a desire not to talk about the issue but "leaving the door open" for future discussion fosters rapport with clients and sometimes paradoxically leads to later disclosure. An AHC counselor remarks:

> Whether the kid says they don't want to talk about it or . . ."I have it under control," they do need to talk about it and that issue needs to be addressed. Sometimes it's up to the clinician to help make those kinds of determinations. Yes, we're not going to talk about this now but this is really a problem and we need to really explore this, maybe at some other point in time.

A clinician gave another example, related to substance abuse, of how mismatches are utilized:

> [K]ids indicate that they are high users and indicate that it is not an issue for them . . . [or] bring up this whole thing about people worry about them or they worry about their friends or they worry about other people . . . it allows one to get into the conversation "why are you worried about them or why do you think they are worried about you?" You kind of mark that. It's a good lead-in.

Sometimes Adquest serves as a vehicle for young persons to later raise issues in therapy that they were unwilling to raise earlier. Clients vary greatly in how much trust and confidence they must develop in the therapist and in the therapeutic relationship before they will disclose intensely painful information. In one instance, a client's Adquest responses provided the opening for her to raise an issue she hid earlier in treatment. Her counselor recalls: "I had a kid just last week apologizing to me for lying on the Adquest because she was incested by her brother and she profusely apologized for not checking it on the Adquest, lying to the intake worker. . . . It's interesting how many people don't check that because they're not ready for it."

A ROAD MAP FOR PRACTITIONERS

Just as Adquest can provide structure for exploration of multiple risks with highly vulnerable and potentially overwhelmed clients, it also provides structure to the treatment planning process. Clinicians report that it is extremely useful in structuring treatment planning and ensuring that they have a grasp of each client's entire story, including inconsistencies and mismatched information.

Practitioners also invent their own clinical uses for Adquest–uses not envisioned by its developers. Some clinicians find it useful to address all the Adquest areas with clients in the first intake session. Most others scan Adquest looking for "trigger items" indicating urgent clinical issues, earmarking most other issues for later discussion.

Clinicians also report that by reading through Adquest responses between the first few sessions and marking areas that don't require immediate attention helps confirm or challenge their diagnostic assessments and the treatment formulations that emerged during the intake process. While clinicians will not typically review each Adquest answer with an adolescent, some practitioners report doing just that with clients who are especially nonverbal. For instance: "With kids that are really quiet and don't talk and are only going to respond to questions, it's really helpful. [If] you know they're not spontaneously going to talk, then I might go through it, piece by piece and really try to engage them in talking about it."

Patterns of response to Adquest also provide some suggestive information about a client's mental status. Clinicians remark that when, as occurs infrequently, an individual will answer all questions "yes" or "no" or leave Adquest entirely blank such response patterns can be a good indication of the client's depressed mood, unwillingness to engage, cognitive limitations or learning disabilities. For clinicians, the undifferentiated client response to Adquest–rare as it is–is a useful place to begin further exploration about what is happening in an adolescent's life.

Adquest has also proven to be helpful when used as a comparison against other persons' accounts of an adolescent's behavior. When adults accompany adolescents and complete the shortened but parallel questionnaire, clinicians report looking for discrepancies on questions, as this can be a clue to what may be going on in the home. Differences can explain more about an adolescent's relationship with a parent or guardian. Parents may over-exaggerate or be blind to their adolescent's substance use, sexual abuse history, or sexual activity. Though an adolescent's responses on Adquest are not discussed with a parent, by comparing parent and adolescent responses clinicians are given insight that they may not otherwise be privy to.

A SECOND SET OF EYES

While clinicians have described Adquest as a "bridge to engagement," a second overarching metaphor that they proffer is Adquest as a "second set of eyes." One aspect of the function described by this metaphor is that Adquest can be used as a "memory check." A second function is that it can "sharpen the focus" of the interpersonal interview with another data source.

Likewise, in clinical team meetings all team members have access to the Adquest responses of the client whose assessment and treatment is being discussed. Here Adquest serves as an independent source of information for other team members and contributes to team considerations about a worker's initial diagnostic assessment and treatment formulations. As such, it promotes a clinical dialogue among team members.

Despite the fact that practitioners expressed a welcoming attitude toward having an independent source of data–*a second set of eyes* and a *second voice*– some concern lingered that their clinical assessment might seem contradicted by Adquest responses. Such contradictions between the written assessment and Adquest might *expose* them to criticism regarding the quality of their assessments, particularly during treatment planning team meetings. For example, one clinician said: "In a non-confrontational way, it's taken in the spirit . . . If someone were to say "you've missed that," then you're obviously going to be . . . [silence]." Another responded: "Yeah, someone in team, the psychiatrist or team leader, might grab it." Yet another suggested that practitioners also find ways to preemptively avoid exposure: "People say 'did you consider that?' . . . When I've gone through Adquest and I've seen these red flag questions that I didn't get a chance to . . . [fully] explore with the kid before I am presenting, I will just indicate in my treatment plan: 'Will explain.'"

However, most comments supported the view that while these team discussions also highlight differences in members' clinical approaches they provide a common base of information for assessing levels of risk. Although they value their autonomy, clinicians report that allowing other team members to see and interpret their clients' Adquest responses takes some of the burden off their shoulders for making clinical decisions entirely alone.

TAKING A QUICK SCAN

As was described earlier, most practitioners also report that they scan Adquest during the intake process as a way of looking for "trigger items" indicating urgent clinical issues, earmarking most other issues for later discussion. At times they report this helps them assess the adolescent's immediate needs. At other times, however, scanning was also used for case-finding purposes by some clinicians responsible for a particular specialized clinical service.

Each clinical team at AHC is composed of a diverse group of practitioners who have individual interests, different personal styles and treatment approaches and specialized areas of practice. Despite AHC's holistic emphasis, there is always the danger that a clinician who is a treatment specialist will focus on information relevant to their area of expertise and ignore other salient factors in the adolescent's life. This use of Adquest–potentially problematic because it militates against the intent of Adquest–emerged in the metaphor of "taking a quick scan."

One specialist said: "I look at the sexual abuse, rape, forced to have sex, violence, witness to domestic violence questions." Another commented: "I like to go to substance abuse." Similarly, other clinicians report that they sometimes focus on that section of Adquest most related to their specialty as a way of case finding even before meeting the client for the first time.

Fortunately, in the treatment teams Adquest brings this tension to the foreground and can be used to develop alternative perspectives with other team members through dialogue and discussion. Across differences that may arise from practitioners' specializations or unique personal styles, Adquest provides a "common language" for clinical assessment and discussion. Practitioners report that prior to implementation of Adquest, each clinician explored risk in her or his own idiosyncratic way and different clinicians focused upon different aspects of the adolescent's experience. Adquest offers a common informational base for all team members to use in assessing risk.

CONCLUSION

Of the approximately twenty AHC practitioners who are currently utilizing Adquest as a bridge to engagement, only one was involved in its original development and design. Nevertheless, these practitioners report that this practitioner-designed, indigenous instrument enhances their ability to engage high-risk urban adolescents. Clinicians have been able to use it creatively despite some concerns that, by offering a different perspective from interviewing alone, Adquest might at times leave them somewhat exposed.

Using Adquest helps practitioners make these adolescent clients feel comfortable, develop trust, and create a genuine clinical dialogue that reflects both the concerns of the adolescent and the clinician's assessment of their risks. These practitioners report that Adquest enables them to create a road map for treatment, i.e., to address adolescents' immediate concerns and to keep the conversation open so that they can circle back to the most loaded issues later, furthering their therapeutic work. Adquest offers a structure to iterate overall risks and vulnerabilities without overwhelming the client, which clinicians can utilize when they need to.

Contrary to the commonly held view among researchers and academics that social work practitioners are averse to research integration in practice and, most particularly, to using assessment instruments–these clinicians have found ways for this indigenous assessment instrument to support their interpersonal work. And, faced with the challenge of engaging high risk adolescents, it offers them a second pair of eyes–helping them assess risks and vulnerabilities holistically while freeing them to focus on what is most relevant to the adolescent.

Implementation of Adquest in a way that encourages experimentation and creativity–rather than uniform intake practices–has resulted in uses that its developers did not imagine, could not have imagined. Clinicians can tailor their use of Adquest to fit each practice situation.

Perhaps most important of all is the rich array of metaphors that emerged from this practitioner-led, practice-based research inquiry. These metaphors show that when practitioners are encouraged to innovate and share their creative experiences, many stereotypes about practice culture dissolve. If we are to genuinely understand how to better serve vulnerable populations, much more needs to be heard from practitioners about their own experiences in integrating innovations into practice.

REFERENCES

Achenbach, T. M., Howell, C. T., Quay, H. C., & Conners, C. K. (1991). National survey of problems and competencies among four-to-sixteen-year-olds. *Monographs of the Society for Research in Child Development.*

American Psychiatric Association. (2000). Global Assessment of Functioning Scale [GAF] Diagnostic and Statistical Manual, Fourth Edition, p. 34.

Balassone, M. L. (1991). A research methodology for the development of risk assessment tools in social work practice. *Social Work Research and Abstracts*, 27 (2), 16-23.

Becker, F. W. Jr., & Becker, N. E. (1986). Productivity in mental health organizations: The need for normalcy. *Journal of Mental Health Administration*, 13 (1), 38-40.

Berkman, B., Rehr, H., & Rosenberg, G. (1980). A social work department develops and tests a screening mechanism to identify high social risk situations. *Social Work in Healthcare*, 5 (4), 373-85.

Bloom, M., Fischer, J., & Orme, J. (1995). *Evaluating practice: Guidelines for the accountable professional* (2nd ed.). Englewood Cliffs, NJ: Prentice-Hall.

Blumenfield, S., & Epstein, I. (2001). Introduction: Promoting and maintaining a reflective professional staff in a hospital-based social work department. *Social Work in Health Care*, 33 (3/4), 1-13.

Chapman, M. V., & Richman, J. M. (1998). Promoting research and evaluation of practice in school based programs: Lessons learned. *Social Work in Education*, 20 (3), 203-208.

Diaz, A., Peake, K., Surko, M., & Bhandarkar, K. (2004). Including "at-risk" adolescents in their own health and mental health care: A youth development perspective. *Social Work in Mental Health*, 3(1/2), 3-22.

Epstein, I. (1995). Promoting reflective social work practice: Research strategies and consulting principles. In E. J. Mullen, and J. L. Magnabosco (Eds.), *Practitioner-Researcher Partnerships: Building Knowledge From, In, and For Practice.* 83- 102. Washington, DC.

Epstein, I. (2001). Using available clinical information in practice-based research: Mining for silver while dreaming of gold. *Social Work in Health Care*, 33 (3/4), 15-32.

Guterman, N. B., & Cameron, M. (1997). Assessing the impact of community violence on children and youths. *Social Work*, 42 (5), 495-505.

Pasahow, C. (1989). Assessing intimacy: The utility of a modified pair inventory as a diagnostic and treatment tool. Unpublished doctoral dissertation, City University of New York, Hunter College School of Social Work.

Peake, K., & Epstein, I. (2004). Theoretical and Practical Imperatives for Reflective Social Work Organizations in Health and Mental Health: The Place of Practice-Based Research. *Social Work in Mental Health*, 3(1/2), 23-37.

Peake, K., Epstein, I., Mirabito, D., & Surko, M. (2004). Development and Utilization of a Practice-Based Adolescent Intake Questionnaire (Adquest): Surveying which risks, worries, and concerns urban youth want to talk about. *Social Work in Mental Health*, 3(1/2), 55-82.

Rubin, A., & Babbie, E. (1989). *Research methods for social work.* Belmont, CA: Wadsworth.

Savaya, S. R., & Spiro, S. (1997). Reactions of practitioners to the introduction of a standard instrument to monitor clinical outcomes. *Journal of Social Service Research,* 22 (4), 39-55.

Savaya, S. R. (1998). The potential and utilization of an integrated information system at a family and marriage counseling agency in Israel. *Evaluation and Program Planning,* 21, 11-20.

Schon, D. (1983). *The reflective practitioner: How professionals think in action.* New York: Basic Books.

Sherman, T., & Zimmerman, M. (2002). Screening for Posttraumatic Stress Disorder in a general psychiatric outpatient setting. *Journal of Clinical & Consulting Psychology,* 70 (4), 961-966.

Springer, D. W., Abell, N., & Hudson, N. M. (2002). Creating and validating Rapid Assessment Instruments for practice and research: Part I. *Research in Social Work Practice,* 12 (3), 408-439.

Tripodi, T., & Epstein, I. (1980). *Research techniques for clinical social workers.* New York: Columbia University Press.

Wolock, I., & Schlesinger, E. G. (1986). Social work screening in New Jersey Hospitals. *Health and Social Work,* 11 (1), 15-24.

Which Adolescents Need to Talk About Safety and Violence?

Michael Surko
Dianne Ciro
Erika Carlson
Nyanda Labor
Vincent Giannone
Elizabeth Diaz-Cruz
Ken Peake
Irwin Epstein

SUMMARY. Exposure to violence has harmful psychological effects on adolescents, and when asked, inner-city adolescents will talk openly about violence in their lives. In response to a clinical self-assessment questionnaire, prospective adolescent mental health clients revealed

Michael Surko, PhD, is Coordinator, Center for Excellence (CfE), Mount Sinai Adolescent Health Center (AHC). Dianne Ciro, CSW, is Clinical Social Worker, AHC. Erika Carlson, BS, is Program Evaluator, CfE. Nyanda Labor, MPH, is Evaluation and Policy Researcher, CfE. Vincent Giannone, PsyD, is Senior Psychologist, AHC. Elizabeth Diaz-Cruz, BA, is Program Assistant, Ryan White Program, AHC. Ken Peake, DSW, is Assistant Director, AHC. Irwin Epstein, PhD, is Helen Rehr Professor of Applied Social Work Research in Health, Hunter College School of Social Work. Mount Sinai Adolescent Health Center is located at 320 East 94th Street, New York, NY 10128.

[Haworth co-indexing entry note]: "Which Adolescents Need to Talk About Safety and Violence?" Surko, Michael et al. Co-published simultaneously in *Social Work in Mental Health* (The Haworth Social Work Practice Press, an imprint of The Haworth Press, Inc.) Vol. 3, No. 1/2, 2004, pp. 103-119; and: *Clinical and Research Uses of an Adolescent Mental Health Intake Questionnaire: What Kids Need to Talk About* (ed: Ken Peake, Irwin Epstein, and Daniel Medeiros) The Haworth Social Work Practice Press, an imprint of The Haworth Press, Inc., 2005, pp. 103-119. Single or multiple copies of this article are available for a fee from The Haworth Document Delivery Service [1-800-HAWORTH, 9:00 a.m. - 5:00 p.m. (EST). E-mail address: docdelivery@haworthpress.com].

http://www.haworthpress.com/web/SWMH
© 2004 by The Haworth Press, Inc. All rights reserved.
Digital Object Identifier: 10.1300/J200v03n01_06

high rates of exposure to physical, sexual, and community violence: 73.5% had witnessed violence, 43.6% had been a victim of violence, 26.4% had had their bodies touched in a way that made them feel uncomfortable, 24.4% had been threatened with a weapon, and 11.1% had experienced forced sex. Clients also expressed substantial worry about their own and their friends' dangerous behaviors. Desire to talk to a counselor about safety was significantly related to overall safety risk (p < .001), and over three-quarters of adolescents either wanted or needed to talk with a counselor. Age and gender differences in patterns of vulnerability and type of counseling need were explored. *[Article copies available for a fee from The Haworth Document Delivery Service: 1-800-HAWORTH. E-mail address: <docdelivery@haworthpress.com> Website: <http://www.HaworthPress.com> © 2004 by The Haworth Press, Inc. All rights reserved.]*

KEYWORDS. Adolescent, safety, violence, mental health, help-seeking, risk

Many American adolescents grow up in violent environments (Kreiter, Krowchuk, Woods, Sinal, Lawless, & Durant, 1999). Homicide is the second leading cause of death for young people aged 15-24 and suicide is the third leading cause of death for young people aged 10-24 (Centers for Disease Control and Prevention, 2002). In the U.S. in the year 2000, 10.6% of all firearm deaths occurred among those aged 19 years or younger. Adolescents aged 15-24 commit suicide at a rate of 11.9 per 100,000; this rate is second only to adults age 75 and over (Centers for Disease Control and Prevention, 2002).

Adolescents face other serious threats to their safety as well as their psychological and emotional well-being. The most recent Youth Risk Behavior Survey by the Centers for Disease Control and Prevention (2002) revealed that 17.4% had carried a weapon in the 30 days preceding the survey, and in the 12 months preceding the survey, 33.2% reported having been in a physical fight, 9.5% had been physically hurt on purpose by their boyfriend or girlfriend, and 8.8% had attempted suicide. In addition, 7.7% had been forced to have sexual intercourse in their lifetime.

Exposure, both direct and indirect, to such violence has been found to be associated with fears of injury, danger, and the unknown; withdrawn behavior, somatic complaints, and posttraumatic symptoms (Cooley-Quille, Boyd, Frantz, & Walsh, 2002); use of violence against others (Durant, Altman,

Wolfson, Barkin, Kreiter, & Krowchuk, 2000); and lasting posttraumatic effects such as anger, anxiety, depression, and low self-esteem (Boney-McCoy & Finkelhor, 1996; Slovak, 2002; Spenciner Rosenthal, 2000).

Kahn, Kazimi, and Mulvihill (2001) found that the more adolescents were exposed to gun violence, the more they wanted to talk about their own safety. Adolescents generally want and need to talk about behavioral and health issues including safety and violence with health care providers but often do not because they are not asked about them (Klein & Wilson, 2002). Some health care providers may not ask because they do not feel adequately trained to deal with adolescent issues, and others may not have enough time for exploration of psychosocial and behavioral issues with adolescents (Ackard & Neumark-Sztainer, 2001).

Many clinicians and other adults understand that the most important resource for children and young people in learning to understand and cope with violence is open and trusting communication with parents and other reliable adults (American Academy of Pediatrics, 1994; Sweatt, Harding, Knight-Lynn, Rasheed, & Carter, 2002). Nonetheless, therapists often lack systematic knowledge of their adolescent clients' exposure to community violence and fail to ask about it (Guterman & Cameron, 1999).

Clinicians seeking to work effectively with adolescents to ensure their physical and emotional safety need to gain an accurate and contextual understanding of the real safety threats and exposures that adolescents face. They also need to establish an ongoing dialogue concerning safety on which to base trust and understanding from which they can develop an effective intervention (Diaz, Peake, Surko, & Bhandarkar, 2004).

Although public and professional awareness of the impact of violence on adolescents has increased, relying entirely upon published research alone can be misleading to the clinician. Many investigators have focused on single experiences of victimization or risk behaviors of respondents. The former is too narrow a focus, and the latter often places blame on the victim. Few researchers have examined multiple exposures to violence, their impact on adolescent risk behaviors and the developmental context in which this interaction takes place (Green, Goodman, Krupnick, Corcoran, Petty, Stockton, & Stern, 2000). In addition, developing a phenomenology of adolescent vulnerability and understanding the meanings that adolescents themselves ascribe to their behaviors and experiences is key to effective intervention (Zaslow & Takanishi, 1993).

Thinking along similar lines, Lerner (1995) advocates working together with adolescents to develop qualitative understandings of their "development-in-context" as a means of building understanding and commitment to jointly planned change efforts. This perspective highlights the importance of adolescents' worries about violence and their need to talk about safety and is important in helping vulnerable adolescents begin to discuss their experiences and concerns (or lack of concerns) regarding safety.

The present article presents research findings extracted from a clinical intake questionnaire (Adquest) designed by clinicians to solicit information about prior experiences of trauma and present safety (e.g., from physical violence, accidental injury, sexual abuse, or assault) among adolescents seeking mental health counseling. Equally important from a clinical point of view, the instrument is intended to open an ongoing dialogue with prospective clients about their "development-in-context" as a means of building a helping relationship and planning for constructive change.

METHOD

Practice Context and Population Served

Mount Sinai Adolescent Health Center (AHC) is a comprehensive health center for inner-city youth who make more than 20,000 mental health visits annually in a confidential setting, where clients are seen regardless of their health insurance status or ability to pay. The study sample consisted of 759 adolescents presenting for mental health intake between 4/27/99 and 4/9/02. Of these, 36.0% were male and 64.0% were female. Ranging in age from 10 through 21, these urban adolescent applicants for mental health services come largely from low-income households in New York City (Diaz et al., 2004). The majority identified themselves as either Hispanic/Latino (44.7%) or African-American (29.8%), with 10.2% giving multiple responses for race/ethnicity, 6.0% identifying as White, 4.5% as West Indian/Caribbean, 2.8% as Other, and 1.6% as Asian/Pacific Islander.

Adquest

Adquest is an indigenous, context-specific instrument designed by practitioners for practitioners. The 80-item adolescent self-report asks about life areas such as school and education, work, safety, health, sexuality, substance abuse, and personal/family life. It was intended to enhance adolescent engagement in psychotherapy by asking young persons who are requesting counseling services to reflect on their own lives, problems, needs, worries and reasons for seeking counseling, and what they want to talk about (Peake, Epstein, Mirabito, & Surko, 2004).

Conceptualization of Safety Items

Adquest safety items were assigned to four categories by consensus among a group of ten AHC practice-based researchers: environmental risk (e.g., direct victimization, witnessing of violence, availability of firearms), behavioral risk (physical fighting with boyfriend/girlfriend), worries about safety (e.g., worry about hurting self or others), and expressed desire to talk about safety with a counselor. In this article, responses to questions relating to the first three categories are generally treated as independent variables; age and gender as mediating variables; and desire/or need to talk about safety as dependent variables. Correlates of race/ethnicity and experience of racism are discussed in a separate study by Surko, Ciro, Blackwood, Nembhard, and Peake (2005).

Wanting Versus Needing to Talk

As noted by Diaz et al. (2004), adolescents who present with substantial areas of vulnerability and risk often do not initially share the clinician's assessment of risk or of priorities for change. It is, therefore, important to track both the level of risk and the adolescent's openness to engaging in a dialogue about the issue. When an adolescent is open to talking about safety issues, clinicians have a range of options for intervention around safety-related issues, including insight-oriented work around personal and family history and present behavior; more concrete problem-solving around behavioral issues (e.g., possible positive and negative results of joining a gang to be safe in a dangerous neighborhood); and psychoeducation and health education around issues such as substance use, relationship, and domestic violence.

In anticipation of the analysis of Adquest data across multiple problem areas, Peake and colleagues (2004) developed a typology of need for counseling based on the adolescent's level of risk exposure and her/his expressed or implied desire to talk to a counselor about it. Accordingly, a Safety Risk Scale (SRS) was developed to quantitatively measure the extent of exposure to safety risk reported by adolescents in our clinical sample. High and low levels were used on an aggregate measure of safety risk, in juxtaposition with the desire to talk about safety, to identify four categories of need for and openness to engagement with a therapist on the issue of safety.

We created the SRS by summing the number of risk indicators adolescents had across the categories of environmental and behavioral risk and worries about safety. Of these, two items were dropped (fighting with boyfriend/girlfriend and worry about friends/associates) due to low intercorrelation with other items. Internal consistency for the resulting nine-item scale was lower (Cronbach alpha = .67) than the generally accepted standard of reliability (.80) for preplanned Rapid Assessment Instruments (Springer, Abell, & Hudson, 2002), but was regarded as clinically adequate to initially identify adolescents with relatively high and relatively low degrees of risk.

SRS median scores were then used to split the sample into high and low safety risk groups; adolescents with scores of 0-3 were assigned to the "low" risk group (54.2% of the sample) and those with scores of 4-9 were assigned to the "high" risk group (45.8% of the sample). This division was then juxtaposed with the expressed or implicit desire to talk, resulting in four clinically relevant groups: Low-Risk/No-Talk, Low-Risk/Talk, High-Risk/Talk, and High-Risk/No-Talk.

Plan for Analysis

In this article, our analytic strategy involves several stages. First, we offer a "snapshot" of respondent exposure to violence and risk behaviors based on the frequency of responses for all 759 adolescents in our clinical sample (e.g., what percentage of our total population experienced forced sex?). Second, we consider gender and age differences associated with exposure to violence and engagement in risk behaviors (e.g., what percentages of males and females experienced forced sex?). Third, we consider the relationships between exposure to violence and risk behaviors on the one hand, and expressed desire to talk with a counselor about safety on the other (e.g., what proportion of respondents who experienced forced sex express a desire to talk about safety with their counselor?). Fourth, we consider gender and age differences in desire to talk about safety and the mediating effects of gender and age on the relationships between exposure to risk and desire to talk about safety (e.g., are males who experienced forced sex more or less likely than females to want to talk about safety with their counselors?). Finally, we describe the gender and age distributions of the mental health counseling applicants who fall into each of the four typological categories on the SRS. The clinical and program implications of these findings conclude the article.

FINDINGS

Safety and Violence "Snapshot"

When asked directly about their exposure to environmental safety risks, adolescents in our clinic populations reported as follows (see Table 1): 73.5% had witnessed violence, 43.6% had been a victim of violence, 26.4% had had their bodies touched in a way that made them feel uncomfortable, 25.9% re-

TABLE 1. Proportion of Adolescents Reporting Safety Risk Indicators (N = 759)

SAFETY RISK INDICATORS	% (n)
Environmental Risks	
Witnessed violence	73.5 (546)
Victim of violence	43.6 (326)
Touched in uncomfortable ways	26.4 (198)
Could get gun	25.9 (190)
Threatened with a weapon	24.4 (182)
Had forced sex	11.1 (82)
Behavioral Risks	
Physical fight with boyfriend/girlfriend	9.0 (59)
Worries About Safety	
Worry do dangerous things	62.8 (469)
Worry about friends/associates	61.2 (455)
Worry about hurting self or others	48.7 (361)
Often feel unsafe	41.4 (309)

ported they could get a gun if they wanted to, 24.4% had been threatened with a weapon, and 11.1% had experienced forced sex. With regard to the risks posed by their own behavior, 9.0% of respondents reported having physical fights with their boyfriend or girlfriend.

Behaviors aside, prospective AHC clients reported the following safety-related worries: 62.8% worried that things they themselves did were dangerous, 61.2% worried about friends or associates they "hung out" with, 48.7% worried about hurting themselves or others, and 41.4% said that they felt unsafe sometimes, often, or always.

Given the general level of risk experienced by these young persons, it is not surprising that 70.9% wanted to talk about it very much, somewhat, or said that they didn't know, and only 29.1% *didn't* want to talk to a counselor about safety. Following the recommendation by Peake and colleagues (2004), "don't know" responses on desire to talk about safety were grouped with affirmative responses because the need to detect and address safety risks with this population makes desirable a moderate bias toward over-inquiring rather than asking too little. Moreover, this assumption was found to have empirical support in that adolescents responding "don't know" on questions regarding violence, sexual abuse, forced sex, etc., generally expressed a similar or greater level of wanting to talk about safety in comparison to those answering "yes" to having experienced these events (Peake et al., 2004).

Gender and Age Factors Associated with Safety Risk Indicators

The relationships between gender and safety risk indicators are summarized in Table 2. Compared to males, females reported significantly higher exposure to being touched in a way that made them uncomfortable (34.9% vs. 11.2%, respectively) and being forced to have sex (15.1% vs. 4.1%, respectively), while males reported higher rates of witnessing or being a victim of violence, being threatened with a weapon and being able to get a gun. No significant gender differences were observed in proportion reporting physical fights with his or her boyfriend/girlfriend.

A significantly greater proportion of females reported worries about hurting themselves or others and about friends or associates they "hang out" with. No significant difference was observed between males and females on worry about one's own dangerous behavior or on feeling unsafe. Although the ma-

TABLE 2. Proportion of Adolescents Reporting Safety Risk Indicators, by Gender

SAFETY RISK FACTORS	Male	Female	
	(N = 272)	(N = 484)	
	% (n)	% (n)	χ^2
Environmental Risks			
Witnessed violence	84.0 (225)	67.7 (320)	23.369***
Victim of violence	49.4 (132)	40.4 (193)	5.720*
Touched in uncomfortable ways	11.2 (30)	34.9 (167)	49.587***
Could get gun	35.4 (93)	20.6 (97)	19.037***
Threatened with a weapon	38.4 (103)	16.6 (79)	44.245***
Had forced sex	4.1 (11)	15.1 (71)	20.836***
Behavioral Risks			
Physical fight with boyfriend/girlfriend	10.1 (23)	8.5 (36)	.496
Worries About Safety			
Worry do dangerous things	66.7 (178)	60.7 (290)	2.638
Worry about friends/associates	55.3 (147)	64.6 (307)	6.307*
Worry about hurting self or others	38.7 (103)	54.2 (257)	16.381***
Often feel unsafe	37.8 (101)	43.4 (207)	2.188

$*p < .05, **p < .01, ***p < .001$

jority of applicants wanted to talk to a counselor about safety, a significantly greater proportion of females indicated interest in talking with their counselor about it than males (74.9% vs. 63.5% of males, $\chi^2(1) = 10.755$, $p = .001$).

With regard to age, all indicators of environmental safety risk increased as adolescents got older (see Table 3). For example, 36% of late adolescents report having been a victim of violence as compared to 54.6% of late adolescents. Similarly, 16.7% of early adolescents report having been threatened with a weapon compared to 36% of late adolescents. When asked about having been forced to have sex, 6.4% of early adolescents responded yes; by mid-adolescence this percentage had nearly doubled (12.4%).

TABLE 3. Proportion of Adolescents Reporting Safety Risk Indicators, by Stage of Adolescence

SAFETY RISK FACTORS	STAGE OF ADOLESCENCE			
	Early[a]	Middle[b]	Late[c]	
	(N = 255)	(N = 302)	(N = 200)	
	% (n)	% (n)	% (n)	χ^2
Environmental Risks				
Witnessed violence	63.1 (159)	78.2 (229)	79.7 (157)	21.125***
Victim of violence	36.0 (91)	42.8 (127)	54.6 (107)	15.710***
Touched in uncomfortable ways	17.3 (44)	27.9 (83)	35.5 (70)	19.622***
Could get gun	16.3 (40)	29.2 (86)	33.2 (64)	18.845***
Threatened with a weapon	16.7 (42)	23.3 (69)	36.0 (71)	22.813***
Had forced sex	6.4 (16)	12.4 (37)	15.0 (29)	9.064*
Behavioral Risks				
Physical fight with boyfriend/ girlfriend	11.3 (24)	5.2 (14)	12.1 (21)	7.990*
Worries About Safety				
Worry do dangerous things	65.3 (164)	65.3 (194)	56.1 (111)	5.352
Worry about friends/ associates	63.6 (159)	62.2 (184)	57.1 (112)	2.078
Worry about hurting self or others	41.0 (103)	50.3 (149)	56.2 (109)	10.570**
Often feel unsafe	42.2 (106)	35.9 (107)	48.5 (95)	7.819*

Note: Early adolescents were ages 10-14, middle adolescents were 15-16, and late adolescents were 17-21. *$p < .05$, **$p < .01$, ***$p < .001$

Late and early adolescents reported higher rates of fighting with a boyfriend or girlfriend than middle adolescents (see Table 3). Worries about hurting self or others increased from early to late adolescence. Older adolescents also felt unsafe "always," "often," or "sometimes" more frequently than younger adolescents. Despite the differences in exposure and worry, however, no significant differences were found among the three age groups on desire to talk about safety. It appears to be a theme of high clinical salience among all age groups.

Safety Risk Indicators and Desire to Talk About Safety

Next we consider the impact of exposure to environmental and behavioral safety risks and the desire to talk about safety in counseling (see Table 4). Adolescents who had been victims of violence, touched uncomfortably, or forced to have sex reported wanting to talk about safety more than those who had not had such experiences. Similarly, those who worried about their own behavior, worried about their friends, or worried about hurting themselves or others, wanted to talk about safety more than those who did not express such worries. Adolescents who acknowledged safety worries were more likely to want to talk to a counselor about safety than those who did not acknowledge such worries. Fighting with a boyfriend or girlfriend did not have a significant relationship with the desire to talk about safety.

When safety risk, as measured by the SRS, and desire to talk were juxtaposed, 36.6% of AHC's adolescent mental health applicants had both high safety risk and wanted to talk to a counselor about it (see Table 5). In contrast, 9.2% of their service-seeking peers were at high safety risk but did not want to talk with a counselor about safety ($\chi^2(1) = 23.616, p < .001$).

Table 6 demonstrates how gender and age differences are associated with each of the four need categories defined above. A higher proportion of females than males fell into the Low-Risk/Talk category (37.5% vs. 28.2%, $\chi^2(3) = 11.446, p = .01$), whereas males were more likely than females to be in the High-Risk/No-Talk category (12.7% vs. 7.3%, $\chi^2(3) = 11.446, p = .01$). Significant differences were also noted between age groups. A higher proportion of early adolescents fell into the Low-Risk/Talk category compared to late adolescents (38.6% vs. 26.7%, $\chi^2(6) = 13.518, p < .05$), whereas a higher proportion of late adolescents fell into the High-Risk/Talk category compared to early adolescents (46.1% vs. 30.5%, $\chi^2(6) = 13.518, p = .036$). These data reflect previous findings that risk level generally increases with age.

TABLE 4. Proportion of Adolescents Wanting to Talk About Safety, by Presence of Safety Risk Indicators

Safety Risk Indicator	Proportion Wanting to Talk About Safety			
	"Don't Know" if Risk Factor Present	Risk Factor Present	Risk Factor Absent	
	% (n)	% (n)	% (n)	χ^2
Environmental Risks				
Witnessed violence		70.1 (377)	73.1 (141)	.612
Victim of violence	90.4 (47)	72.5 (195)	67.1 (278)	12.674**
Touched in uncomfortable ways	86.7 (13)	85.6 (154)	65.5 (355)	28.168***
Could get gun		67.7 (128)	72.1 (388)	1.311
Threatened with a weapon		75.4 (135)	69.4 (386)	2.358
Had forced sex	100 (10)	83.1 (59)	69.3 (452)	10.034**
Behavioral Risks				
Physical fight with boyfriend/girlfriend	81.3 (13)	81.4 (35)	70.6 (416)	3.036
Worries About Safety				
Worry do dangerous things		78.8 (215)	66.2 (309)	13.207***
Worry about friends/associates		76.4 (343)	62.9 (180)	15.411***
Worry about hurting self or others	81.8 (36)	80.7 (255)	61.1 (229)	34.701***
Often feel unsafe		85.6 (262)	60.4 (262)	55.368***

$^*p < .05, ^{**}p < .01, ^{***}p < .001$

DISCUSSION

These findings indicate that a substantial portion of AHC mental health service applicants routinely experiences serious environmental safety risks. Males reported higher rates of risks related to physical violence (e.g., witnessed violence, threatened with a weapon, could get a gun), whereas females reported higher rates of risk associated with sexual violence or abuse (e.g., had forced sex, touched in uncomfortable ways). A consistent pattern of environmental risk increasing with age may have been due to older adolescents' greater geographical mobility, social interaction, and their spending less time under direct adult supervision.

TABLE 5. Distribution of Adolescents by Safety Risk and by Desire to Talk About Safety

Level of Safety Risk (Number of Risk Indicators)[a]	Desire to Talk about Safety[a]	
	Want to Talk % (n)	Don't Want to Talk % (n)
Low (0-3)	Type II 34.1 (237)	Type I 20.1 (139)
High (4-9)	Type III 36.6 (254)	Type IV 9.2 (64)

[a]N = 694. [b]$\chi^2(1) = 23.616$, $p < .001$

TABLE 6. Gender and Stage of Adolescence by Need-to-Talk Type

	Need-to-Talk Type			
	Type I (Low-Risk No-Talk) % (n)	Type II (Low-Risk Talk) % (n)	Type III (High-Risk Talk) % (n)	Type IV (High-Risk No-Talk) % (n)
Gender[a,b]				
Male	23.4 (59)	28.2 (71)	35.7 (90)	12.7 (32)
Female	18.2 (80)	37.5 (165)	37.0 (163)	7.3 (32)
Stage of Adolescence[c,d]				
Early (10-14)	22.3 (52)	38.6 (90)	30.5 (71)	8.6 (20)
Middle (15-16)	20.4 (57)	35.4 (99)	35.4 (99)	8.9 (25)
Late (17-21)	16.7 (30)	26.7 (48)	46.1 (83)	10.6 (19)

[a]N = 692. [b]$\chi^2(3) = 11.446$, $p = .01$, [c]N = 693, [d]$\chi^2(6) = 13.518$, $p = .036$

The frequency of reported dating violence did not increase with age. Instead, early and late adolescents reported higher rates of dating violence than middle adolescents. This finding surprised us as it ran counter to our practice wisdom. AHC has developed group services to address dating violence; however, these services have been oriented toward middle and late adolescents. Interventions focusing on healthy relationships (including dating relationships) may need to be developed for younger adolescents as well.

Across age groups and genders, the majority of adolescents (62.8%) were worried about their own dangerous behavior, with males expressing more worry of this type than females. These findings run counter to the stereotype of adolescents, particularly males, as "thrill-seeking"or oblivious to the risks they take. The findings suggest that, as practitioners, if we fail to see males as worried about their behaviors we are in danger of missing opportunities to identify and fully engage them. Female rates of worry about unsafe behaviors were also high and this also surprised us. Here, too, we learned that a gender-based stereotype about who engages in risky behaviors might lead clinicians to fail to identify this as an issue for many females.

Females also worried more about friends and associates. This may reflect a greater degree of sociability and a greater capacity for intimacy and closeness with friends among females. A related study of adolescent peer networks found that females in middle school and high school were more integrated into social networks, more likely to have a best friend, and more likely to be in a clique than males (Urberg, Digirmencio, Tolson, & Halliday-Scher, 1995).

Overall, adolescents with high levels of safety risk were more likely to want to talk about safety with their counselors than those with low risk levels. The risk indicators with the greatest influence on desire to talk about safety were those in which the adolescent was a target (being touched in a way that made the adolescent uncomfortable, being a victim of violence, and experiencing forced sex).

Although environmental risk increased with age, no differences were found among age groups with regard to desire to talk about safety. Clinically, our experience is that some adolescents appear to become acclimated to living in dangerous environments and regard the hazards of their daily lives as impervious to change. From their perspective it may appear that there is no use in talking about it. This is not to say, however, that they would not benefit from talking with a trusted adult or professional counselor about safety issues. For AHC adolescents and those elsewhere, the counselor may need to initiate the discussion.

In general, a greater proportion of females wanted to talk about safety than males. Given that females experienced higher rates of sexual violence and victimization whereas males experienced more physical violence, the safety concerns experienced by females may be interpreted by them as more germane to mental health treatment. Alternatively, males may be framing physical violence as a normal part of life and unrelated to mental health symptoms that they might be experiencing, such as depression or anxiety.

From a clinical standpoint, those adolescents with low safety risk scores and no desire to talk about safety are in least need of intervention around safety. Those with low risk exposure but an expressed desire to talk about safety require intervention of some kind but with lesser urgency than the remaining categories. Those with high risk-exposure who indicate that they want to talk about safety with a counselor require immediate and direct intervention. Practitioners must be able to assess immediate need and imminent danger and programs must be equipped to respond immediately and effectively to crises. At AHC we have learned that the reason some community-based programs don't ask about safety and violence is the fear that they will not have the capacity to respond appropriately.

We identified three vulnerable groups of adolescents that may require special efforts to engage in discussion about safety. These are: males in general; males and females responding "don't know" to questions about safety risk; and males and females with high exposure to risk but low willingness to talk about it.

In attempting to reach the males, it may be helpful to keep in mind studies that show that adolescent boys have different communication styles than girls (Maccoby, 1990; Pollack, 1998). Girls tend to talk more easily and spontaneously about their emotions, whereas boys may require other approaches, such as talking more indirectly while participating in an activity they enjoy (Pollack, 1998).

The importance of reaching adolescents answering "don't know" on environmental and behavioral risk questions was demonstrated by the fact that they wanted to talk about safety at rates equal to or greater than those who answered "yes" on these items. This indicates the need for further exploration of "don't know" responses on safety items and suggests that these adolescents may be struggling to make sense of personal violations of some sort. For example, some may be confused about sexual transgressions against them, partially blaming themselves for sexual assault. In instances of incest, they may be reluctant to acknowledge that it took place or fear the consequences of disclosure.

These findings were consistent with our clinical experience and practice wisdom. Adquest's designers anticipated that some adolescents might not recognize that they have been abused, raped, or are in coercive relationships (Peake et al., 2004). Some young people need help to get clear about their experience. Psychoeducation should begin during the adolescent's first contact. Clinic staff, office, and waiting room displays, and posters and pamphlets should clearly signal that adolescents have a right to safety. Furthermore, we have learned that when adolescents appear unclear or ambivalent when asked about traumatic experiences we should predicate our assessment on the assumption that they have likely had them, may need help making sense of them, and may be concerned about the consequences of revealing them.

Finally, perhaps the most vulnerable adolescents are those with high exposure to safety risk who indicate no desire to talk about it at all. These adolescents represent a major clinical challenge. The group likely includes adolescents who have significant concerns about safety but are reluctant to commit to talking with a stranger about the issues. Males were more likely to fall into this group than females.

We believe this group includes many adolescents who are less disposed to engaging with adults for support of any kind and/or are distrustful of institutions. These young persons require more subtle engagement strategies and long-term monitoring to be sure that they are not driven away from treatment. Although it may appear that they present a clinical risk of the practitioner inadvertently joining with them in denial of possibly traumatic or life-threatening experiences, practice experience suggests that their acknowledgment on the Adquest of risk exposure is a positive first step. Though apparently unwilling to talk, they present both an opportunity and challenge to practitioners.

AHC has found that these adolescents often need to be engaged around issues that they find pertinent and practitioners need to be patient and respectful of their perspectives (Elliott, Nembhard, Giannone, Surko, Medeiros, & Peake, 2004). This does not mean that we simply take "no" for an answer. Differences in perspective between practitioner and client can be put on the table, presenting an opportunity for the practitioner to circle back and inquire about later on.

Adolescents with high safety risk scores and no desire to talk about safety are faced with an additional danger. It would be programmatically "easy" to let go of these kids or not serve them well. We need to improve our understanding of them and enhance the services we offer. AHC has not yet systematically tracked the progress of these most vulnerable adolescents through its services.

CONCLUSION

Low-income, urban adolescents often come from communities in which violence is a common occurrence. Although exposure to violence has harmful psychological effects on adolescents, clinicians seeing them rarely ask them directly about their exposure to safety risks in their environment. However, when asked, inner-city adolescents will answer openly about violence in their worlds.

Safety and violence are significant issues for adolescents, and they worry about these issues. Despite this, these issues are often overlooked by clinicians (Guterman & Cameron, 1999). Clinicians need to ask about these issues, and programs need to have available expertise and services to address them. Programs need to visibly signal through psychoeducation and clinic setup (e.g., posters, pamphlets, advertised programming) that safety is an issue for young people that they are willing to address.

Many of the findings of this study of the clinical population affirmed practice wisdom, while others challenged long-held assumptions. Clearly, having available data about safety and violence provides practitioners and programs with the opportunity to examine how well they respond to adolescent needs and to plan for change.

REFERENCES

Ackard, D., & Neumark-Sztainer, D. (2001). Health care information sources for adolescents: Age and gender differences on use, concerns, and needs. *Journal of Adolescent Health, 29*, 170-6.

American Academy of Pediatrics. (1994). *Preventing firearm injuries among children and adolescents: A public health concern.* Elk Grove, IL: Author.

Boney-McCoy, S., & Finkelhor, D. (1996). Is youth victimization related to trauma symptoms and depression after controlling for prior symptoms and family relationships? A longitudinal, prospective study. *Journal of Consulting & Clinical Psychology, 64*(6), 1406-1416.

Centers for Disease Control and Prevention. (2002). Youth risk behavior surveillance–United States 2001. *Morbidity and Mortality Weekly Report, 51*(SS04), 1-64.

Cooley-Quille, M., Boyd, R. C., Frantz, E., & Walsh, J. (2002). Emotional and behavioral impact of exposure to community violence in inner-city adolescents. *Journal of Clinical Child Psychology, 30*(1), 199-206.

Diaz, A., Peake, K., Surko, M., & Bhandarkar, K. (2004). Including "at-risk" adolescents in their own health and mental health care: A youth development perspective. *Social Work in Mental Health, 3*(1/2), 3-22.

Durant, R.H., Altman, D., Wolfson, M., Barkin, S., Kreiter, S., & Krowchuk, D. (2000). Exposure to violence and victimization, depression, substance use, and the use of violence by young adolescents. *Journal of Pediatrics, 137*, 707-713.

Elliott, J., Nembhard, M., Giannone, V., Surko, M., Medeiros, D., & Peake, K. (2004). Clinical uses of an adolescent intake questionnaire: Adquest as a bridge to engagement. *Social Work in Mental Health, 3*(1/2), 83-102.

Green, B.L., Goodman, L.A., Krupnick, J.L., Corcoran, C.B., Petty, R.M., Stockton, P., & Stern, N.M. (2000). Outcomes of single versus multiple trauma exposure in a screening sample. *Journal of Traumatic Stress, 13*, 271-286.

Guterman, N.B., & Cameron, M. (1999). Young clients' exposure to community violence: How much do their therapists know? *American Journal of Orthopsychiatry, 69*(3), 382-391.

Kahn, D.J., Kazimi, M.M., & Mulvihill, M.N. (2001). Attitudes of New York City high school students regarding firearm violence. *Pediatrics, 107*(5), 1125-1132.

Klein, J.D., & Wilson, K.M. (2002). Delivering quality care: Adolescents' discussion of health risks with their providers. *Journal of Adolescent Health, 30,* 190-195.

Kreiter, S.T., Krowchuk, D.P., Woods, C.R., Sinal, S.H., Lawless, M.R., & Durant, R.H. (1999). Gender differences in risk behaviors among adolescents who experience date fighting. *Pediatrics, 104*(6), 1286-1292.

Lerner, R. M. (1995). *America's youth in crisis: Challenges and options for programs and policies.* Thousand Oaks, CA: Sage.

Maccoby, E. (1990). Gender and relationships: A developmental account. *American Psychologist, 45*(4), 513-520.

Peake, K., Epstein, I., Mirabito, D., & Surko, M. (2004). Development and utilization of a practice-based adolescent intake questionnaire (Adquest): Surveying which risks, worries, and concerns urban youth want to talk about. *Social Work in Mental Health, 3*(1/2), 55-82.

Pollack, W. (1998). *Real boys: Rescuing our sons from the myths of boyhood.* New York: Holt.

Slovak, K. (2002). Gun violence and children: Factors related to exposure and trauma. *Health and Social Work, 27*(2), 104-112.

Spenciner Rosenthal, B. (2000). Exposure to community violence in adolescence: Trauma symptoms. *Adolescence, 35*(138), 271-284.

Springer, D.W., Abell, N., & Hudson, W.W. (2002). Creating and validating rapid assessment instruments for practice and research: Part I. *Research on Social Work Practice, 12*(3), 408-439.

Surko, M., Ciro, D., Blackwood, C., Nembhard, M., & Peake, K. (2005). Experience of racism as a correlate of developmental and health outcomes among urban adolescent mental health clients. *Social Work in Mental Health, 3*(3), 235-260.

Sweatt, L., Harding, C.G., Knight-Lynn, L., Rasheed, S., & Carter, P. (2002). Talking about the silent fear: Adolescents' experiences of violence in an urban high-rise community. *Adolescence, 37*(145), 109-117.

Urberg, K.A., Degirmencio, S.M., Tolson, J.M., & Halliday-Scher, K. (1995). The structure of adolescent peer networks. *Developmental Psychology, 31*(4), 540-547.

Zaslow, M.J., & Takanishi, R. (1993). Priorities for research on adolescent development. *American Psychologist, 48*(2), 185-192.

Adolescents Seeking Mental Health Services: Self-Reported Health Risks and the Need to Talk

Daniel Medeiros
Leah Kramnick
Elizabeth Diaz-Cruz
Michael Surko
Angela Diaz

SUMMARY. Inner-city adolescents receiving mental health services often get inadequate medical care. However, when those who seek counseling are asked about their health concerns, they say they want to

Daniel Medeiros, MD, is Director of Mental Health Services, Mount Sinai Adolescent Health Center and is Assistant Professor in Pediatrics and Psychiatry at the Mount Sinai School of Medicine. Leah Kramnick, MSW, is staff social worker, Mount Sinai Adolescent Health Center. Elizabeth Diaz-Cruz, BA, is Program assistant, Mount Sinai Adolescent Health Center. Michael Surko, PhD, is Coordinator of the ACT for Youth Downstate Center for Excellence at the Mount Sinai Adolescent Health Center. Angela Diaz, MD, MPH, is Director, Mount Sinai Adolescent Health Center and Professor of Pediatrics and Division Chief, Adolescent Medicine, Mount Sinai School of Medicine. Mount Sinai Adolescent Health Center is located at 320 East 94th Street, New York, NY 10128.

[Haworth co-indexing entry note]: "Adolescents Seeking Mental Health Services: Self-Reported Health Risks and the Need to Talk." Medeiros, Daniel et al. Co-published simultaneously in *Social Work in Mental Health* (The Haworth Social Work Practice Press, an imprint of The Haworth Press, Inc.) Vol. 3, No. 1/2, 2004, pp. 121-133; and: *Clinical and Research Uses of an Adolescent Mental Health Intake Questionnaire: What Kids Need to Talk About* (ed: Ken Peake, Irwin Epstein, and Daniel Medeiros) The Haworth Social Work Practice Press, an imprint of The Haworth Press, Inc., 2005, pp. 121-133. Single or multiple copies of this article are available for a fee from The Haworth Document Delivery Service [1-800-HAWORTH, 9:00 a.m. - 5:00 p.m. (EST). E-mail address: docdelivery@haworthpress.com].

http://www.haworthpress.com/web/SWMH
© 2004 by The Haworth Press, Inc. All rights reserved.
Digital Object Identifier: 10.1300/J200v03n01_07

discuss them with their therapists. Based on responses to a clinical self-assessment questionnaire (Adquest), adolescent mental health clients reported sleep difficulties, weight and eating concerns, and frequent headaches and stomachaches. Age and gender differences in patterns of vulnerability and willingness to talk were explored. *[Article copies available for a fee from The Haworth Document Delivery Service: 1-800-HAWORTH. E-mail address: <docdelivery@haworthpress.com> Website: <http://www.HaworthPress.com> © 2004 by The Haworth Press, Inc. All rights reserved.]*

KEYWORDS. Adolescent, health issues, risk, headaches, stomachaches, eating, sleep

INTRODUCTION

In 2001, the Surgeon General, David Satcher, released a report on children's mental health services recommending that these services be made more readily available in primary care settings in order to provide better access (Department of Health and Human Services, 2001). Although according to estimates only 20% of children and adolescents with mental illness receive services (Kestenbaum, 2000), estimates also indicate that half of adolescent medical visits are due to psychosocial issues (Rappaport, 2001). In addition, studies of clients receiving mental health services show that these clients often receive inadequate medical care (Lieberman & Rush, 1996; Shore, 1996).

Mount Sinai Hospital's Adolescent Health Center (AHC) provides comprehensive health, mental health, and reproductive services in a confidential, adolescent-centered environment. Located in East Harlem, New York, AHC serves inner-city youth, regardless of their ability to pay (Diaz, Peake, Surko, & Bhandarkar, 2004). In order to better address the medical health needs of adolescents presenting for mental health services at AHC, several questions regarding physical health were integrated into the Adolescent questionnaire (Adquest), a self-report form that is filled out by adolescents during the first mental health appointment they attend (Peake, Epstein, Mirabito, & Surko, 2004). Adquest was designed by practitioners at AHC in order to better engage adolescents by giving them an opportunity to express their concerns and what they were interested in talking about with their clinicians. This study reports findings from the aggregate data of the general section of 'Your Health' of the Adquest.

METHOD

The Adquest is an 80-question survey that adolescents are asked to complete on their first mental health intake appointment. The adolescent is told that the purpose of the Adquest is to "provide the best possible services to you and other young people" (Peake et al., 2004). They are also told that their answers will be reviewed and discussed privately with their therapist. The Adquest was distributed to 759 adolescents seeking mental health services at AHC between 4/27/99 and 4/9/02. There are three health related subsections of the Adquest, all under the heading of 'Your Health.' For the purpose of this article we focus exclusively on the eight questions relating to physical health and the body, numbers 38 through 45, which are in the general section of 'Your Health' (Peake et al., 2004). The health sections of sex and sexuality, and cigarettes, alcohol and drugs are reviewed separately in other articles (Labor et al., 2004; Medeiros et al., 2004). See Table 1 for a breakdown of the questions. Data from 759 mental health services applicants were entered into the Statistical Package for the Social Sciences (SPSS), which then allowed for multiple comparisons.

The analysis of the aggregate data of the Adquest Health Section consisted of several levels. Initial analysis determined the percentages reporting each health risk. The next analysis was derived using gender and age. The third level of analysis examined each health risk and the adolescent's expressed desire to talk about her/his health. The next level determined the effect of age and gender on the desire to talk. Finally, by separating the sample into high and low health risk groups, then dividing the groups into those that did or did not want to talk, we derived four types of clients: low risk/no talk, low risk/yes

TABLE 1. Health Risk Indicators, Worries, and Desire to Talk About Health

Health Risk Factors	N	Proportion Reporting (%)
Health Problems/Worries	343	46.1
Worry About Weight	354	47.3
Binge and Purge	55	7.4
Go Days Without Eating	195	26.1
Worry About Sleep Quantity	373	50.0
Frequent Head/Stomachaches	311	42.1
Health in General–Don't Know/Very Poor/Poor/Average	353	40.3
Want to Talk About Health	554	74.6

talk, high risk/yes talk, and high risk/no talk. In addition to the other two groups who express a desire to talk, we view this last group, high risk/no talk as a vulnerable group that needs to talk, as much as, or more than, the other two groups about their health issues.

Because question #44 provided a scale that is a self-rating of health, it was not used in the above outlined analyses. Question #38, regarding health problems/worries, had a 'don't know' category. Because adolescents who responded 'don't know' to this question were even more interested in talking about their health than those who answered 'yes,' these 'don't know' responses were collapsed into the 'yes' category for the analyses. In addition, in question #45 'don't know' has been collapsed with want to talk 'somewhat' and 'very much' for the analyses for reasons of consistency, as is further explained in Peake et al. (2004).

FINDINGS

Of the 759 adolescents presenting for AHC mental health services, 74.6% reported some desire to talk to their counselor about their health (Table 1). Only 25.4% were not interested in talking about their health, a surprisingly small percentage since adults tend to view adolescents as healthy, and given these adolescents were presenting for mental health services, not for medical services. These findings support the hypothesis that clients in mental health care tend to receive inadequate medical care, and confirm that mental health clinicians need to ask about medical concerns in order to help clients obtain appropriate care.

The most significant health concern that the adolescents reported was inadequate sleep. Several studies have reported on the need for more sleep in adolescence accompanied by a general reduction of sleep time, with the need for "catch up" sleep on weekends (Andrade, Benedito-Silva, Domenice, Arnhold, & Menna-Barreto, 1993; Lee, Mcenany, & Weekes, 1998; Laberge et al., 2001). Therefore, it is concerning that a full 50% of adolescents presenting for mental health services reported inadequate sleep.

Worry about weight was reported by 47.3% of the adolescents. This concern was significantly correlated with gender and will be discussed later. Frequent headaches or stomachaches were reported by 42.1% of the adolescents. Although this question elicited limited information that failed to specify if adolescents were experiencing one specific symptom or both, this result is consistent with other studies. One study of high school adolescents reported 27% experienced recurrent headaches occurring at least weekly, with girls reporting more headaches than boys (37.6% and 21.3%, respectively) (Rhee, 2000).

The prevalence of headaches has been known to increase with age and is affected by the interaction between age and sex (Abu-Arefeh & Russell, 1994; Egger, Angold, & Costello, 1998; Rhee, 2000). This literature demonstrates that with increasing age girls report more frequent headaches than boys; this trend has been found to continue into adulthood. One possible explanation for this age and gender trend may be the association of headaches with internalized emotional difficulties often experienced more by women than men.

Previous studies found that 10% to 25% of adolescents experience recurrent stomachaches and that girls report more frequent stomachaches than boys (Egger, Costello, Erkanli, & Angold, 1999; Garber, Walker, & Zeman, 1991). Our results support this research showing girls reporting stomachaches/headaches more frequently than boys (48.8% and 29.5% respectively, p < .001). These symptoms increased by age group ($\chi2 = 6.869$, p < .05). One possibility is that stomachaches and headaches may be reported more frequently by girls because of their menstrual cycle. In addition, given that stomachaches and headaches may also be symptoms of anxiety and depression in adolescence (Egger et al., 1999; Garber et al., 1991), it is significant that 42% of the adolescents surveyed report they suffer from them frequently.

TRENDS BY GENDER

All of the health questions are significantly associated with gender, with females reporting at higher percentages of health issues than males (see Table 2).

Health problems or worries were reported by 51.8% of the girls and 35.7% of the boys (p < .001). Worry about weight was reported by 57.9% of the girls and 27.9% of the boys (p < .001). Going a day without eating was reported by 34.4% of the girls and 11.9% of the boys (p < .001). Frequent headaches and stomachaches were reported by 48.8% of the girls and 29.5% of the boys (p < .001). Bingeing and purging was reported by 9.3% of the girls and 4.1% of the boys (p < .01). Worry about sleep quality was reported by 54.4% of the girls and 42.6% of the boys (p < .01). Given these gender-based associations, it is expected that girls would rate their health as less well than the boys, and that they would be more interested in talking to their counselors about their health than the boys. Both of these expectations were supported by our data (p < .001).

Furthermore, although weight concerns and disordered eating are frequently found in woman, a sizeable proportion of males in our sample were also worried about their weight (27.9%), going days without eating (11.9%) and exhibiting bingeing or purging behavior (4.1%). This finding is consistent with recent studies documenting body dysmorphia and increasing weight concerns in boys (Braun, Sunday, Huang, & Halmi, 1999; Field et al., 2001;

TABLE 2. Percent Reporting Health Risk by Gender

	Male	Female	χ^2
	N = 269	N = 478	
Health problems/worries	35.7	51.8	17.737***
Worry about weight	27.9	57.9	62.459***
Binge/Vomit	4.1	9.3	6.779 **
Days without eating	11.9	34.4	45.173***
Sleep worry	42.6	54.4	9.642**
Frequent headaches/ stomachaches	29.5	48.8	25.898***
Health in general	30.2	57.0	49.430***
Want to talk	65.9	79.3	16.158***

**p < .01, ***p < .001

Neumark-Sztainer, Story, Falkner, Beuhring, & Resnick, 1999; Siegel, Yancey, Aneshensel, & Schuler, 1999).

AGE TRENDS

On all of Adquest's health questions, respondents showed a trend towards increasing concern with increasing age (see Table 3).

The question of health problems/worries was positively associated with age (p < .001), with 37.8% of the 11-14-year-olds reporting health problems/worries compared to 61.0% of the 17-21 age group. Likewise, worry about weight was positively associated with age (p < .001): 36.0% of 11-14-year-olds were worried about weight compared to 55.8% of 17-21-year-olds. Worry about sleep quality was also highly significant at p < .001 (35.3% of 11-14-year-olds, 62.8% of 17-21-year-olds). Going a day without eating was significant at p < .01, with only 19.4% of 11-14-year-olds answering "yes" to this but 32.8% of 17-21-year-olds doing so.

Frequent headaches or stomachaches was significant at p < .05, with 37.3% of 11-14-year-olds and 49.5% of 17-21-year-olds reporting these symptoms. Bingeing and purging was the only question that was not significant by age (p = .091), although the older age group reported over double the percentage of the youngest age group (10.1% and 4.7%, respectively). Given these trends, it is not surprising that a low rating of health is positively associated with age (p < .001), and that the desire to talk about health is also correlated with increasing age (p < .001).

TABLE 3. Percent Reporting Health Risk by Age

	11-14	15-16	17-21	χ^2
	N = 253	N = 296	N = 199	
Health problems/worries	37.8	43	61	25.986***
Worry about weight	36.0	51.0	55.8	20.411***
Binge/Vomit	4.7	7.8	10.1	4.798
Days without eating	19.4	27.5	32.8	10.695**
Sleep worry	35.3	54.1	62.8	36.758**
Frequent headaches/ stomachaches	37.3	41.1	49.5	6.869*
Health in general	36.9	48.0	59.8	20.994***
Want to talk	66.4	75.9	82.8	16.157***

* p < .05, **p < .01,***p < .001

DESIRE TO TALK TO COUNSELOR ABOUT THEIR HEALTH

All of the health concern questions were directly associated with an expressed desire to talk with a counselor about health (see Table 4).

This association was highly significant at p < .001 for having health problems or worries, worries about weight, going days without eating, worries about sleep and having frequent headaches/stomachaches. Bingeing and purging behavior was directly associated with wanting to talk at p < .01.

Desire to talk about health was significantly different based on both age and gender (see Table 5). Females wanted to talk more than males (p < .001), and there was an increase in desire to talk as age increased (p < .001).

Because all the health concern questions were significantly associated with wanting to talk, we decided to use the health questions to create a "health risk scale." Using the six health questions (questions #38 through #43) we ran a Chronbach alpha to assess internal consistency, with a resulting alpha of .63. Given this was not a preplanned scale, the resulting alpha was considered acceptable for further analysis, demonstrating adequate consistency. Running the scale demonstrated a highly significant association with desire to talk (Tau C = .330, p < .001). We can conclude by this finding that adolescents having a higher health risk score want to talk about their health more than adolescents at lower risk.

Using the median on the health risk scale, the sample was then divided into high and low risk groups, with scores of 0-2 in the low risk group (61.5% of the

TABLE 4. Percentage and Number Desiring to Talk by Health Risk Type

Type of Health Risk	Has Health Risk		
	Yes	No	χ^2
	% (N)	% (N)	
Health problems/worries	54.1 (297)	45.9 (252)	50.583***
Worry about weight	85.0 (300)	65.0 (253)	38.789***
Binge/Vomit	92.7 (51)	73.1 (501)	10.308**
Days without eating	87.6 (170)	70.1 (382)	23.280 ***
Sleep worry	87.0 (322)	62.1 (229)	60.717 ***
Frequent headaches/ stomachaches	85.7 (263)	66.4 (282)	34.961***
Health in general	54.6 (302)	45.4 (251)	44.158***

**p < .01, ***p < .001

TABLE 5. Percentage and Number Reporting Desire to Talk by Gender and Age

Gender			Age			
Male	Female	χ^2	11-14	15-16	17-21	χ^2
% (N)	% (N)		% (N)	% (N)	% (N)	
65.9 (176)	79.3 (376)	16.158***	36.9 (166)	48.0 (223)	59.8 (164)	20.994***

sample) and scores of 3-6 in the high risk group (38.5% of the sample). Comparing the two risk groups in regards to desire to talk yields four groups: Low risk/no talk (Type I), low risk/yes talk (Type II), high risk/yes talk (Type III), and high risk/no talk (Type IV): see Table 6.

Of particular concern is that 3.4% of the sample fell into the high risk/no talk group (Type IV), a group that is seen as especially vulnerable and needing to talk as much as, if not more than, the two other groups who express a desire to talk.

GENDER DIFFERENCES IN REGARDS TO VULNERABILITY

Table 7 shows the distribution of the four types noted above based on gender. There is a highly significant difference in the distribution based on gender

TABLE 6. Health Risk and Desire to Talk by Percentage and Number

Risk Level	Desire to Talk About Health	
	Yes	No
	% (N)	% (N)
Low (0-2)	39.4 (293) Type II	22.1 (164) Type I
High (3-6)	35.1 (261) Type III	3.4 (25) Type IV

TABLE 7. Health Risk, Desire to Talk by Gender

Gender	Type I	Type II	Type III	Type IV
	% (N)	% (N)	% (N)	% (N)
Male	32.2 (86)	47.2 (126)	18.7 (50)	1.9 (5)
Female	16.4 (78)	35.1 (167)	44.3 (211)	4.2 (20)

$\chi^2 = 60.854$, p < .001

at p < .001, with females being twice as likely to be in the most vulnerable group (Type IV) than the males (3.4% versus 1.9%).

Although all the other findings in the paper demonstrate that females want to talk more than males, there is clearly a subgroup of females at high risk who resist talking about their vulnerability. Identifying this subgroup (both for males and females) is important as it is likely that a more intensive effort will be needed to engage them regarding their health issues.

AGE TREND IN REGARDS TO VULNERABILITY

Table 8 shows the distribution of the four types based on increasing age. There is a highly significant difference in the distribution based on increasing age at p < .001. Although with increasing age the percentage who are considered high risk increases (Type III and Type IV, 26.3% of 11-14-year-olds and 54.5% of 17-21-year-olds), the percent of adolescents who are at high risk who DO NOT want to talk about their risk drops in half (4.4% of 11-14-year-olds versus 2.0% of 17-21-year-olds). This is consistent with the general understanding of cognitive development in adolescence, in which adolescents move from concrete to abstract thinking, becoming more insightful with increasing age.

TABLE 8. Health Risk, Desire to Talk, by Age

Stage of Adolescence	Type I % (N)	Type II % (N)	Type III % (N)	Type IV % (N)
Early (11-14)	29.1 (73)	44.6 (112)	21.9 (55)	4.4 (11)
Middle (15-16)	20.7 (61)	41.2 (121)	34.7 (102)	3.4 (10)
Late (17-21)	15.2 (30)	30.3 (60)	52.5 (104)	2.0 (4)

χ^2 = 47.633, p < .001

DISCUSSION

Fifty percent of the adolescents we surveyed reported inadequate sleep. This finding is of concern given the need for increased sleep in adolescence. Indeed, adolescent sleep patterns are different from those of other age groups. Adolescents tend to get sleepy later at night, and their best sleep occurs in the morning hours. Social structures, however, do not support this sleep pattern. Many schools begin early in the morning so that the time to prepare for and travel to school requires that adolescents wake up very early and results in chronic sleep deprivation. Adolescents then need to catch up on sleep whenever they have time, usually on weekends (Carskadon, 1990; Carskadon, Labyak, Acebo, & Seifer, 1999; Carskadon, Wolfson, Acebo, Tzischinsky, & Seifer, 1998). In addition, sleep disturbance is a symptom of several mental disorders including Major Depressive Episode, Manic Episode, Posttraumatic Stress Disorder, and Generalized Anxiety Disorder (American Psychiatric Association [APA], 1994). Primary sleep disorders are also listed in the Diagnostic and Statistical Manual of Mental Disorders (DSM IV) such as Primary Insomnia and Primary Hypersomnia (APA, 1994).

A considerable percentage of boys in our study responded positively to disordered eating behavior and weight concern. This finding is significant and may reflect a societal trend towards a more sculpted and muscular body ideal for males. Indeed, recent studies of adolescent boys and body image find that while girls often desire to be thinner, boys desire to be bigger and more muscular (Field et al., 2001; Neumark-Sztainer et al., 1999).

Of most concern is the 3.4% of the sample of adolescents who are identified as having a high health risk score but who report that they do not want to talk about their health with their therapist (Type IV). We found that these teens were twice as likely to be female than male, and twice as likely to be in the younger age group than the older age group. This is clinically important as these adolescents may require more intensive effort to engage them regarding their health risks.

Given the high percentage of adolescents reporting inadequate sleep, somatic complaints, and disordered eating behavior, it is important that mental health providers adequately assess the medical needs of adolescents seeking therapy.

CONCLUSION

This study demonstrates that adolescents who seek mental health counseling have physical health concerns as well. Moreover, when asked, adolescents report wanting to talk about their health risks. Sleep difficulties was the most frequent concern, reported by half of the adolescents surveyed. Worry about weight and concerns about eating were also important. Females reported more health risks than males, and these risks increased with age. When the data was broken down into a high and a low risk group based on a health risk scale, four subtypes of adolescent clients were defined based on their desire to talk. Type IV, which is 3.4% of the sample, is of most concern and clinical importance. These adolescents may require more intensive efforts to engage in treatment around their health risks.

Based on the results of this study we can conclude that adolescents receiving mental health services should be assessed for health problems by their therapists and should have access to health care. Efforts should be made to provide adolescents with a medical home where they are comfortable and can receive high quality health care and therapists need to monitor and explore the health vulnerabilities of their adolescent clients.

REFERENCES

Abu-Arefeh, I., & Russell, G. (1994). Prevalence of headache and migraine in school-children. *BMJ, 309,* 765-769.

American Psychiatric Association. (1994). Diagnostic and statistical manual of mental disorders (4th ed.). Washington, DC: American Psychiatric Association.

Andrade, M.M., Benedito-Silva, A.A., Domenice, S., Arnhold, I.J.P., & Menna-Barreto, L. (1993). Sleep characteristics of adolescents: A longitudinal study. *Journal of Adolescent Health, 14,* 401-406.

Braun, D.L., Sunday, S.R., Huang, A., & Halmi, K.A. (1999). More males seek treatment for eating disorders. *International Journal of Eating Disorders, 25,* 415-424.

Carskadon, M.A. (1990). Patterns of sleep and sleepiness in adolescents. *Pediatrician, 17,* 5-12.

Carskadon, M.A., Labyak, S.E., Acebo, C., & Seifer, R. (1999). Intrinsic circadian period of adolescent humans measured in conditions of forced desynchrony. *Neuroscience Letters, 260*, 129-132.

Carskadon, M.A., Wolfson, A.R., Acebo, C., Tzischinsky, O., & Seifer, R. (1998). Adolescent sleep patterns, circadian timing, and sleepiness at a transition to early school days. *Sleep*, 8871-881.

Department of Health and Human Services. (2001). Report of the surgeon general's conference on children's mental health: A national agenda. Retrieved from Department of Health and Human Services on August 25, 2002 at *http://surgeongeneral. gov/cmh/childreport.htm.*

Diaz, A., Peake, K., Surko, M., & Bhandarkar, K. (2004). Including "At-Risk" Adolescents in Their Own Health and Mental Health Care: A Youth Development Perspective. *Social Work in Mental Health, 3*(1/2), 3-22.

Egger, H.L., Angold, A., & Costello, E.J. (1998). Headaches and psychopathology in children and adolescents. *Journal of the American Academy of Child & Adolescent Psychiatry, 37*, 951-958.

Egger, H.L., Costello, E.J., Erkanli, A., & Angold, A. (1999). Somatic complaints and psychopathology in children and adolescents: Stomachaches, musculoskeletal pains, and headaches. *Journal of the American Academy of Child & Adolescent Psychiatry, 38*, 852-860.

Field, A.E., Camargo, C.A., Taylor, C.B., Berkey, C.S., Roberts, S.B., & Colditz, G.A. (2001). Peer, parent, and media influences on the development of weight concerns and frequent dieting among preadolescent and adolescent girls and boys. *Pediatrics, 107*, 54-60.

Garber, J., Walker, L.S., & Zeman, J. (1991). Somatization symptoms in a community of children and adolescents: Further validation of the children's somatization inventory. Psychological Assessment. *Journal of Consulting & Clinical Psychology, 3*, 588-595.

Kestenbaum, C. (2000). How shall we treat the children in the 21st century. *Journal of the American Academy of Child & Adolescent Psychiatry, 39*, 1-10.

Laberge, L., Petit, D., Simard, C., Vitaro, F., Tremblay, R.E., & Montplaisir, J. (2001). Development of sleep patterns in early adolescence. *Journal of Sleep Research, 10*, 59-67.

Labor, N., Medeiros, D., Carlson, E., Pullo, N., Seehaus, M., Peake, K., & Epstein, I. (2004). Adolescents' Need to Talk About Sex and Sexuality in an Urban Mental Health Setting. *Social Work in Mental Health, 3*(1/2), 135-153.

Lee, K.A., Mcenany, G., & Weekes, D. (1998). Gender differences in sleep patterns for early adolescents. *Journal of Adolescent Health, 24*, 16-20.

Lieberman, J.A., & Rush, A.J. (1996). Redefining the role of psychiatry in medicine. *American Journal of Psychiatry, 153*, 1388-1397.

Medeiros, D., Carlson, E., Surko, M., Munoz, N., Castillo, M., & Epstein, I. (2004). Adolescents' Self-Reported Substance Risks and Their Need to Talk About Them in Mental Health Counseling. *Social Work in Mental Health, 3*(1/2), 171-189.

Neumark-Sztainer, D., Story, M., Falkner, N.H., Beuhring, T., & Resnick, M.D. (1999). Sociodemographic and personal characteristics of adolescents engaged in weight loss and weight/muscle gain behaviors: Who is doing what? *Preventive Medicine, 28,* 40-50.

Peake, K., Epstein, I., Mirabito, D., & Surko, M. (2004). Development and utilization of a practice-based adolescent intake questionnaire (Adquest): Surveying which risks, worries, and concerns urban youth want to talk about. *Social Work in Mental Health, 3*(1/2), 55-82.

Rappaport, N. (2001). Psychiatric consultation to school-based health centers: Lessons learned in an emerging field. *Journal of the American Academy of Child & Adolescent Psychiatry, 40,* 1473-1475.

Rhee, H. (2000). Prevalence and predictors of headaches in U.S. adolescents. *Headache, 40,* 528-538.

Shore, J.H. (1996). Psychiatry at a crossroad: Our role in primary care. *American Journal of Psychiatry, 153,* 1398-1403.

Siegel, J.M., Yancey, A.K., Aneshensel, C.S., & Schuler, R. (1999). Body image, perceived pubertal timing, and adolescent mental health. *Journal of Adolescent Health, 25,* 155-165.

Adolescents' Need to Talk About Sex and Sexuality in an Urban Mental Health Setting

Nyanda Labor
Daniel Medeiros
Erika Carlson
Nancimarie Pullo
Mavis Seehaus
Ken Peake
Irwin Epstein

SUMMARY. For many adults, adolescent sexuality is problematic. For adolescents, it may be problematic, powerfully alluring, or simply a part of becoming an adult. Either way, and irrespective of whether they have

---

Nyanda Labor, MPH, is Evaluation and Policy Researcher, Center for Excellence, Mount Sinai Adolescent Health Center (AHC). Daniel Medeiros, MD, is Director of Mental Health Services, AHC, and Assistant Professor in Pediatrics and Psychiatry, Mount Sinai School of Medicine. Erika Carlson, BS, is Program Evaluator, Center for Excellence, AHC. Nancimarie Pullo, MSW, and Mavis Seehaus, MPH, MSW, are Social Workers, and Ken Peake is Chief Operating Officer, AHC, 320 East 94th Street, New York, NY 10128. Irwin Epstein, PhD, is the Helen Rehr Professor of Applied Social Work Research, Hunter College School of Social Work, 129 East 79th Street, New York, NY 10021.

[Haworth co-indexing entry note]: "Adolescents' Need to Talk About Sex and Sexuality in an Urban Mental Health Setting." Labor, Nyanda et al. Co-published simultaneously in *Social Work in Mental Health* (The Haworth Social Work Practice Press, an imprint of The Haworth Press, Inc.) Vol. 3, No. 1/2, 2004, pp. 135-153; and: *Clinical and Research Uses of an Adolescent Mental Health Intake Questionnaire: What Kids Need to Talk About* (ed: Ken Peake, Irwin Epstein, and Daniel Medeiros) The Haworth Social Work Practice Press, an imprint of The Haworth Press, Inc., 2005, pp. 135-153. Single or multiple copies of this article are available for a fee from The Haworth Document Delivery Service [1-800-HAWORTH, 9:00 a.m. - 5:00 p.m. (EST). E-mail address: docdelivery@haworthpress.com].

http://www.haworthpress.com/web/SWMH
© 2004 by The Haworth Press, Inc. All rights reserved.
Digital Object Identifier: 10.1300/J200v03n01_08

ever had sex, young persons seeking mental health counseling in an urban mental health clinic express a strong desire to talk about sex and sexuality. Significant gender and age differences are noted in desire to talk about sexuality and mediated by involvement in sexual risk behaviors. Having experienced forced sex is directly related to desire for counseling about sex and sexuality. The findings presented in this article compel clinicians to engage *all* adolescents in meaningful dialogue about sex and sexuality. *[Article copies available for a fee from The Haworth Document Delivery Service: 1-800-HAWORTH. E-mail address: <docdelivery@haworthpress. com> Website: <http://www.HaworthPress.com> © 2004 by The Haworth Press, Inc. All rights reserved.]*

KEYWORDS. Adolescent, sex, sexual health, sexuality, help-seeking, risk, vulnerability

While sexuality is a natural and healthy part of life, adolescent sexuality is a highly charged, emotional issue for many adults. As a result, there is more of a public and professional consensus about what is sexually unhealthy for teenagers than there is about what is sexually healthy (Boonstra, 2001; Hafner, 1995). Societal concern about the consequences of adolescent sexual behavior, and their costs, fuels many public policy debates. These debates are too frequently sources of more heat than light (Kirby, 2001; Manlove, Terry-Humen, Romano Papillo, Franzetta, Williams, & Ryan, 2002).

Commenting on this, Hafner (1995) observes that the public discourse on adolescent sexuality has often focused on which, if any, sexual behaviors are appropriate for adolescents, rather than on the inherent complexity of sexuality. She describes three *constellations* of adult opinion that shape public policies and programs. One constellation denies the existence of adolescent sexuality and sexual behavior. A second acknowledges that adolescent sexuality exists but advocates abstinence as the only acceptable adolescent sexual activity. A third constellation acknowledges the powerful reality of adolescent sexuality, encourages adolescents to abstain from sexual intercourse until they are more mature, but recognizes that many adolescents are sexually active and that it is important to provide young people with information about all aspects of sexuality and sexual behavior.

Although there is considerable disagreement among policy makers about adolescent sexuality there is a general consensus regarding the potential negative consequences of adolescent sexual behavior (Hafner, 1995; Kirby, 2001; Manlove et al., 2001). These consequences include unplanned pregnancy, out of wedlock childbearing, sexually transmitted infections (STIs) including AIDS, sexual abuse, date rape, and potential negative emotional consequences of premature sexual behaviors (Hafner, 1995). Adolescents are also more likely than adults to have multiple sexual partners, to engage in unprotected intercourse and to have partners who are at high risk for STIs (Centers for Disease Control and Prevention, 2002; Gittes & Irwin, 1993). Among industrialized nations, the United States has the highest rates of teen pregnancy, childbearing, abortion and STIs (Alan Guttmacher Institute, 2002; Dorach, Singh, & Frost, 2001).

In order to provide young people with information about all aspects of sexuality and sexual behavior, it is important to provide easy access to services where they can talk openly and confidentially about their sexual experiences and concerns. In such a context, they can obtain reproductive health services, access to contraception and condoms, sexual health education, and counseling. This is the treatment philosophy of the Mount Sinai Adolescent Health Center (AHC), with which the authors are affiliated.

In this article, we present findings from the sexual health section of the Adquest, a clinical, self-administered intake questionnaire that was designed to elicit information from adolescents seeking mental health services in order to help counselors engage adolescents in conversations about their sexual health and other concerns (Peake, Epstein, Mirabito, & Surko, 2004). Adquest is intended to open avenues for meaningful discussion by asking adolescents what they are worried about and want to discuss regarding sexual health. Designed to be brief, easy to complete, and colloquial, Adquest responses facilitate the taking of a more detailed sexual history by a social worker at intake. Clearly, however, Adquest is risk-focused and does not explore the psychosocial context of sexual behaviors. Accordingly, it contains no questions about relationship patterns or dating behaviors. Nonetheless, by describing adolescent sexual behaviors and worries for a sample population of AHC mental health service applicants as well as by gender and age, a picture emerges of young persons who very much want to talk about sex and sexuality with their counselors. The interpretation of these findings is limited, however, by the absence of more contextual data. We will return to these limitations and their implications in the Discussion section of the article.

METHOD

Practice Context and Population Served

Mount Sinai Adolescent Health Center (AHC) is a comprehensive health center located in East Harlem in New York City. AHC provides services to young people ages 10 to 21 years regardless of their ability to pay for services.

The center logs more than 20,000 mental health visits annually. The study sample consisted of 759 adolescents presenting for mental health intake between April 1999 and April 2002. Of these, 36.0% were male and 64.0% were female. These urban adolescents seeking mental health services come largely from low-income, minority households in New York City (Diaz, Peake, Surko, & Bhandarkar, 2004). An analysis of race and ethnicity in the AHC mental health service population is discussed in Surko, Ciro, Blackwood, Nembhard, & Peake (2005).

Conceptualization of Sex and Sexuality Items and Plan for Analysis

In this article, the authors analyze responses to the Adquest questions relating to sex and sexuality. A group of AHC practitioner-researchers assigned these questions to five categories: environmental risks, behavioral risks, worries, coping, and desire to talk to a counselor about sex, body, and birth control. *Environmental risks* are conceptualized as conditions occurring outside of the control of a young person, whereas *behavioral risks* are actions taken by a young person. *Worries* include questions and concerns about sexuality expressed by the young person, whereas *coping* refers to how well the individual says he or she is doing regarding sex and sexuality.

As listed in Table 1, Adquest contains eleven questions related to sex and sexuality. The first of these asks respondents to categorize their own sexual identity. Because the issue of sexual identity formation is such a profound one for adolescents, it is excluded from the analysis in this article and is the subject of an Adquest-generated article unto itself (see Ciro, Surko, Bhandarkar, Helfgott, Peake, & Epstein, 2005).

Whereas most of the sexuality questions force a choice between a 'yes' or 'no' response, three offer a 'don't know' category, as the practitioners who designed Adquest thought that in some instances this category would allow identification of some particular concern or risk that might be lost with a forced choice (see Peake et al., 2004). In the sex and sexuality section, the first two of these three questions are "Have you been taught about sex?" and "Have you ever used drugs to make sex easier, longer, or more fun?" As in other Adquest analyses, 'don't know' responses were grouped with 'yes' responses for two reasons. The first is that uncertainty about any of the questions indicates a need for a clinician to probe further. The second is that preliminary cross-tabulation of these items with 'desire to talk' revealed empirically that 'don't know' respondents on these two questions wanted to talk just as much about sexuality as those who checked 'yes.'

The question used as the *dependent variable* in this article is "desire to talk," e.g., "How much do you want to talk to your counselor here about any-

TABLE 1. Adolescent Questionnaire

YOUR HEALTH: SEX AND SEXUALITY

Environmental Risks

Have you been taught about your body and sexuality?

 Yes   No   Don't Know

Behavioral Risks

Have you ever had sex?

 Yes   No

Have you ever been pregnant or gotten someone pregnant?

 Yes   No

Have you ever used drugs or alcohol to make sex easier, longer, or more fun?

 Yes   No

Worries

Have you ever thought about testing for HIV/AIDS?

 Yes   No

Do you ever worry about anything to do with sex, your body, or birth control?

 Yes   No

Do you have any questions or concerns about sex, your body, or birth control?

 Yes   No   Don't Know

Coping

When it comes to sex, your body, and birth control, how would you say you are doing?

1	2	3	4	5
Very poor	Poor	Average	Well	Very well

Desire to Talk

How much do you want to talk to your counselor here about anything to do with sex, your body, or birth control?

1	2	3	4
Not at all	Somewhat	Very much	Don't Know

thing to do with sex, your body, or birth control?" is in the form of a Likert scale. Those who responded 'don't know' to this question were grouped with 'somewhat' and 'very much' responses. This approach was used consistently throughout the Adquest data analysis (see Peake et al., 2004). Moreover, it is clinically important to point out that for the practitioner a 'don't know' response to a question regarding desire to talk about sexuality represents an *opening* for further exploration and discussion.

Finally, for the question 'When it comes to sex, your body and birth control how would you say you are doing?' A self-rating item was created and responses were dichotomized as follows: 'Average,' 'well,' and 'very well,' versus 'very poor,' and 'poor.'

Five analyses are presented. First is a "snapshot" of the responses of the 759 adolescents in our sample. Second is the distribution of responses to questions about behavioral risks and worries by gender and stage of adolescence. Third is the relationship between desire to talk to a counselor and gender and age. The next analysis looks at the relationship between desire to talk and the behavioral risks and worries. In the final analysis we look at the relationships between experiencing forced sex and behavioral risks, worries, and desire to talk to a counselor.

FINDINGS

In presenting a "snapshot" of the sexual risks, worries and coping of the adolescent population applying for mental health services at AHC, three populations are pictured: the entire sample; adolescents who are sexually experienced (i.e., those answering 'yes' to 'Have you ever had sex?'); and those who are not sexually experienced (i.e., those answering 'no' to the same question). In the first analysis the findings are presented for all three groups. For the second and third analyses data were analyzed separately for adolescents who are sexually experienced and those who are not, although the authors present data tables *only* for the sexually experienced adolescents. Data for the fourth and final analyses are presented for the entire sample.

Snapshot

In our sample of 759 adolescents, 51.4% of adolescents reported that they had sexual experience (see Table 2). In terms of behavioral risks, of the sexually experienced adolescents, 22.5% reported that they had been pregnant or gotten someone pregnant and 17.7% reported that they had used drugs to make sex easier, longer, or more fun. It is important to note that a very small proportion of ad-

TABLE 2. Proportion of Adolescents Reporting Sexual Health Indicators

SEXUAL HEALTH INDICATORS	Total Sample N = 759 %(n)	Have Ever Had Sex N = 378 %(n)	Have Never Had Sex N = 359 %(n)	χ^2
Environmental Risks				
Taught about sex	82.0 (602)	84.6 (312)	79.7 (282)	2.949
Behavioral Risks				
Been/gotten someone pregnant	11.6 (86)	22.5 (84)	0.6 (2)	84.406***
Used drugs to make sex easier, longer, or more fun	8.4 (63)	17.7 (67)	1.1 (4)	58.005***
Worries About Sex				
Worry about sex, body, birth control	39.4 (289)	58.2 (216)	19.3 (68)	114.613***
Thought about testing for HIV/AIDS	35.9 (266)	60.0 (225)	10.4 (37)	195.437***
Questions about sex, body, birth control	24.1 (179)	36.0 (135)	27.2 (97)	6.458**
Want to Talk About Sex	67.8 (502)	77.0 (291)	57.7 (203)	31.078***
Coping				
Doing poorly with sex, body, birth control	5.0 (34)	6.3 (23)	3.3 (10)	3.103

*$p < .05$, **$p < .01$, ***$p < .001$

olescents who had never had sex also reported experiencing behaviors associated with having had sex: 0.6% reported that they had been or gotten someone pregnant and 1.1% had used drugs to make sex easier, longer or more fun. This issue is further explored in the Discussion section of this article.

Adolescents with sexual experience reported worries significantly greater than their peers with no sexual experience. For example, 58.2% of the sexually experienced adolescents worried about sex, body, and birth control as compared to 19.3% of adolescents who reported never having had sex. Likewise, 60.0% of those with sexual experience had thought about testing for HIV/AIDS as compared to 10.4% of those who had never had sex. Despite high levels of risk among the sexually experienced youth, very few adolescents in either subgroup reported that they were "doing poorly" regarding sex, their body, or birth control (6.3% of sexually experienced adolescents and 3.3% of those who had never had sex). Nonetheless, the majority of adolescents in each subgroup wanted to talk to a counselor about sex (77.0% of sexually experienced adolescents and 57.7% of those without sexual experience).

Behavioral Risks and Worries by Gender and Stage of Adolescence

Adolescents Who Had Ever Had Sex

In our overall sample, females were about as sexually experienced as males (50.4% of females and 51.9% of males). Among sexually experienced adolescents, there were no significant gender differences regarding behavioral risks, although females worried about sexuality significantly more than males (see Table 3). So, for example, 68.3% of females worried about sex, body, and birth control compared to 39.2% of males; 70.0% of females had thought about testing for HIV/AIDS compared to 41.8% of males; and 42.3% of females had questions about sex, body, and birth control compared to 24.1% of males.

Predictably, the proportion of adolescents with sexual experience increased with age: 25.0% of early adolescents (ages 11-14), 53.4% of middle adolescents (ages 15-16), and 81.2% of late adolescents (ages 17-21). For all sex and sexuality questions except 'questions about sex, body, and birth control,' the trend was for higher risk with increased age. However, the amount of increase in behavioral risks was much greater between the early and middle stages of adolescence than between the middle and late stages (see Table 4). For example, 9.8% of the early adolescents, 17.2% of the middle adolescents and 21.3%

TABLE 3. Proportion of Adolescents with Sexual Experience Reporting Behavioral Risks and Worries, by Gender

SEX AND SEXUALITY QUESTIONS	Male	Female	χ^2
	N = 134	N = 243	
	% (n)	% (n)	
Behavioral Risks			
Been/gotten someone pregnant	19.8 (26)	24.1 (58)	0.864
Used drugs to make sex easier, longer, or more fun	22.4 (30)	15.2 (37)	3.031
Worries About Sex			
Worry about sex, body, birth control	39.2 (51)	68.3 (164)	29.339***
Thought about testing for HIV/AIDS	41.8 (56)	70.0 (168)	28.485***
Questions about sex, body, birth control	24.1 (32)	42.3 (102)	12.433***

*p < .05, **p < .01, ***p < .001

TABLE 4. Proportion of Adolescents with Sexual Experience Reporting Behavioral Risks and Worries, by Stage of Adolescence

SEX AND SEXUALITY QUESTIONS	STAGE OF ADOLESCENCE			χ^2
	Early N = 61 % (n)	Middle N = 157 % (n)	Late N = 160 % (n)	
Behavioral Risks				
Been/gotten someone pregnant	9.8 (6)	21.3 (33)	28.7 (45)	9.154**
Used drugs to make sex easier, longer, or more fun	9.8 (6)	17.2 (27)	21.3 (34)	3.996
Worries About Sex				
Worry about sex, body, birth control	49.1 (28)	57.1 (89)	62.7 (99)	3.306
Thought about testing for HIV/AIDS	30.5 (18)	62.4 (98)	68.6 (109)	26.612***
Questions about sex, body, birth control	27.9 (17)	42.3 (66)	32.9 (52)	5.099

Note. Early adolescents were ages 10-14, middle adolescents were 15-16, and late adolescents were 17-21.
*$p < .05$, **$p < .01$, ***$p < .001$

of the late adolescents reported using drugs to make sex easier, longer or more fun. Similarly, 9.8% of adolescents in the early stage, 21.3% of those in the middle stage, and 28.7% of those in the late stage reported that they had been or gotten someone pregnant. Thinking about testing for HIV/AIDS also followed this pattern. Hence, 30.5% of adolescents in the early stage, 62.4% of those in the middle stage, and 68.6% of those in the late stage had thought about testing for HIV/AIDS.

Adolescents Who Had Never Had Sex

Adolescents without sexual experience also reported much less worries about their sexual health than those who had sexual experience. However, gender and age differences reflected a similar pattern of worries as the sexually experienced adolescents. Females worried more about sex, their bodies, and birth control than males (23.4% females vs. 12.4% males, $\chi^2 = 6.344$, df = 1, $p < .01$) and had more questions about sex, their body, and birth control (33.0% females vs. 17.6% males, $\chi^2 = 9.973$, df = 1, $p < .001$). Middle stage, inexperienced adolescents had the highest level of worry (13.9% early, 25.9% middle, and 22.2% late, $\chi^2 = 7.364$, df = 2, p < .05), but there were no significant age differences regarding 'questions about sex, your body or birth control' ($\chi^2 = 4.422$, df = 2, p = ns). There were no significant differences by age or gender regarding 'thought about testing for HIV/AIDS' (for age, $\chi^2 = 1.548$, df = 2, p = ns; and for gender, $\chi^2 = .016$, df = 1, p = ns). Finally, as shown earlier, a very small proportion of adolescents who indicated that they had never had sex also indicated behaviors associated with having had sex.

Adolescents' Desire to Talk by Gender and Stage of Adolescence

Gender and age significantly influenced adolescents' desire to talk to a counselor about sex, body, and birth control (see Table 5). Females wanted to talk to a counselor more than males; of the sexually experienced adolescents, 81.9% of females and 67.9% of males reported that they wanted to talk about sexuality, while 64.7% of the inexperienced females wanted to talk compared

TABLE 5. Proportion of Adolescents Wanting to Talk to Counselor About Sex, Body, Birth Control by Gender and Stage of Adolescence

	Proportion of adolescents wanting to talk to counselor about sex, body, birth control			
	%(n)	%(n)	%(n)	χ^2
	Gender			
	Male	**Female**		
Adolescents who have **ever** had sex	67.9 (91)	81.9 (199)		9.513**
Adolescents who have **never** had sex	46.2 (60)	64.7 (143)		11.552***
	Stage of Adolescence			
	Early	**Middle**	**Late**	
Adolescents who have **ever** had sex	62.3 (38)	75.8 (119)	83.8 (134)	11.687**
Adolescents who have **never** had sex	48.9 (88)	68.4 (93)	62.9 (22)	12.474**

Note. Early adolescents were ages 10-14, middle adolescents were 15-16, and late adolescents were 17-21.
*p < .05, **p < .01, ***p < .001

to 46.2% of the inexperienced males. Desire to talk to a counselor about sex, body and birth control also increased with advancing age. Among adolescents with sexual experience, 62.3% of those in the early stage, 75.8% in the middle stage and 83.8% in the late stage wanted to talk to a counselor about sexual issues. Among adolescents who had never had sex, 48.9% of those in the early stage, 68.4% in the middle stage, and 62.9% in the late stage wanted to talk to a counselor.

Desire to Talk, Behavioral Risks, and Worries About Sex

As shown earlier, the majority of the young persons in our sample wanted to talk to a counselor about sex, body, and birth control, particularly those who had sexual experience. The desire to talk about sex in counseling was further intensified when respondents reported the presence of behavioral risks and worries (see Table 6). For example, 79.1% of adolescents who had been or gotten someone pregnant reported that they wanted to talk to a counselor about sex, body, and birth control compared to 66.2% of adolescents who had never been pregnant or caused a pregnancy. Worry questions were also strongly correlated with desire to talk. For instance, 94.1% of adolescents who had questions about sex, body, and birth control wanted to talk versus 55.4% who did not have questions, and 90.3% of adolescents who reported that they worried

TABLE 6. Proportion of Adolescents Wanting to Talk to a Counselor About Sex, Body, and Birth Control by Report of Behavioral Risks and Worries

SEX AND SEXUALITY QUESTIONS	Proportion of adolescents wanting to talk about sex, body, birth control		
	Indicator Present % (n)	Indicator Absent % (n)	χ^2
Behavioral Risks			
Been/gotten someone pregnant	79.1 (68)	66.2 (429)	5.749**
Used drugs to make sex easier, longer, or more fun	83.1 (59)	66.2 (443)	8.383**
Worries About Sex			
Worry about sex, body, birth control	90.3 (261)	53.3 (234)	109.682***
Thought about testing for HIV/AIDS	81.6 (217)	60.0 (282)	36.230***
Questions about sex, body, birth control	94.1 (222)	55.4 (277)	109.802***

*$p < .05$, **$p < .01$, ***$p < .001$

about sex, body, and birth control also wanted to talk to a counselor compared to 53.3% of those who did not worry.

The Experience of Forced Sex

In addition to the questions contained within the sexual health section of Adquest, we explored behavioral risks, worries, and desire to talk in relation to one question from the safety section of Adquest: "Have you ever been forced to have sex when you didn't want to?" Accordingly, a comparison of sexual risk factors for adolescents who *had* been forced to have sex and those who *had not* been forced to have sex is presented in Table 7.

Nearly 11.0% of our total sample reported having experienced forced sex. These adolescents had more than twice the rates of behavioral risks than adolescents who had not experienced forced sex. More specifically, 22.0% of those who had experienced forced sex had been or gotten someone pregnant as compared with 9.9% who had experienced consensual sex. Likewise, 20.7% of those who had experienced forced sex reported using drugs or alcohol to make sex easier, longer, or more fun as compared to 8.0% who had not. Similarly, worries about sex, body, and birth control were significantly higher among this group than among those who had not had forced sex (64.2% vs. 36.3%, respectively); they were more likely to have thought about testing for

TABLE 7. Proportion of Adolescents Who Had Experienced Forced Sex Reporting Behavioral Risks, Worries, and Desire to Talk to a Counselor

SEX AND SEXUALITY QUESTIONS	Had experienced forced sex	Had not experienced forced sex	χ^2
	% (n)	% (n)	
Behavioral Risks			
Been/gotten someone pregnant	22.0 (18)	9.9 (64)	10.478**
Used drugs to make sex easier, longer, or more fun	20.7 (17)	8.0 (52)	13.824***
Worries About Sex			
Worry about sex, body, and birth control	64.2 (52)	36.3 (232)	23.523***
Thought about testing for HIV/AIDS	54.9 (45)	33.1 (214)	15.103***
Questions about sex, body, and birth control	48.8 (39)	29.9 (194)	11.580***
Want to Talk About Sex	85.2 (69)	66.3 (428)	11.927***

$*p < .05, **p < .01, ***p < .001$

HIV/AIDS (54.9% vs. 33.1%, respectively); and they were more likely to have questions about sex, body, and birth control (48.8% vs. 29.9%, respectively). Finally, significantly more adolescents who had experienced forced sex wanted to talk to a counselor than those who had not (85.2% vs. 66.3%, respectively).

DISCUSSION

Aggregating Adquest intake information from AHC mental health service applicants reveals that over half of them had sexual experience, and that the majority of applicants wanted to talk to a counselor about sex, body, and birth control. This was true whether or not they were sexually experienced. In general, females were more likely to want to talk to their counselors about sexual health concerns than males, and older adolescents more than younger ones. Nonetheless, over 90% of these adolescents reported that they were coping well with sexual issues, suggesting that the majority of these adolescents viewed their own experiences, concerns, and questions about sexuality as "normative." At the same time, these were issues that they wanted to address in counseling.

Too often, health care providers fail adolescents with regard to sexual health services by not discussing sexual health and risky behavior. While young people generally view health care providers as credible sources of health-related information, many health professionals who provide care to adolescents do not discuss sexual or other related health risks with their patients. Our results are consistent with studies that demonstrate that adolescents want to talk about their sexual behaviors and concerns, yet, too often, are not asked (CDC, 2002; Klein & Wilson, 2002; Schoen, Davis, Scott Collins, Greenberg, Des Roches, & Abrams, 1997). And sadly, it is the most high-risk adolescents who are likely to be ignored (Klein & Wilson, 2002). Some health professionals have reported that they do not feel adequately trained to deal with adolescent issues, and others may not have enough time for discussions with adolescents (Ackard & Neumark-Sztainer, 2001).

By engaging adolescents in dialogue, healthcare providers can help determine why some adolescents have sex and engage in risky behaviors, and help them make decisions that result in healthy responsible sexual behavior. In a multi-dimensional study entitled *Protecting Teens: Beyond Race, Income, and Family Structure*, Blum and his co-investigators found that for all racial and ethnic groups the most significant and proximate predictor of an adolescent having sexual intercourse was his or her having been in a romantic relationship within the previous 18 months. By contrast, the most powerful protective factors for almost all racial and ethnic groups were the perceived personal and social costs of having sex or getting pregnant or causing a pregnancy (Blum, Beuhring, & Rinehart, 2000).

The finding that whether or not a teenager has ever had sexual intercourse is largely explained by that individual's own perceptions about the costs and benefits of having sex is in stark contrast to findings regarding other major risk behaviors. For example, cigarette smoking, drug and alcohol use, weapons-related violence, suicidal thoughts and attempts are predicted by more external factors, such as problems with school or peer influences such as the number of friends who regularly smoke or drink (Blum et al., 2000; Dailard, 2001).

Consequently, Blum and his colleagues argue that "sex doesn't really fit in with the other risky behaviors," suggesting that "[w]hile we tend to lump sexual activity together with other risk factors, it is fundamentally different than drug use or weapon carrying–behaviors we hope to prevent altogether. In contrast, sexual activity is a normative behavior, which we merely seek to delay rather than prevent. As a result, we need to remove it from this collective framework" (Blum et al., 2000). Though evidence-based, the foregoing shift from a *risk paradigm* to considering adolescent sexuality from the dual standpoints of *developmental mastery* and *harm reduction* present many challenges to politicians, policy makers, and service providers who might prefer to ignore the complexity of these issues and their intervention implications.

Recent studies of risk and protective factors that influence adolescent sexual risk-taking have shown a complex web of antecedents of sexual risk-taking. These include community variables, family variables, and variables intrinsic to the adolescents themselves (Kirby, 2001). At the community level, community disadvantage (e.g., low levels of education, employment, and income) and disorganization (e.g., the crime rate) are predictive of sexual risk behaviors and outcomes such as teen pregnancy. Within the family, variables such as level of education, income, family structure, family dynamics and attachment, family values about sexual behavior and contraceptive use, and family sexual behavior significantly influence adolescent sexual behavior (Kirby, 2001). Among teens themselves, variables including age, hormone levels, attachment to school and religious institutions, engagement in other kinds of risk behaviors, emotional well-being, relationships with romantic partners, past history of sexual abuse, and their own sexual beliefs have been shown to affect their sexual and contraceptive behavior (Kirby, 2001).

Adolescents in our sample who had sexual experience worried more and wanted to talk to their counselors more than those who had no sexual experience. This strongly suggests that those who have been sexually active may be struggling to understand how healthy sexuality can fit into their lives and they are open to seeking guidance regarding these concerns.

Females and males in our sample were equally likely to be sexually experienced, but significantly more females than males worried and wanted to talk to a counselor about sexual concerns. This finding parallels those from other studies that indicate that adolescent females are much more likely than adolescent males to have a health "home" and to visit their physicians at least yearly (Klein, Wilson, McNulty, Kapphahn, & Collins, 1999). It also parallels other studies that indicate that females are more interested in discussing sexual health concerns than males (Ackard & Neumark-Sztainer, 2001). Whether better insight into sexual health concerns leads to seeking health care or having consistent health care increases insight into sexual health concerns is an area for further study. We do not know if females perceive more consequences related to their sexual behavior than do males. One might hypothesize that they are more concerned about unwanted pregnancy or contracting STIs and have questions or concerns about reproduction. Another possible explanation could be that more females responded in the affirmative to the questions because it asked whether they worried about sex, body, and birth control, and females may be more concerned than males about body image and birth control.

A few of the adolescents who reported that they had never had sex also reported behaviors associated with having sex, for example, been or gotten pregnant and used drugs to make sex better. We see similar responses in our findings on forced sex: A few adolescents report that they have never *had* sex but that they *had been forced to have sex*. These apparent ambiguities may imply that the adolescents did not consider forced sex as having sex, which, if true, the authors would view as a positive distinction. Certainly, practitioners need to help adolescents who have experienced forced sex to distinguish between coercion and choice. It also suggests that practitioners should carefully explore the contexts in which an adolescent's sexual experiences occur–even for those adolescents who do not initially report having experienced coercive sex.

For the adolescents in this study who were sexually experienced, the percent experiencing a behavioral risk (e.g., pregnancy, using drugs with sex) increased from early to late adolescence. This finding may just represent a cumulative risk based on length of sexual experience and exposure to risk. Determining how the age of first sexual experience and the context in which it occurred influences the ability to make informed decisions regarding sexual behavior is also an area for further study. However, although rates of reported pregnancy and use of drugs with sex were higher in the older, sexually experienced adolescents, these young persons were also significantly more likely to want to be tested for HIV/AIDS and to want to talk to their counselors about their sexual health. Thus, although they have experienced more behavioral risks, they also are more aware of the potential consequences of their sexual behaviors and are more interested in seeking guidance regarding these issues.

Increasing age had a significant association with behavioral risks, worries, and desire to talk among those adolescents who reported that they had ever had sex. For those who had not, it had a positive association with worry and desire to talk about it. In general, rates of sexual risk exposure increased with age, with the biggest increase occurring between early (ages 10-14) and middle adolescence (ages 15-16). This may be an artifact of the Adquest questions, which are in a *lifetime ever* format (e.g., "Have you *ever* had sex?"). Alternatively, it may be that this trend reflects other circumstances such as relaxation of family rules, and/or increased pressure, desire, and opportunity. For instance, it is possible that this is a reflection of transitioning from middle school to high school, a period when adolescents are exposed to and influenced by older peers in their school environment, a place where they spend the majority of their time on a daily basis. Most likely, the associations are due to a combination of factors.

It is important that adolescents receive accurate information about sexuality that is appropriate for their stage of development. Early adolescence marks the beginning of puberty, when adolescents experience physical changes and the initiation of a struggle for independence (Neinstein, 1996). This stage is also marked by adolescents' ability to think concretely and experiment with some sexual behaviors, but have limited sexual intercourse of any kind (Hafner, 1995). During this time, adolescents may be more interested in concrete information about bodily changes. The transitions during middle adolescence are very dramatic; sexuality and sexual expression become very important and the ability to think abstractly increases (Hafner, 1995). Also, the scope and intensity of adolescents' feelings and the importance of peer group values increase (Neinstein, 1996). All these changes make it a prime time for experimenting with relationships and sexual behaviors, as well as having questions and concerns. During late stage, physical maturity is complete and many adolescents understand the consequences of their actions and behavior and struggle with the complexities of identity, values, and ethical principles (Hafner, 1995). Clinicians engaging in discussions with adolescents during this later stage of development may have to focus more on psychosocial aspects of sexuality.

Among adolescents who had never had sex, our findings indicate that middle adolescents were the most worried. This finding may reflect a change in thinking from concrete to more abstract allowing a better understanding of sexual consequences, greater exposure to sexual health information, greater peer pressure to become sexually active and greater attraction to sexual/romantic relationships. Only more rigorous research and multi-variate analysis can answer such questions. These are beyond the scope of Adquest.

Finally, our data show a significant association between having experienced forced sex and other sexual risk behaviors, worries, and desire to talk to a counselor about them. Some adolescents appear to distinguish between consensual and forced sex, while others do not. Either way, AHC mental health clients who have experienced forced sex are more likely to have higher pregnancy rates and to use drugs to make sex easier, longer or more fun. It is unclear from our study, however, which occurred first, the forced sex or the behavior risks (such as drug use). Hence, increased drug use and other behavioral risks may be a reaction to the trauma of forced sex. However, reports also show that use of drugs or alcohol increases an adolescent's chances of experiencing sexual violence (National Center on Addiction and Substance Abuse, 1999). Regardless of which occurred first, teens who have experienced forced sex are significantly more likely to express worry about sexual matters and desire to talk to a counselor about sexual health. Responsive clinicians must find a sensitive and non-stigmatizing way to surface and answer the sexual health questions and concerns of these potentially traumatized young persons in an affirming and empowering manner.

While analysis of existing Adquest data regarding client sexuality was highly productive, it does have some limitations. For example, Adquest asks whether the adolescent has ever had sex, but it does not ask about sexual and romantic relationships, as it is a risk-focused assessment. Not only can we not determine which adolescents in our sample were sexually active at the time Adquest was completed or which ones might be considering becoming sexually active, we also have no sense of the social context in which they may be making these decisions. The implication of this for AHC clients is that *all* of them *need* to be engaged in dialogue about their sexual health. A revision of the Adquest instrument may be necessary to allow for further exploration of adolescents' sexual behavior in the context of current sexual activity, romantic relationships, and other life circumstances or events.

CONCLUSION

This complex set of findings supports the view that the majority of adolescents–even among those who might be viewed as high risk–want to be asked directly about their behaviors (Diaz et al., 2004; Klein & Wilson, 2002; Schoen et al., 1997). These findings are contradictory to the view of adults who deny the existence of sex and sexuality in the lives of urban adolescents. Instead, they support the view that many adolescents are sexually active and that it is important to provide all adolescents with information about all aspects of sexuality and sexual behavior. For clinicians who are comfortable enough to ask adolescents about sex and can cope non-judgmentally with the answers they receive, asking can open a meaningful clinical dialogue. It gives permission to the adolescent to talk about something that is both normative and highly salient. For young persons who are engaged in sexually risky behaviors, who have been forced to have sex against their will, or both, the importance of engaging them in a discussion about their worries and concerns cannot be overstated.

From a service-delivery standpoint, our study indicates: a need to provide adolescents with an opportunity to talk and for them to receive accurate information about various topics that can influence their decision-making when it comes to sex and their bodies; that discussions should be appropriate for the stage of development of the adolescent; and that male adolescents require different methods of engagement than female adolescents. For clinicians, we suggest a shift in the discussion of adolescent sex and sexuality from a pathology focus to a more holistic approach that relates sexuality to all facets of a young person's life. For example, most clinic intake questionnaires ask about sexual orientation, sexual activity including number of partners, history of STIs, sexual abuse, etc. Clinicians should be able to engage adolescents in discussion about sexuality in the context of the adolescent's relationships with their family, friends, boyfriend, or girlfriend; what sexuality means to the adolescent; the adolescent's values; as well as the kinds of decisions the adolescent is going to make.

Whether through health, mental health, or school settings, AHC connections with adolescents present a wide array of opportunities to engage adolescents in dialogue about sex and sexuality. Clearly, adolescents want and need to talk about it. Perhaps the more fundamental question is whether practitioners are willing and able to do so.

REFERENCES

Ackard, D., & Neumark-Sztainer, D. (2001). Health care information sources for adolescents: Age and gender differences on use, concerns, and needs. *Journal of Adolescent Health, 29*, 170-6.

Alan Guttmacher Institute. (2002). *Teenagers' sexual and reproductive health: Facts in brief.* Washington, DC: Alan Guttmacher Institute.

Blum, R., Beuhring, T., & Rinehart, P.M. (2000). *Protecting teens: Beyond race, income, and family structure.* Princeton, NJ: Robert Wood Johnson Foundation.

Boonstra, H. (2001). The 'Add Health' Survey: Origins, purposes, and design. *The Guttmacher Report on Public Policy, 4*(3). Washington, DC: Alan Guttmacher Institute.

Centers for Disease Control and Prevention. (2002). Sexually transmitted diseases treatment guidelines. *Morbidity and Mortality Weekly Report, 51*(RR-6).

Ciro, D., Surko, M., Bhandarkar, K., Helfgott, N., Peake, K., & Epstein, I. (2005). Lesbian, gay, bisexual, sexual orientation questioning adolescents seeking mental health services: Risk factors, worries, and desire to talk about them. *Social Work in Mental Health,* 3(3), 213-234.

Dailard, C. (2001). Recent findings from the 'Add Health' Survey: Teens and sexual activity. *The Guttmacher Report on Public Policy, 4*(4). Washington, DC: Alan Guttmacher Institute.

Darroch, J., Singh, S., & Frost, J. (2001). Differences in teenage pregnancy rates among five developed countries: The roles of sexual activity and contraceptive use. *Family Planning Perspectives, 33,* 244-50.

Diaz, A., Peake, K., Surko, M., & Bhandarkar, K. (2004). Including at-risk adolescents in their own health and mental health care: A youth development perspective. *Social Work in Mental Health,* 3(1/2), 3-22.

Gittes, E.B., & Irwin C.E. (1993). Sexually Transmitted Diseases in Adolescents. *Pediatric Review, 14*(5), 180-189.

Hafner, D. (Ed.) (1995). *Facing facts: Sexual health for America's adolescents.* New York, NY: Sexuality Information and Education Council of the United States.

Kirby, D. (2001). *Emerging answers: Research findings on programs to reduce teen pregnancy.* Washington, DC: The National Campaign to Prevent Teen Pregnancy.

Klein, J., & Wilson, K. (2002). Delivering quality care: Adolescents' discussion of health risks with their providers. *Journal of Adolescent Health, 30,* 190-195.

Klein, J., Wilson, K., McNulty, M., Kapphahn C., & Collins K. (1999). Access to medical care for adolescents: Results from the 1997 Commonwealth Fund Survey of Health of Adolescents Girls. *Journal of Adolescent Health, 25*(2), 120-130.

Manlove, J., Terry-Humen, E., Romano Papillo, A., Franzetta, K., Williams, S., & Ryan, S. (2002). *Preventing teenage pregnancy, childbearing, and sexually transmitted diseases: What research shows.* Washington, DC: Child Trends.

National Center on Addiction and Substance Use. (1999). *Dangerous liaisons: Substance abuse and sex.* New York, NY: National Center on Addiction and Substance Use at Columbia University.

Neinstein, L. S. (1996). *Adolescent health care: A practical guide.* (3rd ed.). Baltimore, MD: Williams & Wilkins.

Peake, K., Epstein, I., Mirabito, D., & Surko, M. (2004). Development and utilization of a practice based, adolescent intake questionnaire (Adquest): Surveying which risks, worries, and concerns urban youth want to talk about. *Social Work in Mental Health,* 3(1/2), 55-82.

Schoen, C., Davis, K., Scott Collins, K., Greenberg, L., Des Roches, C., & Abrams, M. (1997). *The Commonwealth Fund Survey of the Health of Adolescent Girls.* New York: The Commonwealth Fund.

Surko, M., Ciro, D., Blackwood C., Nembhard, M., & Peake, K. (2005). Experience of racism as a correlate of developmental and health outcomes amoung urban adolescent mental health clients. *Social Work in Mental Health,* 3(3), 235-260.

Adolescents' Need to Talk About School and Work in Mental Health Treatment

Elizabeth Diaz-Cruz
Daniel Medeiros
Michael Surko
Ruth Hoffman
Irwin Epstein

SUMMARY. School-aged adolescents spend much of their time in school. As a result, it is important for mental health practitioners who work with adolescents to address their clients' educational concerns and risks. Based on data "mined" from an adolescent intake questionnaire (Adquest), this study explores how adolescents view their educational

Elizabeth Diaz-Cruz, BA, is Program Assistant, Mount Sinai Adolescent Health Center. Daniel Medeiros, MD, is Director of Mental Health Services, Mount Sinai Adolescent Health Center and is Assistant Professor in Pediatrics and Psychiatry, Mount Sinai School of Medicine. Michael Surko, PhD, is Coordinator, ACT for Youth Downstate Center for Excellence, Mount Sinai Adolescent Health Center. Ruth Hoffman, CSW, is Social Work Preceptor, Mount Sinai Adolescent Health Center, 320 East 94th Street, New York, NY 10128. Irwin Epstein, PhD, is the Helen Rehr Professor of Applied Social Work Research, Hunter College School of Social Work, 129 East 79th Street, New York, NY 10021.

[Haworth co-indexing entry note]: "Adolescents' Need to Talk About School and Work in Mental Health Treatment." Diaz-Cruz, Elizabeth et al. Co-published simultaneously in *Social Work in Mental Health* (The Haworth Social Work Practice Press, an imprint of The Haworth Press, Inc.) Vol. 3, No. 1/2, 2004, pp. 155-169; and: *Clinical and Research Uses of an Adolescent Mental Health Intake Questionnaire: What Kids Need to Talk About* (ed: Ken Peake, Irwin Epstein, and Daniel Medeiros) The Haworth Social Work Practice Press, an imprint of The Haworth Press, Inc., 2005, pp. 155-169. Single or multiple copies of this article are available for a fee from The Haworth Document Delivery Service [1-800-HAWORTH, 9:00 a.m. - 5:00 p.m. (EST). E-mail address: docdelivery@haworthpress.com].

http://www.haworthpress.com/web/SWMH
© 2004 by The Haworth Press, Inc. All rights reserved.
Digital Object Identifier: 10.1300/J200v03n01_09

155

life and their need to address educational risks clinically. Likewise, the world of work, also important to adolescents, is discussed. Overall, adolescents are concerned about their educational risk factors, want to be employed, and want to talk about both with clinicians in a mental health context. *[Article copies available for a fee from The Haworth Document Delivery Service: 1-800-HAWORTH. E-mail address: <docdelivery@haworthpress.com> Website: <http://www.HaworthPress.com> © 2004 by The Haworth Press, Inc. All rights reserved.]*

KEYWORDS. Adolescent, education, risk, employment, help-seeking

INTRODUCTION

Much of an individual's orientation to adult life is formed by his or her adolescent experience with school and work. Consequently, it is essential that parents, teachers, community members and mental health practitioners who interact with adolescents accurately assess school and employment risk factors of teens in order to gain a better understanding of their needs, delays, and future orientation.

Truancy and academic failure are two major determinates of school dropout. Dropout, in turn, is correlated with fewer employment options, higher rates of criminal activity, alcohol, tobacco and illicit drug use, and mental health and health problems (Martin, Tobin, & Sugai, 2002; McEvoy & Welker, 2002; Barrowman, Nutbeam, & Tresidder, 2001; Reyes, Gillock, Kobus, & Sanchez, 2000; Swaim, Beauvais, Chavez, & Oetting, 1997; Rumberger, 1995).

For those who remain in school, Maguin and Loeber have shown that poor academic performance is caused by cognitive deficits and attention problems, and is highly correlated with the frequency, onset and intensity of delinquent offending behaviors for both adolescent boys and girls (1996). Poor academic performance can also be related to a poor adjustment from junior to high school (Reyes et al., 2000). The difficulty of this transition is often due to a change in school atmosphere, since junior high and elementary schools tend to be smaller and are centered on homeroom work and activity. High schools by contrast are most often large, impersonal, and decentralized. During such transitions, it is particularly important that mental health practitioners and school personnel are aware of risk factors associated with this adjustment period.

Discussing school truancy with adolescents is essential for the mental health practitioner. The reasons underlying an adolescent's decision to skip school can give one a great deal of insight into his or her life in and out of school. For example, in their study of school truancy motivation, Bimler and Kirkland found 73 reasons for skipping school (2001). Reasons included parents who don't value education, poor social and academic skills, problems with family, avoidance of violence, substance use, physical abuse, criminal activity, and a negative view of future life possibilities. Consequently, exploration of patterns of truancy and its causes can yield significant insight into an adolescent's biopsychosocial situation.

In this broader context, studies on the effects of part-time employment on adolescents enrolled in school have produced mixed results. In an in-depth study on the effects of adolescent employment, Safron, Schulenberg, and Backman found strong inverse correlations between numbers of hours worked and grade point averages, college plans, and maintenance of healthy lifestyles. Additionally, hours worked was positively associated with drug use (2001). And, in a study of adolescent females, Rich and Kim found that while employment during school enrollment did not increase the likelihood of pregnancy, each month of employment increased the hazard of the first intercourse experience by 1% (2002).

Alternatively, positive correlates of moderate adolescent employment have been shown to include increased involvement in extracurricular activities, positive peer social interaction, improved rates of future employment, and an improved orientation to the work world (Schoenhals, Tienda, & Schneider, 1998; Mael, Morath, & McLellan, 1997; Safyer, Leahy, & Colan, 1995).

Mining data from a clinical intake questionnaire for adolescents (Adquest), the present study seeks to better understand the worlds of school and work in the lives of these young persons. In so doing, we hope to demonstrate how knowledge of adolescent risk factors associated with education and work, such as truancy, class failure, and problems at work can create therapeutic engagement opportunities. Similarly, with work. Moreover, assessing the desire of teenagers to talk about school and/or work may debunk some of the clinical myths that presuppose that low-income adolescents have little insight into or interest in discussing issues related to their own education. In the present study, the sample consists of adolescents from a large urban inner-city, with many under-performing schools. Adolescents were asked in Adquest to rate their own schools. Adolescents who self-rate their schools as poor may be aware of the consequences of poor education. Additionally, they may also be aware of possible discriminatory policies which lead to under-funded schools in inner-cities. It is critical that counselors discuss with adolescents any feelings of academic or career hopelessness as well as societal disenfranchisement.

While the present study draws no conclusions as to the cause of school failure, truancy, or difficulties with employment, it sheds light on the importance of these issues for adolescents seeking mental health services. More specifically, it describes the prevalence of academic and employment risk factors in this population, their correlations with other high-risk activities, and the desire of these teens to talk about school and work. For mental health practitioners, the findings demonstrate the importance of asking adolescents about their school and work lives in assessing their overall cognitive, psychological, and social functioning.

METHOD

Mount Sinai Hospital's Adolescent Health Center (AHC) is a freestanding, adolescent-specific, out-patient health center which serves persons ages 10-21, the majority of whom reside in the East Harlem and the Bronx sections of New York City. Clients are seen regardless of their health insurance status for short- and long-term individual, family and group treatment. Adolescents make over 20,000 mental health visits annually and are seen by certified social workers, psychologists and child and adolescent psychiatrists. Upon their initial mental health intake visit, adolescents complete an 80-item self-report risk assessment questionnaire (Adquest) developed by mental health practitioners at AHC (Peake, Epstein, Mirabito, & Surko, 2004). The Adquest was developed as a practice-based research instrument with two main goals: To assess youth for risk, and to help engage patients into mental health treatment primarily by asking directly what the adolescent wishes to discuss with a counselor. Adolescents complete the Adquest in a room separate from their parents, and upon its distribution are assured that, like the counseling services, Adquest responses are confidential.

The Adquest is divided into several sections that aim to assess for an array of risk factors relating to adolescent life. These involve: School and work, safety and violence, health, sex and sexuality, and substance use. Responses from 759 adolescent mental health service applicants collected between 4/27/99 and 4/9/02 were entered into the Statistical Package for the Social Sciences (SPSS), which formed a data-base that allowed for multiple explorations of AHC client experience. The present article addresses adolescents' school and work risks and their desire to talk about these in mental health treatment.

School and work data were analyzed on five different levels. The first level of analysis or "snapshot" describes the prevalence of school and work risks and aspirations for all 759 responses, including by grade level. The second level involves the cross-tabulation of responses to school and work questions by selected demographics–e.g., age and gender. Because race is recognized as a critical variable in many areas in the lives of adolescents, the overall impact of race and ethnicity on adolescent risks assessed in the Adquest is discussed in a paper devoted to that subject (Surko, Ciro, Carlson, Labor, Giannone, & Diaz-Cruz et al., 2004). The third level of analysis explored in this paper involves the relationship between school and work risk factors, and adolescents' desire to talk about these issues with their mental health counselor. The next level of analysis expands on the third level by considering the desire to talk about school and work issues by age and gender (e.g., Of those females who are failing a class, what proportion wish to talk about school with a counselor? And, how do these compare with males in similar circumstances?).

Practice wisdom tells us that we must view an adolescent's school and work life in the context of other areas of his or her life. Therefore, the final level of analyses looked at the effects of other risk factors on school and work risks and whether these other risks affect the desire to talk about school and work. To do this, we employ three original risk scales that were developed using other content areas of the Adquest: a health risk scale (Medeiros, Kramnick, Diaz-Cruz, Surko, & Diaz, 2004), a safety risk scale (Surko, Ciro, Carlson, Labor, Giannone, & Diaz-Cruz et al., 2004) and a substance use risk scale (Medeiros, Carlson, Surko, Munoz, Castillo, & Epstein, 2004). These previously developed risk scales measure an adolescent's risk as pertaining to physical health issues, experience with violence in the home, neighborhood and school, and exposure to and participation in substance use. In this final analysis, questions such as "What proportion of adolescents who were categorized as having high substance risk were failing or skipping classes?" were explored.

For the purpose of our study, those adolescents who were currently enrolled in school when they completed the Adquest were included in analysis of education risk factors. Similarly, only those adolescents who responded that they were currently working were analyzed for employment risk factors.

Adquest asks four education and four employment risk questions (see Table 1). Additionally, respondents are asked to separately rate their desire to talk about school and their desire to talk about work issues on a three-item Likert scale. Consistent with other Adquest data analyses, when respondents were asked if they were currently failing a class, those who answered "don't know" were collapsed with those who responded "yes." These two categories were collapsed because both practice wisdom and prior empirical analysis (Peake et al., 2004) suggest that they are indeed failing a class, and that they are equally as interested in talking with a counselor about school as those who readily acknowledge failing.

Table 1. Proportion of Adolescents Reporting Educational and Work Issues and Desire to Talk

	% (N)
Educational issues	
Failing Classes	64.7 (438)
Skipping school	51.0 (347)
Rate school: Good/Very Good	52.0 (353)
Doing in school:	
Very Poor/ Poor	21.2 (157)
Well/Very Well	40.1 (297)
Want to talk education	81.7 (611)
Work issues	
Want to work	93.4 (555)
Currently working	20.1 (137)
Problems with work	22.1 (27)
Problems balancing work	37.4 (46)
Talk about work	64.6 (84)

Another item on the Adquest asked adolescents to rate the quality of their school on a five-item Likert scale, ranging from "very bad" to "very good." For the purposes of analysis, these groups were collapsed into two categories, "good/very good," and "average and below." We decided to collapse these items in such a fashion for two reasons. First, those who rated their school above average responded similarly to the desire to talk about school item. Secondly, the schools that the majority of AHC clients attend are some of the worst in the country. Even an "average" rating for these schools refers to a school that is, in reality, sub-par academically.

Likewise, desire to talk indicators were collapsed into two categories. Originally, there were four options for the school and employment desire to talk indicators. Those who responded "don't know," "somewhat," and "very much" were collapsed into the "yes" category. Those who responded that they did not want to talk to a counselor at all about school and work issues remained in the "no desire to talk" category.

FINDINGS

Our descriptive "snapshot" of the educational performance of adolescents presenting at AHC for mental health services demonstrates that educational problems are apparent for many (see Table 1). Fifty-one percent reported skipping school and 64.7% reported that they were failing classes. Only about half (52%) rated their school as good or very good. Additionally, only 40.1% of these adolescents reported doing well/very well in school, and 21.2% reported doing poorly or very poorly. Given the high rate of school problems reported, it is not surprising that 81.7% indicated that they wanted to talk to a counselor about school.

Only 20.1 % of adolescents said that they were currently working, although 93.4% reported that they want to work. Of those who were working, 22.1% reported problems with work and 37.4% reported having problems balancing work and school. Of those who were working, 64.6% wanted to talk about employment with their counselors.

Grade Level and Education Risk Factors

Table 2 shows a snapshot of education risk questions based on grade level.

Rates of failure are highest in the eighth and ninth grades (74.7% and 76.6%, respectively). The percent skipping school peaked in the ninth grade (62.3%). On the other hand, seventh graders rated their schools most negatively, with 58.1% rating their schools average to bad. Adolescents who were in the beginning or the end of their secondary education were most likely to re-

TABLE 2. Grade Level and Educational Risks

EDUCATION ISSUES	Grade						
	≤ 6	7	8	9	10	11	12
	%	%	%	%	%	%	%
	(N)	(N)	(N)	(N)	(N)	(N)	(N)
Failing classes	42.1 (8)	67.7 (42)	74.7 (62)	76.6 (118)	65.9 (87)	60.5 (69)	50 (34)
Skipping school	38.9 (7)	36.1 (22)	41.7 (35)	62.3 (96)	49.2 (65)	49.1 (56)	57.4 (39)
Rate school: avg./bad	52.6 (10)	58.1 (36)	50.6 (43)	55.6 (85)	48.5 (63)	42.6 (49)	31.3 (21)
Doing with school: well/very well	68.4 (13)	32.3 (20)	41.7 (35)	35.9 (56)	40.9 (54)	41.7 (48)	52.9 (36)
DESIRE TO TALK							
Talk education	73.7 (14)	78.7 (48)	70.6 (60)	80.0 (124)	87 (114)	88.8 (103)	76.1 (51)

port doing well or very well in school: 68.3% of those in the sixth grade or below and 52.9% of those in the twelfth grade indicated as much. Early and mid-high school students were the most likely to report wanting to talk about education: 80.0% of ninth graders, 87.0% of tenth graders, and 88.8% of eleventh graders. Given that eleventh grade is when students need to begin to plan their post high school career, in choosing to either continue with higher education or work, it is logical so many eleventh graders would want to talk to their counselors about their education.

Gender

There were few significant differences based on gender regarding educational and work related issues. Females reported doing well or very well in school significantly more than males (43.6% versus 33.7%, $\chi^2 = 8.42$, $p < .05$), although there were no significant gender differences in adolescents self-reporting of failing classes or skipping school. Males were more likely to categorize their schools as average to bad than females (52.9% versus 45.4%, $\chi^2 = 3.49$, $p < .05$). Despite this, females were more likely to want to talk to their counselors about education than males (84.1% versus 77.2%; $\chi^2 = 5.39$, $p < .05$). There were no significant gender differences in proportion presently working, proportion wanting to work, those with work-related problems, or desire to talk about work.

Age

There were significant differences among early, middle, and late adolescents on proportion failing classes, proportion skipping school, and rating of school. Accordingly, the percent reporting failing classes was highest in the younger age groups: 66.1% of early adolescents reported failing a class, 69.4% of middle adolescents versus 50.4% of late adolescents ($p < .01$). Fewer young adolescents reported skipping classes (41.5%) than older adolescents (55.3% middle and 58.6% late, $p < .01$). More early adolescents and middle adolescents rated their school as average or poor than did late adolescents (52.2% for early and 52.0% for middle, versus 36.3% for late, $p < .01$). However, no significant age differences were observed in adolescents' assessments of how well they were doing in school or in their desire to talk to a counselor about education.

Although the majority of respondents wanted to talk to a counselor about work, early adolescents were less likely than middle and late adolescents to want to work (78.0%, versus 88.8% and 87.6% for middle and late respectively, $p < .01$). Likewise, as expected, with increasing age, an increased proportion of adolescents were working (11.2% early, 17.8% middle, 37.3% late, p < .001). In fact, early adolescents were less likely to want to talk about work even if they were working (43.5% early, 70.7% middle, 70.5% late, p < .05).

Desire to Talk About School and Work

As noted in Table 1, the majority of adolescents had a strong desire to talk about issues related to school and education with a counselor (81.7%). However, desire to talk about school or education was not significantly related to self-reports of failing classes, skipping school, assessment of school, or performing poorly in school. In contrast, however, desire to talk about work was significantly associated with responses to work questions.

As shown in Table 3, not surprisingly, adolescents wanting to work wanted to talk about work more than did those who didn't want to work (83.6% versus 21.6%, respectively). However, more adolescents currently not working wanted to talk about work than did adolescents who were currently working (79.3% versus 64.6%, p < .001). Significantly more adolescents experiencing problems balancing work wanted to talk about work than did those not experiencing such problems (75.6% versus 54.7%, p < .05). Even more significantly, 96.2% of adolescents reporting problems with work wanted to talk about work, as opposed to 53.8% for those reporting no problems at work (p < .001).

As noted in Table 4, few age and gender differences were noted in regards to educational risks and the desire to talk about education. Among adolescents rating their schools as average to bad, females were more likely to want to talk about education than males (84.6% versus 74.0%, $\chi^2 = 5.49$, p < .05). Among those failing classes, skipping school, or doing poorly in school, there were no

TABLE 3. Proportion of Adolescents Wanting to Talk About Work in Relation to Work Issues

	Yes % (N)	No % (N)	χ^2
Want to work	83.6 (455)	21.6 (8)	82.329***
Currently working	64.6 (84)	79.3 (414)	12.458***
Problems balancing work	75.6 (34)	54.7 (41)	5.24*
Problems with work	96.2 (25)	53.8 (50)	15.668***

*p < .05, **p < .01, ***p < .001

TABLE 4. Proportion of Adolescents Reporting Educational and Work Issues and Desire to Talk, by Stage of Adolescence

	STAGE OF ADOLESCENCE[1]			
	Early	Middle	Late	
	% (N)	% (N)	% (N)	χ^2
Educational Issues				
Failing classes	66.1 (150)	69.4 (179)	50.4 (69)	14.72**
Skipping school	41.5 (95)	55.3 (142)	58.6 (82)	13.37**
Rate school: avg./bad	52.2 (120)	52.0 (133)	36.2 (50)	10.78**
Doing with school: well/very well	40.2 (94)	39.8 (109)	39.8 (70)	1.22
Talk education	77.9 (183)	86.1 (235)	80.9 (148)	5.92
Work Issues				
Want to work	78.0 (149)	88.8 (207)	87.6 (106)	14.78**
Currently working	11.2 (23)	17.8 (46)	37.3 (62)	40.48***
Problems with work	18.2 (4)	15.4 (6)	30.4 (17)	3.27
Problems balancing work	30.4 (7)	30.8 (12)	46.4 (26)	3.11
Talk about work	43.5 (10)	70.7 (29)	70.5 (43)	6.1*

[1]*Note.* Early adolescents were ages 10-14, middle adolescents were 15-16, and late adolescents were 17-21.
*$p < .05$, **$p < .01$, ***$p < .001$

significant gender differences in desire to talk about education. However, among those failing classes, middle adolescents were more likely to want to talk about education (with 88.2% wanting to talk) than were early or late adolescents (77.3% and 80.9% wanting to talk, respectively, $\chi^2 = 6.98$, p < .05). No significant age-related differences were observed in desire to talk about education among adolescents who reported skipping school, rated their school as average or bad, or said they were doing poorly in school. Likewise, there were no significant age- or gender- related differences in regards to work risks and the desire to talk about work.

Other Risks Related to School and Work

Three original risk scales were developed from other sections of the Adquest. These involved health, safety, and substance use risk respectively. These scales were then cross-tabulated with educational/employment questions to determine whether they were associated with educational and/or work problems. Remarkably, only one educational risk item was significantly associated with substance risk, e.g., skipping school. Of those adolescents who scored high in substance risk, 62.6% reporting skipping school as compared to 40.9% of those scoring low in substance risk ($\chi^2 = 20.32$, p < .001). Although safety risk was not associated with educational risk items, adolescents who scored high on this scale reported wanting to work significantly more (89.8% versus 83.3%, $\chi^2 = 7.11$, p < .05) and wanting to talk significantly more about work with a counselor than those with low safety risk (81.0% versus 71.3%, $\chi^2 = 8.46$, p < .01).

Most striking was the finding that several educational and work problems and concerns were significantly associated with health risk (see Table 5).

So, for example, adolescents who were in the high health risk group reported problems balancing work significantly more than those who rated low (47.4% versus 28.8%, respectively, p < .05). This makes sense intuitively, but for reasons less clear those with high health risk rated their school as average or bad significantly less often than those (42.8% versus 51.2%, respectively, p < .05) who rated low on health risk scale. These high health risk scorers were also significantly more likely to report skipping school (58.1% versus 46.6%,

TABLE 5. Health Risk and Educational/Work Issues

	Low Health Risk	High Health Risk	χ^2
	% (N)	% (N)	
Educational Issues			
Failing classes	64.4 (268)	65.1(170)	.04
Rate school: Avg./bad	51.2 (216)	42.8 (110)	4.50*
Skipping school	46.6 (196)	58.1 (151)	8.54**
Doing with school: Poor	19.4 (89)	24.1 (68)	3.83
Talk education	76.8 (354)	89.5 (257)	19.24***
Work Issues			
Want to work	92.8 (348)	94.5 (207)	.67
Problems with work	23.1 (15)	21.1 (12)	.07
Problems balancing work	28.8 (19)	47.4 (27)	4.51*
Want to talk about work	64.2 (43)	65.1 (41)	.01

*p < .05, **p < .01, ***p < .001

respectively p < .01). Finally, high health risk adolescents were significantly more likely to want to talk to a counselor about education (89.5% versus 76.8%, p < .001).

DISCUSSION

The findings of this study highlight the importance of school and work to adolescents presenting for mental health services. Over four-fifths of the adolescents surveyed wanted to talk to a counselor about school. Although this is logical in view of the number of hours adolescents spend in school, the salience of school is not always recognized by mental health practitioners. For adolescents, school is not only an educational institution. It is a prime location for sorting out psycho-social issues such as peer and dating relationships, for exploring new social roles and for providing alternative adult role models.

In this clinical population, more than half of the adolescents surveyed reported skipping school and failing classes and less than half said they were doing well in school. Given the level of school problems reported, it is critical that mental health clinicians serving adolescents obtain a detailed picture of each client's school life, including an understanding of the school's reputation for safety and academic strength, location and community involvement, class size, as well as an understanding of the client's typical school day and their impression of their personal history of school successes and failures. Given that adolescents who are skipping and failing classes do not have a greater desire to talk about school issues it is imperative that clinicians explore education issues with each school attending client. Adquest just begins this exploration.

Of particular clinical concern are periods of transition which may carry a potential of increased vulnerability. For instance, the highest level of skipping school was reported in 9th grade, when adolescents transition from junior high schools to high school. High schools tend to be larger with less monitoring, and students are expected to act more autonomously and responsibly than in junior high school. However, at the same time, new high school students are coming into contact with older adolescents and may be more easily influenced to act out such as by skipping school or experimenting with drugs. Our findings are consistent with those of Reyes et al., who reported that adolescents, in general, who are transitioning from middle to high schools, are likely to encounter a number of adjustment difficulties (2000). In that regard, the AHC clinical sample may be more vulnerable to such difficulties. This may be illustrated in our finding linking substance risk and truancy.

Another critical transition period identified in this clinical sample of urban adolescents seeking mental health services appears to be 11th grade. Adolescents in this grade are highest in percent wanting to talk to their counselors about education. Clearly, it is during 11th grade that students have to seriously consider their post-high school options: Continued education or employment. Clients at this time may need extra support while taking college placement exams, applying to schools, exploring career options and their vocational strengths, especially if they come from home environments with little educational/vocational success.

Of particular concern is the fact that a large proportion of adolescents rate their schools as below average. Adolescents are savvy as to the repercussions of poor education. Students may feel highly disenfranchised and marginalized in attending schools which they deem as substandard (in terms of teaching staff, resources, or the physical condition of the school). It is critical that clinicians address such issues with the adolescents with whom they work. These have educational as well as a host of self-esteem and intra-personal implications. Students may be more compelled to drop-out of school, or not make education a priority, if they feel as though their schools are not up to par academically. They may believe that investing their time into a system that invests little into them is fruitless.

Although only one in five adolescents in this study population was working, nine out of ten wanted to, and those not working were most likely to want to talk to a counselor about work. It is encouraging that so many of these adolescents were motivated to work, and points to the need for society to provide youth with opportunities for work success. These work opportunities need to be provided in the form of peer education programs, internships, and summer youth employment since traditional avenues of employment are not necessarily open to hiring low-income, minority youth under eighteen and may not be flexible regarding work/school schedules.

Those youth who were working and having problems with work were also more likely to want to talk about work. The pressure of balancing work and school, especially if the youth feels the need to work to generate money for family support, can lead to failure at both school and work. Providing appropriately structured employment opportunities could prevent this, which is even more critical given budgetary constraints that threaten to cut government sponsored youth employment opportunities. Penny-wise, pound-foolish cuts that reduce the availability of appropriate opportunities for youth employment will only increase the chance of early career failure, which can then have longer-lasting effects.

Finally, of interest is that adolescents who scored high in the health risk scale were significantly more likely to report skipping school, having problems balancing work and school, and wanting to talk to a mental health counselor about school. The relationship between the stresses of school/work on health, and health issues causing absenteeism from work/school are areas for further study and for clinical intervention. It is important that the mental health practitioner be cognizant of these relationships and discuss health concerns with adolescents who present with school and work problems so appropriate referrals for medical services can be made.

CONCLUSION

This study highlights the significance of school and work to adolescents presenting for mental health services. Additionally, it emphasizes the necessity that mental health clinicians working with adolescents explore school and school issues as a critical component of their clients' world, both academically and socially. Finally, this study provides powerful evidence that urban, low-income, and minority youth are motivated to work and need to be provided with appropriate work opportunities. As a result, mental health providers may need to more actively step out of their traditional roles of counseling to include greater advocacy for their young clients in order to maximize educational and work opportunities so essential to mental health and the assumption of positive and successful adult roles.

REFERENCES

Barrowman, C., Nutbeam, D., & Tresidder, J. (2001). Health risks among early school leavers: Findings from an Australian study examining the reasons for, and consequences of, early school drop out. *Health Education, 101*(2), 74-82.

Bimler, D., & Kirkland, J. (2001). School truants and truancy motivation sorted out with multidimensional scaling. *Journal of Adolescent Research, 16*(1), 75-102.

Mael, F.A., Morath, R.A., & McLellan, J.A. (1997). Dimensions of adolescent employment. *The Career Development Quarterly, 45*(4), 351-368.

Maguin, E., & Loeber, R. (1996). How well do ratings of academic performance by mothers and their sons correspond to grades, achievement test scores, and teachers' ratings? *Journal of Behavioral Education, 6*(4), 405-425.

Martin, E.J., Tobin, T.J., & Sugi, G.M. (2002). *Preventing School Failure, 47*(1), 10-17.

McEvoy, A., & Welker, R. (2000). Antisocial behavior, academic failure and school climate: A critical review. *Journal of Emotional & Behavioral Disorders, 8*(3), 130-140.

Medeiros, D., Carlson, E., Surko, M., Munoz, N., Castillo, M., & Epstein, I. (2005). Adolescents' self-reported substance risks and their need to talk about them in mental health counseling. *Social Work in Mental Health, 3*(1/2), 155-169.

Medeiros, D., Kramnick, L., Diaz-Cruz, E., Surko, M., & Diaz, A. (2004). Adolescents seeking mental health services: Self-reported health risks and the need to talk. *Social Work in Mental Health, 3*(1/2), 121-133.

Peake, K., Epstein, I., Mirabito, D., & Surko, M. (2004). Development and utilization of a practice-based, adolescent intake questionnaire (Adquest): Surveying which risks, worries, and concerns urban youth want to talk about. *Social Work in Mental Health, 3*(1/2), 55-82.

Reyes, O., Gillock, K.L., Kobus, K., & Sanchez, B. (2000). A longitudinal examination of the transition into senior high school for adolescents from urban, low-income, and predominantly minority backgrounds. *American Journal of Community Psychology, 28*(4), 519-544.

Rich, L.M., & Kim, S.B. (2002). Employment and the sexual reproductive behavior of female adolescents. *Perspectives of Sexual and Reproductive Health, 34*(3), 127-134.

Saffron, D.J., Schulenberg, J., & Bachman, J.G. (2001). Part-time and hurried adolescence: The links among work intensity, social activities, health behaviors, and substance use. *Journal of Health & Social Behavior, 42*(4), 425.

Safyer, A.W., Leahy, B.H., & Colan, Neil B. (1995). The impact of work on adolescent development. *Families in Society, 76*(1), 38.

Schoenhals, M., Tienda, M., & Schneider, B. (1998). The educational and personal consequences of adolescent employment. *Social Forces, 77*(2), 723-761.

Surko, M., Ciro, D., Blackwood, C., Nembhard, M., & Peake, K. (2005.) Experience of racism as a correlate of developmental and health outcomes among urban adolescent mental health clients. *Social Work in Mental Health, 3*(3), 235-260.

Surko, M., Ciro, D., Labor, N., Giannone, V., Diaz-Cruz, E., Peake, K., & Epstein, I. (2004). Which adolescents need to talk about safety and violence? *Social Work in Mental Health, 3*(1/2), 101-117.

Swaim, C., Beauvai, F., Chavez, E.L., & Oetting, E.R. (1997). The effect of school dropout rates on estimates of adolescent substance use among three racial/ethnic groups. *American Journal of Public Health, 87*(1), 51-55.

Adolescents' Self-Reported Substance Risks and Need to Talk About Them in Mental Health Counseling

Daniel Medeiros
Erika Carlson
Michael Surko
Nicole Munoz
Monique Castillo
Irwin Epstein

SUMMARY. Although adolescents seeking mental health services may not consider them related, the prevalent co-morbidity of substance use and mental health problems makes it imperative that practitioners find ways of engaging troubled youth about substance issues. Based on their

---

Daniel Medeiros, MD, is Director of Mental Health Services, Mount Sinai Adolescent Health Center and is Assistant Professor in Pediatrics and Psychiatry, Mount Sinai School of Medicine. Erika Carlson, BS, is Program Assistant and Michael Surko, PhD, is Coordinator, ACT for Youth Downstate Center for Excellence, Mount Sinai Adolescent Health Center. Nicole Munoz, MWS, CASAC, and Monique Castillo, MSW, are Staff Social Workers, Mount Sinai Adolescent Health Center, (320 East 94th Street, New York, NY 10128). Irwin Epstein, PhD, is the Helen Rehr Professor of Applied Social Work Research (Health), Hunter College School of Social Work, 129 East 79th Street, New York, NY 10021.

[Haworth co-indexing entry note]: "Adolescents' Self-Reported Substance Risks and Need to Talk About Them in Mental Health Counseling." Medeiros, Daniel et al. Co-published simultaneously in *Social Work in Mental Health* (The Haworth Social Work Practice Press, an imprint of The Haworth Press, Inc.) Vol. 3, No. 1/2, 2004, pp. 171-189; and: *Clinical and Research Uses of an Adolescent Mental Health Intake Questionnaire: What Kids Need to Talk About* (ed: Ken Peake, Irwin Epstein, and Daniel Medeiros) The Haworth Social Work Practice Press, an imprint of The Haworth Press, Inc., 2005, pp. 171-189. Single or multiple copies of this article are available for a fee from The Haworth Document Delivery Service [1-800-HAWORTH, 9:00 a.m. - 5:00 p.m. (EST). E-mail address: docdelivery@haworthpress.com].

http://www.haworthpress.com/web/SWMH
© 2004 by The Haworth Press, Inc. All rights reserved.
Digital Object Identifier: 10.1300/J200v03n01_10

responses to a clinical self-assessment questionnaire (Adquest), this study shows that mental health service applicants are willing to disclose their substance use behaviors and are open to talking about them to intake workers. Age and gender differences in substance use patterns and willingness to talk are explored. *[Article copies available for a fee from The Haworth Document Delivery Service: 1-800-HAWORTH. E-mail address: <docdelivery@haworthpress.com> Website: <http://www.HaworthPress.com> © 2004 by The Haworth Press, Inc. All rights reserved.]*

KEYWORDS. Adolescent, tobacco, alcohol, marijuana, drugs, risk, co-morbidity

INTRODUCTION

Among adolescents, a high prevalence of co-morbidity exists between substance use and mental health problems. For example, Clark et al. (1997) found that in clinical populations of adolescents, the co-morbidity of substance abuse disorders and conduct disorders was as high as 95% in some samples. And, among samples of adolescents with diagnosed substance use disorders, 28% to 48% exhibited major depression. Additionally, these authors found that adolescents with alcohol or mixed substance use disorders had significantly higher rates of disruptive behavior, mood, and anxiety disorders. Finally, in a clinical sample of adolescents with alcohol dependence, they showed that only 11% had neither diagnosable conduct disorders nor major depressions (Clark et al., 1997).

In other studies, it was revealed that rates of depression and disruptive disorders among alcohol abusing or dependent adolescents were 3 and 10 times greater than among adolescent alcohol abstainers, respectively (Rohde, Lewinsohn, & Seeley, 1996). Although several studies have focused on primarily White, middle-class adolescents (Grilo, Walker, Becker, Edell, & McGlashan, 1997; Rohde, Lewinsohn, & Seeley, 1996), similar patterns of co-morbidity between substance abuse and psychopathology have been observed among non-White and Hispanic adolescents (Kelder et al., 2001). Because of these high rates of co-morbidity, adolescent mental health providers need effective means to detect and appropriately engage adolescents seeking mental health treatment who also have substance use problems. This may require both mental health counseling and substance abuse treatment.

An important first step in clinical engagement and treatment planning for such youth involves eliciting accurate information about their patterns of and preferences of substance use. Studies testing the veracity of adolescent self-reports of substance use with non-clinical population samples have yielded mixed findings. Nonetheless, they do support the validity and reliability of these reports, consistent with findings in the adult general population (Johnston & O'Malley, 1997; Shillington & Clapp, 2000). However, these studies generally offer participants both anonymity and confidentiality.

In clinical populations, the former is impossible and the latter is absolutely essential. Whatever the method for gathering information, confidentiality is key; in seeking help from clinicians, adolescents are more willing to disclose sensitive information, communicate with, and seek health care from providers who can assure confidentiality (Ford, Millstein, Halpern-Felsher, & Irwin, 1997).

Although adolescents entering mental health treatment have a substantial likelihood of coexisting substance abuse disorders, our clinical experience is that many are initially uninterested in receiving substance-abuse treatment. Their lack of interest can be conceptualized using the "transtheoretical," or "stages of change" model proposed by Prochaska and DiClemente (1983).

According to this model, recovery from any addiction can be seen as a process with successive stages, from *precontemplation*, in which the person has not considered change as an option, has little insight into the problem, and is relatively well-defended; through *maintenance*, in which new behavioral alternatives to substance use take hold, support structures for abstinence or moderation are in place, and the individual either stays in recovery or experiences a *relapse* and reverts to an earlier stage.

Following Prochaska and DiClemente, intervention strategies must be appropriate to the individual's stage in the recovery process. For this reason, in working with substance-using adolescents, it is crucial to comprehend their own understandings of their substance use, in addition to their patterns of use, in order to effectively engage them in treatment of any kind.

In this study, the adolescents seeking mental health services but not explicitly substance abuse services were surveyed about their substance use. Employing the theory posited above, we therefore assumed that many of these adolescents were in the *precontemplation* phase. Moreover, it was unclear whether they would initially disclose their patterns of substance use *and* whether they wanted to talk about their related risk behaviors to a mental health practitioner.

METHOD

Mount Sinai Hospital's Adolescent Health Center (AHC) provides comprehensive health, mental health, and reproductive services in a confidential, adolescent-centered environment. Located in East Harlem, New York, AHC serves inner-city youth, regardless of their ability to pay (Diaz, Peake, Surko, & Bhandarkar, 2004). In order to engage adolescents presenting for mental health services at AHC regarding substance issues, several questions regarding cigarettes, alcohol and drugs were included in the Adolescent Intake Questionnaire (Adquest) that all mental health service applicants were asked to complete (Peake, Epstein, Mirabito, & Surko, 2004). Adquest was designed by practitioners at AHC in order to more effectively engage adolescents by giving them an opportunity to express their concerns in a confidential manner and to indicate what they were interested in talking about with their mental health counselors. In this study, we report on Adquest findings concerning cigarette, alcohol, and drug use drawn from the Health Section of Adquest.

The sample upon which this study is based includes 759 inner-city adolescents seeking mental health services at AHC between 4/27/99 and 4/9/02. The substance use section of the Adquest (Peake et al., 2004) consisted of nine questions, questions 57 through 65 (see Table 1). Question 59, which consists of four parts, reads as follows:

59. Check any of the following that you have tried.
—— Tobacco (cigarettes, snuff, chew)
—— Alcohol (beer, wine, wine coolers, hard liquor)
—— Marijuana (pot, weed, reefer, boom, chronic, blunts, joints)
     other drugs (e.g., crack, cocaine, ecstasy, special K, LSD, acid, glues, heroin, uppers, downers, steroids)

In addition, one item from the Sex & Sexuality section of the Adquest, question 51, "Have you ever used drugs to make sex better?" was also included in data analysis. Thus, together, there were a total of thirteen questions subjected to data analysis and included in this study. Data were entered into the Statistical Package for the Social Sciences (SPSS), which then allowed for multiple comparisons by gender and by age.

More specifically, analysis of the Adquest substance use data involved several levels. Initial analysis determined the percentages reporting each substance risk and provided a "snapshot" of patterns of use within this clinical population. Second, we considered gender and age differences in substance use. The third level of analysis examined different substance use patterns and their associated expression of desire to talk about substance issues with a mental health counselor. The fourth level considered age and gender differences in desire to talk about substance use. Finally, by separating the sample into high and low substance risk groups, then dividing the groups into those that did or did not want to talk, we derived four types of clients: Low risk/no talk, low risk/yes talk, high risk/yes talk, and high risk/no talk and report the clinical

TABLE 1. Substance Risk Indicators, Worries, and Desire to Talk About Drug Use

Substance Risk Factors	N	Proportion Reporting (%)
Environmental Risk		
Been Offered Drugs	387	52.7
Spend Time with Drug User	365	50.0
Behavioral Risk		
Tried Tobacco	312	53.8
Tried Alcohol	401	65.1
Tried Marijuana	280	47.6
Tried Other Drugs	32	6.3
Used Drugs in Last Month	200	27.3
Worried About Drug Use		
Worried About Own Use	127	17.8
Worried About Other's Use	256	35.4
Others Worry About Your Use	250	34.6
How Doing–Very poor/poor	47	6.7
Want to Talk About It		
Want to Talk About Drugs	448	61.8

distributions of each of these sub-types. In comparison with the low and high risk groups who do express a desire to talk about substance use, we view this last group, i.e., those whose self-reported behavior puts them at high risk but indicate no desire to talk to a counselor about it as possibly being most vulnerable. In this context, for practitioners then, the "precontemplative" substance users represent the greatest clinical challenge.

There are some issues to note in regards to data analysis. Question 59 ("Check any of the following drugs you have tried") indicates a response only if the youth checked off a substance or substances they had tried. Only those questionnaires in which the adolescent also responded to both the previous question and the subsequent question were counted; if those two questions were not answered, responses for question 59 were also considered "missing data." Thus, the results presented here could be an overestimate or underestimate of use.

Because question 64 ("In general, when it comes to alcohol and drugs, how would you say you are doing?") is a self-rating scale of how the young person thinks he or she is doing regarding drugs (not binary), it was not used in the data analyses. Question 63 ("Do your friends and family ever worry about your alcohol or drug use?") had "don't know" as a response choice. Adolescents who responded "don't know" to this question had higher rates of wanting to talk about substances than those who answered "yes"; therefore, these "don't know" responses were collapsed into the "yes" category for the analyses. Finally, in question 65 ("How much do you want to talk to your counselor here about anything to do with alcohol or drugs?"), "don't know" responses were collapsed with "somewhat" and "very much" responses for the analyses for reasons of consistency, as explained in Peake et al. (2004).

FINDINGS

The findings are consistent with our general belief that inner-city adolescents seeking mental health services are at significant risk for substance abuse (see Table 1). Hence, our clinical "snapshot" reveals that over 50% of our teens have been offered drugs and 50% have spent time with a drug user.

Studies have consistently reported that family and peer pro-drug attitudes and behaviors are powerful risk factors for adolescent substance abuse. Adolescents with parents who have permissive attitudes towards alcohol and other drug use are more likely to use drugs (Kandel, Kessler, & Margulies, 1978; McDermott, 1984). A strong correlation between parental substance use and adolescent use has also been found (National Center for Children of Alcoholics, 2000). In addition, adolescents are more likely to smoke, drink alcohol and use drugs if they believe that an older sibling has used and are twice as likely to use if an older sibling is encouraging them to use drugs (National Center on Addiction and Substance Abuse, 2002). Finally, research also indicates that association with drug using peers is one of the strongest predictors of adolescent drug use (Guo, Hill, Hawkins, Catalano, & Abbott, 2002; Hawkins, Catalano, & Miller, 1992; Prinstein, Boergers, & Spirito, 2001).

Our initial findings are also consistent with the Gateway Theory originally proposed by Kandel (1975), which suggests that there is typically a progression from legal to illegal drug use among adolescent drug users. Accordingly, AHC mental health service applicants had high rates of at least trying legal drugs such as tobacco and alcohol, with 53.8% having tried tobacco and 65.1% having tried alcohol. However, it is disturbing that such a high percent of these adolescents have also tried an illegal drug: 47.6% have tried marijuana. The risk associated with marijuana use extends beyond the drug itself and includes knowing and buying from a drug dealer, which increases access to other illegal drugs and exposes the adolescent to the associated risk of the drug culture, e.g., violence, drug selling, arrests, etc.

While national studies of adolescent substance use have largely Caucasian samples and report lower rates of lifetime substance use among minority adolescents (Centers for Disease Control and Prevention, 2002; Johnston, O'Malley, & Bachman, 2002), the *majority* of our sample is of minority adolescents. As noted above, our analyses reflect similar rates of substance use as reported in national samples.

Moving from "being offered" and "trying" substances to actual use, more than one-quarter of the AHC sample reported that they used alcohol or drugs during the past month (27.3%). Given that the sample is comprised entirely of adolescents seeking mental health services, this clinical indication of current use (although not assessing abuse/dependence) is consistent with studies showing a high level of co-morbidity between substance disorders and various mental disorders in adolescents, including conduct disorder, oppositional defiant disorder, attention-deficit hyperactivity disorder, depression, and posttraumatic stress disorder (Brown, Gleghorn, Schuckit, Myers, & Mott, 1996; Clark et al., 1997; Simkin, 2002).

A fascinating but unanticipated finding involves our sample's reported worry about other's use. For example, over a third said they worried about other's use and that others worried about their use (35.4% and 34.6%, respectively). These findings show that rates of worry about others use are double the "worry about their own use" (17.8%). A possible explanation of this may be the use of projection (worry about other's use) and denial (not worried regarding own use although others worry about them) as the literature reports both as common defenses in adolescent substance disorders (Noshpitz, 1994). Consistent with this interpretation is that only 6.7% rated themselves as doing "poorly" or "very poorly" with regard to their own alcohol or drug use, although close to two-thirds (61.8%) wanted to talk to their counselor about drugs.

GENDER TRENDS

A surprising finding emerging from this clinical sample of urban, primarily minority adolescents seeking mental health services is that girls are experimenting with substances more than boys (Table 2).

For example, female AHC applicants tried tobacco significantly more than boys (57.9% of girls and 46.1% of boys, p < .01). Likewise, significantly more girls reported having tried alcohol than did boys (68.2% of girls, 59.2% of boys, p < .05). Girls also tried marijuana and other drugs more than boys, but these differences were not statistically significant (marijuana: 48.4% of girls vs. 46.2% of boys; other drugs: 6.7% of girls vs. 5.6% of boys). These gender-based differences in experimentation with substances existed despite there be-

TABLE 2. Percent Reporting Substance Risk/Worries/Desire to Talk, by Gender

Substance Risk Factors	Male N = 263	Female N = 469	χ^2
Environmental Risk			
Been Offered Drugs	52.5	52.9	.011
Spend Time with Drug User	48.3	50.9	2.178
Behavioral Risk			
Tried Tobacco	46.1	57.9	7.385**
Tried Alcohol	59.2	68.2	4.937*
Tried Marijuana	46.2	48.4	.265
Tried Other Drugs	5.6	6.7	.201
Tried Drugs in Last Month	27.6	27.0	.027
Worried About Drug Use			
Worried About Own Use	21.3	15.9	3.341
Worried About Other's Use	31.2	37.4	2.888
Others Worry About Your Use	42.2	30.4	10.153**
How Doing–Poor/very poor	8.3	5.8	1.571
Want To Talk About It			
Want to Talk About Drugs	58.3	63.6	1.958

*$p < .05$, **$p < .01$, ***$p < .001$

ing no reported differences between boys and girls in being offered drugs or spending time with a drug user.

We also explored gender differences in relation to having spent time with a drug user or having been offered drugs with rates of trying each drug. Girls were more likely than boys to try tobacco (72.5% vs. 59.1% respectively, $\chi^2 = 5.977$, p < .05, df = 1) and alcohol (84.2% vs. 73.9% respectively, $\chi^2 = 5.093$, p < .01, df = 1) if they had ever spent time with a drug user. Girls were also more likely than boys to try tobacco (77.3% vs. 61.6% respectively, $\chi^2 = 9.017$, p < .01, df = 1) and alcohol (86% vs. 75% respectively, $\chi^2 = 6.336$, p < .01, df = 1) if they had ever been offered drugs. There were no significant differences between girls and boys for trying marijuana or other illegal drugs and having been offered drugs or having spent time with a user. Our findings, then, are suggestive of Kandel's (1978) claim that adolescent girls are more susceptible than boys to the influences of friends, especially in peer-related activities.

Despite the finding that AHC females were experimenting more than males, males reported that others worried about their use significantly more than females (42.2% of males vs 30.4% of females, p < .01). In addition, males reported that they worried about their own use more than did females. The difference (21.3% of males vs. 15.9% of females) did not reach statistical significance, however. Likewise, there was no significant difference between boys and girls in their desire to talk to their counselor about drugs (58.3% of boys vs. 63.6% of girls). For both groups then, well over half wanted to talk with their counselors about substance use .

Other gender-based co-morbidities also exist among adolescents. For instance, although girls attempt suicide more often than boys (F:M = 2:1), boys complete suicide more often than girls (M:F = 5:1) (Shaffer & Pfeffer, 2001). Boys tend to use more lethal methods such as guns (which account for 65% of suicides by boys and 56% of the suicides by girls) (American Academy of Pediatrics, 1992), while the most frequent method of suicide attempt by girls is medication overdose (Shaffer & Pfeffer, 2001). Furthermore, alcohol was involved in approximately 20% of adolescent male suicides (Knight, 1997), which can effectively lower inhibitions, thus causing boys to carry out their suicidal intent.

AGE TRENDS

Not surprisingly, substance risk-exposure increases significantly as age increases (see Table 3). For example, 36.1% of 10- to 14-year-olds reported being offered drugs compared to 65.1% of 17- to 21-year-olds (p < .001). Similarly, 34.6% of 10- to 14-year-olds reported spending time with a drug user as compared to 58.8% of 17- to 21-year-olds (p > .001).

Experimentation was also significantly associated with increasing age. This was true for tobacco, alcohol, marijuana, and other drug use during the month prior to Adquest completion. The findings in Table 3 make it clear that both risk-exposure and experimentation increase dramatically between early (10 to 14) and mid-adolescence (15 to 16). This sharp increase roughly corresponds to when teens transition from junior high school into high school, clearly a highly vulnerable period in an adolescent's life. At this time young persons often attend larger school settings, are exposed to a wider circle of potential acquaintances, interact with older and more experienced adolescents and have less parental supervision. Notwithstanding the above, our clinical findings make it clear that urban, junior high school students are already at significant risk, and that prevention strategies will need to begin before children even reach junior high school.

A more positive finding perhaps is that AHC service applicants worry more about their own substance use with increasing age (p < .001). In addition, they

TABLE 3. Percent Reporting Substance Risk/Worries/Desire to Talk, By Age

			STAGES OF ADOLESCENCE	
SUBSTANCE RISK FACTORS	Early	Middle	Late	χ^2
	N = 244	N = 294	N = 195	
	(10-14)	(15-16)	(17-21)	
Environmental Risk				
Been Offered Drugs	36.1	58.5	65.1	43.147***
Spend Time with Drugs User	34.6	57.0	58.8	38.014***
Behavior Risk				
Tried Tobacco	37.4	58.5	64.2	28.314***
Tired Alcohol	42.6	70.6	80.6	63.100***
Tried Marijuana	24.7	53.6	62.6	55.717***
Tried Other Drugs	1.9	6.9	10.3	9.375**
Used Drugs in Last Month	12.0	32.1	39.1	45.746***
Worried About Drug Use				
Worried About Own Use	9.0	18.5	27.2	24.139***
Worried About Other's Use	28.3	37.0	41.2	8.473*
Others Worry About Your Use	35.7	37.6	29.1	3.928
How Doing–poor/very poor	5.4	7.0	7.8	1.077
Want to Talk It				
Want to Talk About Drugs	57.1	65.8	61.5	4.201

*$p < .05$, **$p < .01$, ***$p < .001$

also worry more about others' use with increasing age ($p < .05$). On the other hand, these patterns may simply reflect the reality that adolescents and their friends are at greater risk of substance use and abuse as they get older. To add to the complexity of the picture, there were no age-based trends with regard to their experience of others worrying about them, how they felt they were doing in relation to alcohol/drug use, or their desire to talk to their counselor about substance use.

DESIRE TO TALK ABOUT SUBSTANCES

For AHC mental health service applicants, most questions indicating substance use were significantly associated with desire to talk to a counselor about it ($p < .001$) (see Table 4). This was true of those who said they had been offered drugs and/or had spent time with a drug user. This was true as well for worry about one's own use, worry about another's use, and others worry about one's own use (p < .001). Self-reports about how poorly the adolescent is doing with alcohol and drugs was also associated with desire to talk (p < .05).

There was an increasingly powerful association between seriousness of substance experimentation and desire to talk to a counselor about substance use, which is consistent with Gateway Theory. Thus, the level of significance of the association with desire to talk increased from p < .05 for tobacco, to p < .01 for alcohol, to p < .001 for marijuana and for reported use of drugs in the last month. There was no significant difference in desire to talk based on report of trying other drugs, which may be due to the relatively small sample size of those who reported using other drugs (6.3% of the sample). As reported earlier, desire to talk about substances was not associated with either gender or age.

Because the substance use questions correlated so highly with desire to talk, we decided to use the questions to construct an additive Substance Risk-Exposure Scale (SRES) after discarding question 64, which is a self-rating scale. Using the ten remaining questions (questions 57 through 63), a Cronbach's alpha was computed to assess internal consistency of the scale, which

TABLE 4. Percentage and Number Desiring to Talk, by Presence of Drug Risk/Worry Indicator

SUBSTANCE RISK FACTOR	Proportion Wanting to Talk About Drugs (%)		
	Risk Factor Present	Risk Factor Absent	χ^2
	% (N)	% (N)	
Environmental Risk			
Been Offered Drugs	70.3 (268)	52.2 (178)	25.080***
Spend Time with Drug User	71.0 (255)	52.1 (187)	27.853***
Behavioral Risk			
Tried Tobacco	68.2 (210)	60.1 (158)	4.068*
Tried Alcohol	68.7 (272)	55.7 (118)	10.188**
Tried Marijuana	73.2 (202)	56.1 (170)	18.350***
Tried Other Drugs	78.1 (25)	62.0 (292)	3.345
Used Drugs in Last Month	79.6 (156)	55.0 (289)	36.390***
Worries About Drug Use			
Worried About Own Use	76.2 (96)	58.5 (338)	13.728***
Worried About Other's Use	77.2 (196)	53.3 (245)	39.569***
Others Worry About Your Use	40.3 (176)	59.7 (261)	16.142***
How Doing–Poor/very poor	78.3 (36)	60.6 (393)	5.645*

*p < .05, **p < .01, ***p < .001

yielded an alpha of .8044. This is a very respectable measure of the reliability of the index, especially since these questions were not initially designed to be a substance risk scale.

There was a significant relationship ($p < .001$) between the SRES and adolescents' desire to talk. Thus, by using this scale we can reasonably predict that the greater the substance risk exposure, the more adolescents will want to talk about substance issues with mental health practitioners.

Again, using the SRES, the sample was divided into low- and high-risk groups, with scores of 0-3 indicating low risk (48.8% of the sample) and scores of 4-10 indicating high risk (51.1% of the sample). This was done based on dividing the sample as close to the median SRES score as possible. Comparing the two risk groups in regards to the desire to talk yielded four groups: Low risk/no talk (Type I), low risk/yes talk (Type II), high risk/yes talk (Type III), and high risk/no talk (Type IV) (see Table 5).

Of particular concern is that 13.7% of the sample fell into the high risk/no talk group, a group that is seen as vulnerable and needing to talk as much as, if not more than, the other two groups who want to talk to their counselors about substance issues.

GENDER AND AGE TRENDS IN REGARDS TO VULNERABILITY

When the four types are analyzed based on gender, there is no significant difference in vulnerability between males and females, with 15.4% of males and 12.8% of females being high risk/no talk (Type IV) (see Table 6).

In contrast, when the four types are divided by age, a troubling pattern is revealed. Predictably, as age increases, risk increases. However, as age increases, a higher proportion of adolescents at high risk report that they *do not want to talk* about their substance risk ($p < .001$).

Although it is unclear why this trend exists, a possible explanation is that as age increases, substance experimentation is normalized and thus the desire or

TABLE 5. Substance Risk Scale and Desire to Talk, by Percent

	Desire to Talk	
	Yes	No
Low Risk (0-3)	24.6 (117) Type II	24.2 (115) Type I
High Risk (4-10)	37.5 (178) Type III	13.7 (65) Type IV

$\chi^2 = 26.262$, $p < .001$

TABLE 6. Substance Risk, Desire to Talk, by Gender and Age

	Type I	Type II	Type III	Type IV
	% (N)	% (N)	% (N)	% (N)
Gender[a]				
Male	26.5 (43)	27.2 (44)	30.9 (50)	15.4 (25)
Female	23.1 (72)	23.4 (73)	40.7 (127)	12.8 (40)
Age[b]				
10-14	31.5 (46)	38.4 (56)	21.2 (31)	8.9 (13)
15-16	20.8 (41)	23.3 (44)	44.7 (88)	12.2 (24)
17-21	21.2 (28)	12.9 (17)	44.7 (59)	21.2 (28)

[a] $\chi^2 = 4.436$, $p = .218$, [b] $\chi^2 = 46.695$, $p < .001$

willingness to talk about substances decreases. Although early substance experimentation increases the risk of substance addiction (Bruner & Fishman, 1998; Hawkins, Catalano, & Miller, 1992), present Adquest data cannot determine if these older, "precontemplative" adolescents began experimentation at an early age and are already in an advanced stage of addiction and denial.

FURTHER EXPLORATIONS OF SUBSTANCE-RELATED RISKS

One item from the Sex and Sexuality section of the Adquest–"Have you ever used drugs to make sex better?"–also related to substance use and warranted further analysis. Of adolescents who reported using drugs to make sex better, 51.6% reported worrying about their own drug use (p < .001, $\chi^2 = 53.329$, df = 2), 71.7% wanted to talk about drugs (p < .05, $\chi^2 = 7.857$, df = 2), and 19.4% reported that they were doing "poor" or "very poor" with drugs in general (p < .001, $\chi^2 = 17.604$, df = 2). These findings suggest that using drugs to enhance sex might be a particularly sensitive indicator of adolescent risk.

Next, we explored self-reports of substance use among adolescents who had spent time with a drug user (Table 7) and had been offered drugs (Table 8).

Of adolescents who had spent time with a drug user, 80.7% had tried alcohol, 68% had tried tobacco, 64.2% had tried marijuana, and 44.5% had used drugs in the month preceding the survey (p < .001 for all items). Likewise, there were significant associations between having been offered drugs and having tried drugs (see Table 8).

Table 7. Time Spent with User and Lifetime Drug User

| | Proportion Having Spent Time with a User | | |
	Risk Factor Present	Risk Factor Absent	χ^2
	% (N)	% (N)	
Tried Tobacco	68.0 (219)	35.5 (89)	61.648***
Tried Alcohol	80.7 (272)	46.0 (126)	80.258***
Tried Marijuana	64.2 (212)	25.0 (63)	89.390***
Tried Other Drugs	10.1 (28)	1.7 (4)	14.963***
Used Drugs in Last Month	44.5 (161)	10.2 (37)	108.188***

*$p <. 05$, **$p < .01$, ***$p < .001$

TABLE 8. Offered Drugs and Lifetime Drug Use

| | Proportion Having Been Offered Drugs | | |
	Risk Factor Present	Risk Factor Absent	χ^2
	% (N)	% (N)	
Tried Tobacco	72.0 (237)	29.3 (73)	104.009***
Tried Alcohol	82.3 (284)	42.5 (114)	104.823***
Tried Marijuana	65.4 (223)	22.4 (55)	105.460***
Tried Other Drugs	10.5 (29)	1.3 (3)	18.003***
Used Drugs in Last Month	41.8 (161)	11.3 (39)	85.171***

*$p < .05$, **$p < .01$, ***$p < .001$

Of adolescents who had been offered drugs, 82.3% of adolescents had tried alcohol, 72% had tried tobacco, 65.4% had tried marijuana, and 41.8% had used drugs in the month preceding the survey ($p < .001$ for all items).

Finally, because one Adquest item asked about substance use in the last month, which is most likely to capture those teens who may have a substance use problem, we cross-tabulated answers to this question with questions regarding worry about own use, others worry about your use, and the rating of how they were doing regarding drugs (see Table 9).

All of these questions were highly associated with use in the past month at $p < .001$, with worry of own use/tried to cut down being the most strongly associated ($\chi^2 = 116.327$). While it may appear obvious that adolescents who are worried about their own use are likely to have used drugs in the past month, this powerful relationship demonstrates that many of these adolescents at risk are willing to disclose their risk status in an intake questionnaire. Whether they are willing to talk about their problems with a counselor depends, in part, on the counselor's clinical skills in their subsequent face-to-face meetings.

DISCUSSION

A limitation of this study is that adolescents are being asked to self-report their drug use/risks. As with most self-reports of "high-risk" issues, it is likely that there is an underreporting of these issues. Given that these numbers are probably underestimates, the percentage of adolescents seeking mental health services who are using substances is concerning. The Adquest begins to address some of these concerns by defining the process of asking questions about substance risk/use as being part of appropriate mental health care.

As indicated earlier, Adquest does not ask about the sequence of drug involvement. Nonetheless, our analysis lends partial support to the Gateway Theory as originally proposed by Kandel (1975). More specifically, the percent of adolescents who reported trying the legal drugs (alcohol and tobacco) was higher than the percentage trying illegal drugs (marijuana and other drugs) and the relationship between drug use and the desire to talk to a counselor about drugs became stronger as adolescents progress from tobacco, to alcohol, to marijuana. Ideally, however, clinical evaluations at AHC attempt to reconstruct a client's history of involvement with substance use when Adquest information "triggers" a counselor's awareness of a possible drug problem.

Additionally, although Adquest responses do not substitute for a clinical diagnosis of substance abuse, our findings indicate that drug use in the past month is highly correlated with worry about one's own use, others' worry about the adolescent's use, and his/her self-assessment of doing poorly with

TABLE 9. Used Drugs in the Past Month

	Risk Factor Present	Risk Factor Absent	χ^2
	% (N)	% (N)	
Worried About Own Use	42.5 (85)	8.2 (42)	116.327***
Others Worry About Your Use	53.0 (106)	27.4 (143)	41.739***
How Doing–poor/very poor	13.5 (27)	4.0 (47)	20.363***

$*p < .05$, $**p < .01$, $***p < .001$

alcohol and/or drugs. In this regard, it is valuable for clinicians to recognize that adolescents who report recent use have some insight regarding their drug use as being problematic, which can make it easier for the clinicians to ask the "tough" questions that are required in order to make an appropriate assessment for substance disorders.

More broadly, it is clear from our findings that the environmental risks of spending time with a drug user and being offered drugs highly influences the decision to try drugs. Especially noteworthy is that with similar exposure to these external pressures, girls were trying tobacco, alcohol, marijuana, and other drugs more than boys. At the same time, boys thought others worried about their drug use *more* than did girls. Thus, although clinicians, teachers, family members, and friends may be highly sensitized to drug use in boys, our findings strongly suggest the need for clinicians to be more acutely aware of the vulnerability to drug use and abuse of girls who are seeking mental health services.

For boys as well as girls, this study raises serious issues that mental health practitioners need to be aware of in order to better serve urban adolescent clients. First, a sizeable proportion of our youngest age group (10-14-year-olds) has already experimented with tobacco, alcohol and marijuana. The implication of this is that drug prevention strategies need to begin prior to adolescence and clinicians need to become used to asking substance use questions in their assessment of pre-teens. Second, constructing an original Substance Risk-Exposure Scale, we found that nearly 14% of AHC mental health services applicants scored high on substance risk but did not want to talk to a counselor about alcohol and drug issues. For these highly vulnerable adolescents, clinicians are challenged to find new approaches to client engagement.

Because these adolescents are seeking mental health services and are not presenting for substance treatment, they are initially seen as in the stage of precontemplation regarding changing substance use behaviors. Filling out the Adquest is an initial step that can help them assess their current substance use. By linking their current substance use to other concerns these adolescents may express in their Adquest responses, clinicians may be able to move them from a stage of precontemplation to contemplation, and ultimately to a point where they can commit to a change in their substance use behaviors (action stage).

Finally, we note with particular concern that with increasing age, the proportion of teens at high substance risk increases as their desire to talk about alcohol and drug use decreases. Given that these youth may see drug use as more "normal" as they get older and feel less compelled to talk about their use than younger teens, clinicians may need to rely more heavily on motivational interviewing strategies to engage older adolescents who are at greater risk.

CONCLUSION

Inner-city adolescents are often faced with momentous decisions regarding substance use that can drastically affect their future health and well being. Those seeking mental health services may be at greater risk for substance use and experimentation than their non-clinical peers. Providers need to know adolescents' perceptions and understandings of their own drug use, in addition to their behavioral patterns of use, in order to effectively engage them in discussion and treatment.

The findings from the substance use section of the Adquest are consistent with our belief that urban adolescents are at serious risk for substance abuse. When combined with other risk factors for substance use including using drugs to make sex better, having ever been offered drugs, and having ever spent time with a drug user, the risks increase significantly. In turn, the risks are intensified for certain age and gender groups. More generally, our findings are consistent with studies showing a high level of co-morbidity between substance disorders and various mental disorders in adolescents such as depression and post-traumatic stress disorders.

Arguably, the most positive finding in this troubling exploration of Adquest information is that the majority of AHC applicants want to talk to a mental health counselor about drugs and expressed worry about their own or another's use. As a result, practitioners working with this population must integrate their own understanding of mental health counseling to routinely include drug prevention and treatment.

REFERENCES

American Academy of Pediatrics, Committee on Adolescence. (1992). Firearms and adolescence. *Pediatrics*, 89, 784-787.

Brown, S.A., Gleghorn, A., Schuckit, M.A., Myers, M.G., & Mott, M.A. (1996). Conduct disorder among adolescent alcohol and drug users. *Journal Studies on Alcohol*, 57, 314-24.

Bruner, A.B., & Fishman, M. (1998). Adolescents and illicit drug use. *JAMA*, 280, 597-598.

Centers for Disease Control and Prevention (2002). Youth Risk Behavior Surveillance, United States 2001. *MMWR*, 51, 1-64.

Clark, D.B., Pollock, N., Bukstein, O.G., Mezzich, A.C., Bromberger, J.T., & Donovan, J.E. (1997). Gender and comorbid psychopathology in adolescents with alcohol dependence. *Journal of American Academy of Child & Adolescent Psychiatry*, 36, 1195-1203.

Diaz, A., Peake, K., Surko, M., & Bhandarkar, K. (2004). Including at-risk adolescents in their own health and mental health care: A youth development perspective. *Social Work in Mental Health,* 3(1/2), 3-22.

Ford, C.A., Millstein, S.G., Halpern-Felsher, B.L., & Irwin, C.E. (1997). Influence of physician confidentiality assurances on adolescents' willingness to disclose information and seek future health care: A randomized control trial. *JAMA,* 278(12), 1029-1034.

Grilo, C.M., Walker, M.L., Becker, D.F., Edell, W.S., & McGlashan, T.H. (1997). Personality disorders in adolescents with major depression, substance use disorders, and coexisting major depression and substance use disorders. *Journal of Consulting & Clinical Psychology,* 65(2), 328-32.

Guo, J., Hill, K.G., Hawkins, J.D., Catalano, R.F., & Abbott, R.D. (2002). A developmental analysis of sociodemographic, family, and peer effects on adolescent illicit drug initiation. *Journal of the American Academy of Child & Adolescent Psychiatry,* 41, 838-45.

Hawkins, J.D., Catalano, R.F., & Miller, J.Y. (1992). Risk and protective factors for alcohol and other drug problems in adolescence and early adulthood: Implications for substance abuse prevention. *Psychological Bulletin,* 112, 64-105.

Johnston, L.D., & O'Malley, P.M. (1997). The recanting of earlier reported drug use by young adults. *National Institute for Drug Abuse Research Monographs, 176,* 59-80.

Johnston, L.D., O'Malley, P.M., & Bachman, J.G. (2002). *Monitoring the Future national results on adolescent drug use: Overview of key findings, 2001.* (NIH Publication No. 02-5105). Bethesda, MD: National Institute on Drug Abuse.

Kandel, D.B. (1975). Stages of adolescent involvement in drug use. *Science,* 190, 912-914.

Kandel, D.B. (1978). Longitudinal Research on Drug Use: Empirical Findings and Methodological Issues. New York: Hemisphere-Wiley.

Kandel, D.B., Kessler, R.C., & Margulies, R.S. (1978). Antecedents of adolescent initiation into stages of drug use: A developmental analysis. *Journal of Youth & Adolescence,* 7, 13-40.

Kelder, S.H., Murray, N.G., Orpinas, P., Prokhorov, A., McReynolds, L., Zhang, Q., & Roberts, R. (2001). Depression and substance use in minority middle-school students. *American Journal of Public Health,* 91, 761-766.

Knight, J. (1997). Adolescent substance use: Screening, assessment, and intervention. *Contemporary Pediatrics* 14, 49-72.

McDermott, D. (1984). The relationship of parental drug use and parents' attitude concerning adolescent drug use to adolescent drug use. *Adolescence,* 19(73), 89-97.

National Center for Children of Alcoholics. (2000). *Children of addicted parents: Important facts.* Rockville, MD: Author.

National Center on Addiction and Substance Abuse. (2002). *Center on Addiction and Substance Abuse 2002 Teen Survey.* Washington, DC: Author.

Noshpitz, J.D. (1994). Self-destructiveness in adolescence: Psychotherapeutic issues. *American Journal of Psychotherapy,* 48, 347-363.

Peake, K., Epstein, I., Mirabito, D., & Surko, M. (2004). Development and utilization of a practice-based adolescent intake questionnaire (Adquest): Surveying which risks, worries, and concerns urban youth want to talk about. *Social Work in Mental Health,* 3(1,2), 55-82.

Prinstein, M.J., Boergers, J., & Spirito, A. (2001). Adolescents' and their friends' health-risk behavior: Factors that alter or add to peer influence. *Journal of Pediatric Psychology,* 26, 287-298.

Prochaska, J.O., & DiClemente, C.C. (1983). Stages and processes of self-change of smoking: Toward an integrative model of change. *Journal of Consulting & Clinical Psychology,* 51(3) 390-395.

Rohde, P., Lewinsohn, P.M., & Seeley, J.R. (1996). Psychiatric comorbidity with problematic alcohol use in high school students. *Journal of the American Academy of Child & Adolescent Psychiatry,* 35, 101-109.

Shaffer, D., & Pfeffer, C.R. (2001). Practice parameter for the assessment and treatment of children and adolescents with suicidal behavior. *Journal of American Academy of Child & Adolescent Psychiatry,* 40, 24S-51S.

Shillington, A.M., & Clapp, J.D. (2000). Self-report stability of adolescent substance use: Are there differences for gender, ethnicity and age? *Drug and Alcohol Dependence,* 60, 19-27.

Simkin, D.R. (2002). Adolescent substance use disorders and comorbidity. *Pediatric Clinics of North America,* 49, 463-477.

Adolescents' Self-Reported Risk Factors and Desire to Talk About Family and Friends: Implications for Practice and Research

Vincent Giannone
Daniel Medeiros
Jennifer Elliott
Caroline Perez
Erika Carlson
Irwin Epstein

SUMMARY. Adolescents entering an urban mental health program completed Adquest, an 80-item self-report inventory asking about im-

Vincent Giannone, PsyD, is Senior Psychologist, Mount Sinai Adolescent Health Center (AHC) and Assistant Clinical Professor in Pediatrics, Mount Sinai School of Medicine. Daniel Medeiros, MD, is Director of Mental Health Services, AHC and Assistant Professor in Pediatrics and Psychiatry, Mount Sinai School of Medicine. Jennifer Elliott, MSW, and Caroline Perez, MSW, are social workers for Project Impact, AHC. Erika Carlson, BS, is Program Evaluator, AHC, (320 East 94th Street, New York, NY 10128). Irwin Epstein, PhD, is the Helen Rehr Professor of Applied Social Work Research, Hunter College School of Social Work, 129 East 79th Street, New York, NY 10021.

[Haworth co-indexing entry note]: "Adolescents' Self-Reported Risk Factors and Desire to Talk About Family and Friends: Implications for Practice and Research." Giannone, Vincent et al. Co-published simultaneously in *Social Work in Mental Health* (The Haworth Social Work Practice Press, an imprint of The Haworth Press, Inc.) Vol. 3, No. 1/2, 2004, pp. 191-210; and: *Clinical and Research Uses of an Adolescent Mental Health Intake Questionnaire: What Kids Need to Talk About* (ed: Ken Peake, Irwin Epstein, and Daniel Medeiros) The Haworth Social Work Practice Press, an imprint of The Haworth Press, Inc., 2005, pp. 191-210. Single or multiple copies of this article are available for a fee from The Haworth Document Delivery Service [1-800-HAWORTH, 9:00 a.m. - 5:00 p.m. (EST). E-mail address: docdelivery@haworthpress.com].

http://www.haworthpress.com/web/SWMH
© 2004 by The Haworth Press, Inc. All rights reserved.
Digital Object Identifier: 10.1300/J200v03n01_11

portant areas in their life such as school and education, work, health, sexuality, substance abuse, personal and family life. This article examines how much adolescents wanted to talk about family and friends with their counselors, gender and age differences in this desire, and how that is mediated by behavioral risk factors. Irrespective of the existence of coping problems and behavioral risks, adolescents expressed a strong desire to discuss family, and, to a lesser extent, friends, in counseling. From a clinical standpoint, this finding highlights Adquest's limitations because it is based on an individual, behavioral risk paradigm rather than on more systemic factors in the lives of these adolescents. Implications regarding the use of practice-based research to facilitate reflective practice are discussed. *[Article copies available for a fee from The Haworth Document Delivery Service: 1-800-HAWORTH. E-mail address: <docdelivery@ haworthpress.com> Website: <http://www.HaworthPress.com> © 2004 by The Haworth Press, Inc. All rights reserved.]*

KEYWORDS. Adolescent, mental health, family, friends, risk, coping

The importance of interpersonal relationships is noted throughout the literature on adolescent development. It is during this period that peers and other social groups begin to take precedence over the family. Nonetheless, for better or for worse, present or absent the family remains highly significant. This complex developmental transition can be understood in a number of ways. During this period, underlying biological changes are occurring in tandem with cognitive skill development and new social expectations. As a result, adolescent behavior is notoriously unpredictable.

The focus of this paper is upon adolescents' self-reported behavioral risk factors and concerns about family and friends. While the paper explores gender differences and age-graded changes in adolescents' perceptions of family and friends, we recognize adolescents' developmental need to have concomitant changes in significant others in their environment, within families and other social institutions such as schools (Arnett, 1993; Eccles, Midgley, Wigfield, Buchanan, Reuman, Flanagan, & Mac Ivers, 1993).

In this article, we will develop a number of themes concerning our empirical understanding of a clinical population of urban youth. We go on to reflect upon how the practice-based research model and the data-mining strategy that we have employed has brought to light a number of unformulated assumptions that govern our therapeutic interventions (Peake & Epstein, 2004).

This article is part of a larger practice-based research effort to better understand the issues in the lives of urban adolescents that bring them into mental health treatment. This understanding is based on answers to a set of questions about areas of their lives that we believe are important to them through a self-administered intake questionnaire (Adquest). While colloquial and intended to be user-friendly, the questions in Adquest were primarily influenced by theories that focus on adolescent risk-taking and experimentation. A principal assumption that guided Adquest's development was that risk factors are central to understanding adolescent behavior and helping adolescents better cope with problematic issues in their lives (National Research Council, 1993; Jessor, 1991). Throughout Adquest are questions reflecting the premise that mental health treatment should be guided by questions asking young people how they are dealing with important risk factors in their lives, which of these are most serious, and how much they want to discuss them in treatment.

By aggregating and analyzing individual responses at intake, this and preceding articles seek generalizations about the lives of urban adolescents seeking mental health services (Peake, Epstein, Mirabito, & Surko, 2004). Although gender and developmental stage are factored into the analysis, the larger project in which this paper is contained maintains an individual focus on risk-factor management by the adolescent. However, this is only one of many ways to conceptualize adolescent development. Nonetheless, the view of adolescents as individuals coping with a myriad of internal and external changes has an extensive history in the area of developmental psychology (Arnett, 1999).

Early theorists of adolescent development presumed that this was a time of individual "stress and storm" in response to internal biological changes (Arnett, 1999). Psychoanalytic theorists postulated that adolescence represents an important transition point for the individual in which there is a consolidation of previous developmental achievements. Some authors, notably Anna Freud (1998), suggested that the line between normality and pathology is difficult to draw in adolescence, as extreme mood changes and lability are normal during this phase of emotional development. She also believed that increased conflicts with parents and others is normal rather than pathological, describing a peaceful transition from dependence during childhood to the independence of adulthood as indicative of psychological problems rather than of adolescent mental health. In response, Freud recommended that therapists involve parents in their work with adolescents. In so doing, she emphasized the need to provide parents with guidance for "weathering the storm" that is a normal phase of their adolescent's development (Freud, 1998).

Others theorized that what may be viewed as a *stormy* period in development is actually related to changes in cognitive capacity and functioning which requires the adolescent to question established shibboleths and to engage in independent thought experiments that are the beginning of abstraction and formal reasoning (Keating, 1990).

The assumptions of early theorists of adolescent development have been challenged by empirical research. Studies indicate that most young people make a relatively smooth transition from childhood to adulthood even though personal problematic issues do arise during adolescence, and interpersonal conflicts do occur over rules, curfew, and friends (Arnett, 1999; Steinberg, 1990; Powers, Hauser, & Kilner, 1989).

More specifically, Eccles et al. (1993) have commented that with regard to school and family, conflicts are usually over issues that involve a "goodness of fit" between the adolescent's needs and the environmental response to these. This is a more *transactional* rather than individual paradigm which focuses on the adolescent *within* a family and points to the necessity for the family to change and develop along with the adolescent. This transactional view emphasizes the importance of interplay between the changing developmental requisites of the adolescent and his parents. Moreover, developmental theorists note that in the homes of adolescents, parents are also moving through life-cycle changes and dealing with a host of salient challenges in their own lives (Carter & McGoldrick, 1989; Garcia Preto, 1989).

While it is not the primary focus of this article, one cannot ignore how social class, racial and ethnic factors may also contribute to family stressors that, in turn, impact on developmental needs of the adolescent (National Research Council, 1993; Boyd-Franklin, 1989). This point of view contains within it offers a more *systemic* notion of how the environment can contribute to the "stress and storm" of adolescence. The systematic perspective considers adolescents as embedded in complex and multi-layered systems, which can facilitate or inhibit positive growth and development (Cauce, Domenech-Rodriquez, Paradise, Cochran, Shea, Srebnik, & Baydar, 2002; National Research Council, 1993; Eccles et al., 1993; Boyd-Franklin, 1989).

As adolescents become more psycho-socially aware and develop a more complex understanding of themselves, they become more oriented towards an expanding social world. Although attempting to separate themselves from family, family remains important (in both positive and/or negative ways) in promoting or constricting adolescent growth and development. At the same time, the adolescent is devoting increased attention to the world outside the family, especially peers and friends. Just as the family is an important factor in the lives of healthy adolescents, so are friends.

Although parents don't always view it this way, the role of friends in the lives of adolescents can be seen as a positive and important protective factor (Savin-Williams & Berndt, 1990; Sullivan, 1953). Young persons who have satisfying and harmonious friendships manifest self-esteem, empathy, and sensitivity to others. However, as with any complex social dynamic and community, there are important variables that will affect the outcome of this interaction between adolescents and their peer-group. Hence, the choice of friends is important, and adolescents tend to choose their friends based on a number of different variables (Savin-Williams & Berndt, 1990).

Conceptualizing friendship or peer relationships as a unidimensional aspect (i.e., either positive or negative) of a young person's life is overly simplistic. Relationships in any adolescent's life may serve many different purposes and represent a means of experimentation with different social roles and responsibilities. Well-adjusted adolescents tend to have supportive friends, while adolescents with difficulties tend to associate with individuals who have similar difficulties and may reinforce problematic behaviors (Savin-Williams & Berndt, 1990).

In this paper, adolescents' relationships with friends and family are considered essential to understanding adolescent development. Each is seen as a potential source of resiliency or a potential source of risk. As a risk factor, it is thought that lack of friends, difficulties with friends, or value conflicts with friends and associates is an important aspect of understanding an adolescent's adjustment.

On the other hand, families generate strengths and risks in and of themselves as well as in response to adolescent peer relations (Eccles et al., 1993; Steinberg, 1990). How a family deals with this normative period of change and development can facilitate or inhibit an adolescent's adjustment within the community. As clinicians, the authors of this paper recognize and work with the multiple dimensions and complexities involved in adolescent clients' family and social connections. However, information provided by Adquest limits our understanding of respondents' lives to individual risk factors, worries, and concerns and the desire to talk about these. Nonetheless, in this paper, a systemic perspective was used to analyze and interpret Adquest-generated findings.

THEORETICAL ASSUMPTIONS UNDERLYING ADQUEST

Adquest was designed as an initial assessment instrument to survey prospective adolescent mental health clients about how well they are negotiating various developmental tasks in their lives. It attempts to do so by asking young persons to reflect on and respond to various sets of questions that ask about a number of potentially problematic life events involving sexuality, safety, family, school, and health among others. In doing so, it emphasizes risk factors and life events that may confront or be available to urban adolescents. These risky life events are individual (e.g., trying drugs), interpersonal (e.g., spending time with a drug user), and social (e.g., experiencing racism).

Because Adquest employs a self-administered questionnaire format, it emphasizes the adolescent respondent's subjective assessment and perception of her or his own life. This individual focus is an essential part of the underlying structure of the questionnaire. Its construction was heavily influenced by prior research concerning adolescent behavioral risk. This led to a decision to limit the information solicited about families. Consequently, respondents were asked to comment on a very limited number of questions about family or friends, i.e., whether they worried about their families or their friends and how much they wanted to talk about family or friends with a counselor. As an indicator of coping, they were also asked how well they thought they were doing in various aspects of their lives (e.g., school, work, health).

Parents or guardians were also asked to complete a survey about family events and stressors and how they thought the service applicant was doing in various life areas. These data were not included in the present analysis in order to maintain a larger sample size but will be analyzed in subsequent studies when more family data has been accumulated.

Clearly, the empirical findings presented in this chapter reflect the underlying assumptions and limitations of the instrument. It is the authors' intention, however, to use Adquest data to venture beyond its underlying assumptions by expanding its focus from the individual to a more systematic perspective. We attempt to do so by considering the relationship between the many questions concerning individual risk and the very few concerning family and friends. In doing so, we employ a systemic perspective to interpret the limited data that we do have as well as to make suggestions about how Adquest should be modified to take this perspective into account.

METHOD

The Mount Sinai Adolescent Health Center (AHC) is a comprehensive health center for inner city youth. The center has an extensive mental health program, which provides over 20,000 mental health visits annually to adolescents between the ages of 10 and 21 years of age. Clients are seen regardless of their ability to pay or their health insurance status. The study sample consisted of 759 adolescents presenting for a mental health intake session between April 27, 1999 and April 9, 2002. Within this sample, 36.0 % were male and 64.0% were female, the majority of whom come from low-income minority households in New York City (Diaz, Peake, Surko, & Bhandarkar, 2004).

The Adquest is an indigenous, context-specific instrument designed by practitioners for practitioners. The 80-item adolescent self-report inventory asks adolescents about important areas in their life such as school and education, work, health, sexuality, substance abuse, and personal and family life. It was intended to enhance adolescent engagement in psychotherapy by asking young people who are requesting counseling services to reflect upon their own lives, problems, needs, worries, and reasons for seeking counseling. An important aspect of the Adquest is that it also asks the adolescents what areas they feel are important to discuss (Peake, Epstein, Mirabito, & Surko, 2004).

ADQUEST MEASURES CONCERNING FAMILY AND FRIENDS

As indicated earlier, Adquest has numerous questions concerning adolescent risk exposures and behaviors but few that ask directly about family life or concerns. The following three questions are the only ones that do:

71. Do you have any worries about your family or home life? Yes No
72. In general, when it comes to your family/home life, how would you say you are doing? 1. Very poor 2. Poor 3. Average 4. Well 5. Very well
73. How much do you want to talk to your counselor here about your family or home life? 1. Not at all 2. Somewhat 3. Very much 4. Don't know.

With regard to friends and friendship, three parallel questions are asked within Adquest, questions that follow the same general format. These are as follows:

66. Do you have any worries about your friends or associates? Yes No
68. In general, when it comes to friendships how would you say you are doing? 1. Very poor 2. Poor 3. Average 4. Well 5. Very well
69. How much do you want to talk to your counselor here about friends or associates? 1. Not at all 2. Somewhat 3. Very much 4. Don't know

In mining what Adquest has to tell us about these important dimensions of urban adolescent life, our analytic strategy involves a number of different steps. The first is to present a "snapshot" of the 759 respondents in our sample, which gives the percentages of adolescents that express concerns about family or home life and about friends. Included in this picture is the percentage of service applicants that indicate wanting to talk about these issues in counseling.

Response categories to the latter questions require adolescents to give one of four choices when asked if they would want to talk to a counselor about family or friends, i.e., not at all, somewhat, very much, and don't know. Consistent with prior Adquest studies (Peake et al., 2004), this data analysis will follow the practice of combining responses of "somewhat," "very much," and "don't know" as indications that the adolescent wanted to talk about the issue in treatment. To reiterate, the inclusion of the "don't know" response as a positive indicator is based on the empirically supported assumption that in so saying, the adolescent is inviting a clinician to clarify the issue. On the other hand, a response of "no" is honored as a clear statement that, at the present time, the young person has no desire to talk to a counselor about family or friends (Elliott, Nembhard, Giannone, & Surko, 2004). We use this dichotomous measure of desire to talk throughout this article.

After the initial "snapshot," a second level of analysis is presented to reflect on gender and age differences in concern about family or friends. Third, consideration is given to the relationship between self-reported worry about family or friends and desire to talk to a counselor about one or the other. In addition, the relationship between reported coping with family and with friends and the desire to talk is briefly examined. A fourth level of analysis examines how gender and age influence the relationship between worry and desire to talk. A final stage in our analysis utilizes risk scales developed in prior Adquest studies (Medeiros, Kramnick, Diaz-Cruz, Surko, Diaz, & Epstein, 2004; Surko, Ciro, Carlson, Labor, Giannone, Diaz-Cruz, Peake, & Epstein, 2004; Medeiros, Carlson, Surko, Munoz, Castillo, & Epstein, 2004) to examine the relationship between adolescent risk and desire to talk about family or friends.

FINDINGS

"Snapshot" of Friends and Family

Table 1 presents a descriptive "snapshot" of the level of concern that respondents feel about friends and family and their desire to talk to a counselor about them. The results indicate that when asked, 49.9% of the adolescents in our client sample report that they have worries about their friends or associates and 61.8% have worries about their family or home life.

Irrespective of their level of concern, over three-quarters of AHC service applicants want to talk to a counselor about one or the other. More specifically 75.6% want to talk to a counselor about friends and associates and 80.4% want to talk about family or home life.

TABLE 1. Proportion of Adolescents Reporting Worries and Wanting to Talk (N = 759)

Indicator	% (N)
Concerns	
Worry about friends/associates	49.9 (365)
Worry about family/home life	61.8 (453)
Want to talk	
Friends/Associates	75.6 (555)
Family/Home life	80.4 (589)

Gender Trends

Gender is clearly associated with worries about friends and family and with desire to talk about them. For instance Table 2 reveals that females are significantly more likely to report having worries about their friends and associates than males (54.5% versus 41.6 %, respectively). This significant gender difference was also noted in reported worries about family and home life. In this regard, more than two-thirds (67.9%) of the females were worried, as opposed to about half (50.8%) of the males.

This significant gender difference holds for adolescents' desire to talk about friends and family. Four-fifths (80.1%) of the females expressed a desire to discuss their friends and associates in treatment as compared to two-thirds (67.7%) of the adolescent males. Similarly, adolescent females have significantly higher rates of wanting to talk about family than males (86.1% versus 70.2%, respectively). While the differences between the genders are statistically significant in that females evidence a greater worry about and desire to talk about friends or family, it is notable that both genders have a high degree of desire to talk about them both. And, of the two, family appears to be the highest priority.

Stages of Adolescence, Worry, and Desire to Talk About Friends and Family

The findings in Table 3 suggest that as adolescents move through early, middle, and late adolescence, their concern about friends and associates remains at a consistent, level. More specifically, about half of each age group expresses worry about friends or associates. Likewise, while about three-quarters of the sample want to talk to a counselor about friends or associates, there are no significant differences by stage of adolescence. In other words, the de-

TABLE 2. Percentage of Adolescents Reporting Worries and Wanting to Talk, by Gender

Indicator	Male N = 272	Female N = 484	x^2
Concerns			
Worry about Friends/Associates	41.6	54.5	11.15 **
Worry about Family/Home life	50.8	67.9	21.12***
Want to talk			
Friends/Associates	67.7	80.1	14.16***
Family/Home life	70.2	86.1	27.02***

*p < .05, **p < .01, ***p < .001

TABLE 3. Percentage of Adolescents Reporting Worries and Wanting to Talk, by Stage of Adolescence

Stage of Adolescence

Indicator	Early N = 247	Middle N = 290	Late N = 93	x^2
Concerns				
Worry about Friends/Associates	47.8	50.3	52.1	.83
Worry about Family/Home life	50.2	64.1	73.1	25.49***
Want to talk				
Friends/Associates	73.5	78.5	73.6	2.11
Family/Home life	70.9	86.9	82.7	22.57***

*p < .05, **p < .01, ***p < .001

sire to talk about this issue in counseling appears to remain constant and high throughout adolescence.

In contrast, increasing age correlates with an increase in percent expressing concern about family and home life. Thus, half (50.2%) of the early adolescents, slightly less than two-thirds (64.1%) of middle adolescents, and close to three-quarters (73.1%) of late adolescents express worry about their family and home lives. Older adolescents expressed a greater desire to talk to a counselor or about family/home life than early adolescents, but the wish to do so appears to peak during mid-adolescence (70.9% early, 86.9% middle, 82.7% late).

Relationship Between Worry and Desire to Talk

Adquest data strongly suggests that the majority of AHC clients want to talk about their family and home life as well as friends and associates. Considering the relationship between expressed worry and desire to talk (see Table 4), it becomes clear that adolescents who report worrying about friends or family are significantly more likely to want to talk about them in counseling.

Hence, over four-fifths (84%) of those who said that they worried about friends or associates wanted to speak to a therapist about it, compared to two-thirds (66.8%) of those who did not. Likewise, over ninety percent of adolescents who were worried about their family/home life wanted to talk about it compared to less than two-thirds of those who did not (91.3% versus 62.6%, respectively). Although worry was clearly predictive of desire to talk about friends as well as about family, worry about family was clearly a more sensitive predictor of desire to talk.

Gender and Stage of Adolescence in Mediating Worry and Desire to Talk

Next we consider how gender might affect the relationship between worry and desire to talk. As seen in Table 5, gender influences the strength of the relationship between worry and desire to talk, with females expressing a greater desire to talk when worried than males.

For example, 86.9% of females who worried about friends or associates wanted to talk about them in treatment as compared to 77.1% of the worried males. This pattern is even stronger in regards to family/home life. Here, 94.9% of the worried females express desire to talk as compared to 82.8% of worried males. Irrespective of gender differences, what is most striking is the

TABLE 4. Proportion of Adolescents Reporting Wanting to Talk Based on Expressed Worry

	Worry About Friends or Family		χ^2
	Yes % (N)	**No** % (N)	
Want to Talk About Friends	84.0 (304)	66.8 (243)	28.97***
Want to Talk About Family	91.3 (411)	62.6 (174)	89.94***

*p < .05, **p < .01, ***p < .001

high level of worry and desire to talk about friends and family in this client population.

Table 6 suggests that stage of adolescence does not mediate the relationship between worry about friends and desire to talk to a counselor about them. In other words, there is no significant relationship between worry and desire to talk by age group. However, with regard to family and home life, worried middle-stage adolescents again peak in desire to talk about family and home life (82.3% early, 96.2% middle, 93.0% late, respectively).

Coping with Friends and Family and Desire to Talk

As might be expected, there was an inverse relationship between perceived coping and desire to talk about friends or family (Table 7). Thus 70% of the adolescents who felt they were coping well/very well in regards to friendships wanted to talk about these friendships, while 91.4% of those who felt they were coping poorly/very poorly wanted to talk about friends/associates. What is perhaps most striking, however, is that such high levels of those adolescents who say they are coping well with regard to peers still want to talk about this issue.

TABLE 5. Influence of Gender on the Proportion of Worried Adolescents Wanting to Talk

	Male	**Female**	χ^2
	% (N)	% (N)	
Worry/Talk: Friends/Associates	77.1 (84)	86.9 (219)	5.46*
Worry/Talk: Family/Home life	82.8 (111)	94.9 (299)	17.13***

$* p < .05, ** p < .01, *** p < .001$

TABLE 6. Influence of Stage of Adolescence on the Proportion of Worried Adolescents Wanting to Talk

	Stage of Adolescence			
	Early	**Middle**	**Late**	χ^2
	% (N)	% (N)	% (N)	
Worry/Talk: Friends/Associates	78.8 (93)	88.1 (126)	84.2 (85)	4.158
Worry/Talk: Family/Home life	82.3 (102)	96.2 (176)	93.0 (133)	18.827***

$* p < .05, ** p < .01, *** p < .001$

TABLE 7. Relationship Between Coping and Desire to Talk

Coping indicator	Poor/very poor % (N)	Average % (N)	Well/very well % (N)	χ^2
Coping Friends/ Talk Friends	91.4 (85)	82.0 (132)	70.0 (332)	23.94***
Coping Family/ Talk Family	96.1 (197)	80.5 (215)	67.5 (172)	59.03***

* $p < .05$, ** $p < .01$, *** $p < .001$

The relationship between perceived coping and desire to talk about family is stronger than for friends. Over two-thirds (67.5%) of adolescents who felt they were coping well/very well with family/home life wanted to talk about it, whereas almost all (96.1%) of those coping poorly/very poorly expressed a desire to talk with a counselor about family life. The latter finding makes sense. Young persons asking for help who think they are doing poorly with their families would naturally want to talk about this with a counselor. Here again, however, what is most striking is the vast majority of those who report they are coping well with family and home life who indicate that they want to talk about these very issues.

Behavioral Risk and Desire to Talk About Friends and Family

Prior studies based on Adquest data made use of original, behavioral risk scales in areas such as general health (Medeiros, Kramnick et al., 2004), physical safety (Surko et al., 2004) and substance use (Medeiros, Carlson et al., 2004). In this final analysis, these scales were used to determine the extent to which exposure to risk is associated with desire to talk about friends or family life. In considering this question, one might just as easily hypothesize positive, negative, or no relationship at all between these sets of variables. Thus, for example, one might theorize that if adolescents perceived that risk of a particular kind were a *direct* response to problems within the family, one would predict that the higher the risk, the greater the desire to talk about family. Alternatively, if risk-taking or exposure to risk were seen as an expression of rebellion against family, one would predict an *inverse* relationship between risk-taking or exposure and desire to talk about family. Finally, if risk-taking in these other areas were unrelated to family life but perhaps related to peer influences, one might predict no relationship between risk taking and desire to talk about family but a *direct* relationship between risk taking and desire to talk about friends. Moreover, these relationships could differ by type of risk. Only by considering the data that Adquest provides can we begin to answer these questions.

To perform this analysis, each scale was dichotomized into "low" and "high" risk using median scores. Cross-tabulations and Chi-square analysis were then performed to determine whether different kinds of risks were associated with desire to talk about friends or about family life (Table 8). Although with each scale the trend is consistent that those scoring at higher risk were more likely to want to talk, the strength of this relationship varied greatly by type of risk. For instance, there is no significant relationship between substance risk and desire to talk about friends or about family. This finding suggests that for this client population exposure to substance risk is not linked to a desire to talk about friends or family in treatment. However, what is remarkable is the high level of desire to talk about friends or family *irrespective* of their level of risk.

Unlike substance risk, the safety risk scale is directly and significantly associated with desire to talk about friends and desire to talk about family. On this measure, the desire to talk about family is more sensitive ($p < .05$ for talk regarding friends/associates and $p < .01$ for talk regarding family/home life). However, here again the vast majority of those in either safety risk category want to talk about friends and about family.

The health risk scale demonstrates the strongest *direct* relationship between risk and wanting to talk ($p < .001$ for desire to talk about both family and friends). In this regard, desire to talk about family is most sensitively related to

Table 8. Risk Scales and Desire to Talk

Risk Scales	Low % (N)	High % (N)	x^2
Substance Risk:			
Talk Friends	74.7 (174)	78.3 (191)	.86
Talk Family	78.5 (183)	84.4 (205)	2.68
Safety Risk:			
Talk Friends:	71.7 (266)	79.0 (245)	4.85 *
Talk Family:	75.1 (278)	85.2 (264)	10.48**
Health Risk:			
Talk Friends:	70.1 (319)	84.6 (236)	19.66***
Talk Family:	74.5 (339)	89.9 (250)	26.00***

*p < .05, **p < .01, ***p < .001

risk. However, health risk notwithstanding, the most persistent finding remains the desire to talk about friends and family.

DISCUSSION

The young people who presented at the Adolescent Health Center for services evidenced a consistent trend. Regardless of the behavioral risk factors that may have brought them to be seen at the clinic, the majority evidenced a desire to talk about their families and home life, and to a certain extent their friendships. These results are both statistically *and* clinically significant and are an important insight derived from practice-based research. When Adquest was developed a great deal of attention was given to the inquiry into the risk factors in adolescents' lives. The focus on risk factors fit with a number of significant assumptions regarding the focus on the individual adolescent and the need to help the adolescent develop skills to cope with these deficits in either emotional or behavioral functioning (Weisz & Hawley, 2002; National Research Council, 1993; Jessor, 1991). In this model the focus is upon identifying areas of problems with the assumption that this is primarily related to issues of emotional functioning or problem behaviors (Cauce et al., 2002). For example, some authors see the primary task as fostering separation from the family and the development of independence, or developing a sense of identity. The individual is the focus and other social systems are seen as secondary or a possible hindrance. While some attention may be paid to environmental or social factors, the primary focus is on the adolescent.

As noted, the primary focus of our survey is to develop an inventory of risk behaviors as a way of developing a dialogue with the adolescent in order to intervene in their lives (Elliott et al., 2004). Given the high prevalence of potentially harmful and life- threatening consequences of many of these risk factors in our clinical population, it is not surprising that we attend to these factors in our attempts to intervene. The assumption that adolescents are interested in and motivated to explore these issues is a frequently accepted idea although there is limited information about what adolescents are looking for in treatment. In this regard, Cauce et al. (2002) note the cultural divide potential between adolescents and those who seek to provide services.

Adolescents come to therapy with various concerns and questions. While important, the focus on individual risk factors does not reflect the multidimensional aspects that bring adolescents or their families into treatment. The importance of the risk scales in understanding adolescents is highlighted by the acknowledgment that those adolescents who evidence high risk in the areas of safety and health seek an understanding adult with whom to discuss these issues.

Adolescents in our population sample evidence a clear trend of being concerned about their friends and their family/home life. The majority acknowledge a desire to discuss these issues with a therapist. It is not surprising that in our population females were more concerned about their friends than males. It is noted in the literature that females are generally more open in their acknowledgment of interpersonal concerns than males (Cauce et al., 2002). The trend also holds when we focus on the desire to discuss these issues with a therapist. As an adolescent moves from early to late adolescence there is no change in the desire to discuss these issues in therapy, but a trend is noted with their families. The trend may be indicative of the changing relationship that is acknowledged across the life span of adolescents (Weisz & Hawley, 2002; Arnett, 1999; Eccles et al., 1993).

As they move through the life cycle it appears that those in middle adolescence have a greater desire to discuss family concerns. According to developmental literature, this period may be a time when adolescents are dealing with significant internal issues and a concomitant increase in conflicts with their families. While these conflicts may be mundane and focused on curfews, friends and other minor issues, it may be difficult for both the young person and their parents to develop the appropriate skills and behaviors to negotiate these issues (Eccles et al., 1993; Garcia-Preto, 1989). We can see in our population that even those adolescents who feel they are coping well evidence a desire to discuss issues related to their home life. In addition to these mundane issues there is also a heightened awareness of the young person fostered by their changing cognitive skills in their capacity to reflect and think abstractly about their perceptions and the community in which they are living. This ability to reflect on issues also gives rise to changing thoughts about their parents and their circumstances (Hauser & Bowlds, 1990). What previously was viewed from a limited perspective can now be seen more abstractly and in an emotional more complex manner. The idea that a parent is powerless or is severely ill now has a different impact on the adolescents' emotional functioning. Given the number of psychosocial stressors noted in the population we are studying, it can be an important time to facilitate emotional growth and helping these adolescents develop effective coping strategies (Greenspan, 1997). Our survey indicates that middle adolescents may have a window or period of time when these issues are most relevant for the adolescent in our population and potentially most available for intervention. Prior to this time the young person does not have the ability to reflect on these issues and at a later period is less open to discussing these issues. Based upon our survey, we can see that no matter what the difficulty or level of risk, more adolescents indicate a desire to discuss issues than not.

The idea that adolescents may come to therapy with a different set of needs and ideas than the adults in their lives is an important aspect of therapy rarely discussed from the point of view of the adolescent. While complex, these issues were relevant in that we undertook an analysis of the connection between the adolescents' level of concern and their desire to discuss these issues. We tended to focus upon our own conceptual ideas even when given information from adolescents who felt that we focused too much on them and ignored their families. This is especially important with youth from an urban environment where issues related to their families can be quite important in understanding their behavior, values and ideas (Cauce et al., 2002; Eccles et al., 1993). Mirabito (2001) noted in her study that adolescents felt that therapists focused too much on them and not enough on their parents. Given the information and feedback we received from adolescents, it is relevant that we chose to maintain our focus on the importance of individual factors rather than familial and community context issues.

Many of the adolescents presenting for services at our center have family members with significant psychosocial issues and problems, such as HIV/AIDS, substance abuse, poverty, unemployment, etc. These events will and do have a profound impact on mental health and functioning. In a separate parent/caretaker survey we asked about stressful events that are present in the family or had occurred in the past. We will analyze this data at a later date. From the adolescents' point of view, it is more important that we inquire more in depth about concerns and issues that they have about their families, i.e., perception of rules, discipline, and other issues that directly affect the adolescent. On a systematic level this communicates our underlying assumptions that the most salient aspect of treating the adolescents is focusing on his/her risk factors and coping. While we are concerned about contextual issues, in contrast our primary focus is the individual.

An important aspect of the Adquest is the need to place more of a focus on contextual factors. We can see that the adolescent considers issues within their families as important and the desire to discuss these issues comes through for most of the individuals seen at the clinic. However, we are unsure of the specific issues that may be of concern to adolescents. While we were reviewing the literature in the field we found few articles that asked the adolescent what was important to them to discuss in treatment. While we have a better understanding that no matter what the factors are in the life of an adolescent, it is important to acknowledge the issue of family. The fact that there are no differences based on age or gender indicate that this is a rich source to facilitate our understanding of adolescents and engaging young people in treatment. It is unclear from the present results what issues or factors substance abuse contribute to an adolescent's lack of desire to discuss their family, although it indicates that this may be a subsample of our population that has different needs or problems in treatment.

The importance of friendships and adolescents' needs to discuss these issues is significant, although we have tended to focus this article on families due to space limitations. The trends, however, are similar in that adolescents evidence an interest in discussing these issues although the relationships are not as consistent as those noted with their families. The differences indicate that at an early age a significant number of adolescents worry about their friends and associates and this remains consistent throughout the development. The idea that males acknowledge less worry about their associates and friends than females is an area worth exploring. It is well known that males who are members of minority groups in the inner city are at high risk for being victims of violence and other high risk behaviors, whether from external sources or through their own behavior patterns (National Research Council, 1993). It is also noted that the trend related to those who engage in substance abuse behavior and score at a high-risk level do not wish to discuss these issues related to friendship. However, in the areas of health and safety the higher the risk factors the greater the desire to discuss this with a therapist. The importance of this trend is that related to substance abusing, adolescents are also engaging in behaviors that are risk factors in both the areas of safety and health. This issue bears further clarification.

The relationships between family and friends is seen as significant in that both areas are important to adolescents and something that the adolescent sees as important to discuss in treatment. While the data indicates that this is of concern to adolescents, we do not know the specific areas or issues that adolescents would consider important to discuss.

CONCLUSION

Adolescents who are seen for a mental health treatment intake session at the Adolescent Health Center have been the focus of this article. These adolescents are most concerned and worried about their families, and when asked, they will readily identify these concerns on a paper and pencil task.

Given that most treatment emphasizes individual therapy with adolescents, it is important that clinicians expand their inquiry to include the adolescents' worries and concerns about their families. Clinicians may need to shift the focus of therapy to include more frequent collateral sessions with family members or family therapy, in order to more appropriately address the adolescents' concerns regarding their families.

REFERENCES

Arnett, J.J. (1999). Adolescent storm and stress reconsidered. *American Psychologist,* 54(5), 317-326.

Boyd-Franklin, N. (1989). *Black families in therapy: A multisystems approach.* New York, NY: Guilford Press.

Carter, B., & McGoldrick, M. (1989). *The changing family life cycle: A framework for family therapy,* 2nd ed. Boston, MA: Allyn & Bacon.

Cauce, A.M., Domenech-Rodriquez, M., Paradise, M., Cochran, B.N., Shea, J.M. Srebnik, D., & Baydar, N. (2002). Cultural and contextual influences in mental health help seeking: A focus on ethnic minority youth. *Journal of Clinical & Consulting Psychology,* 70(1), 44-55.

Diaz, A., Peake, K., Surko, M., & Bhandarkar, K. (2004). Including at risk adolescents in their own health and mental health care: A youth development perspective. *Social Work in Mental Health,* 3(1/2), 3-22.

Eccles, J.S., Midgley, C., Wigfield, A., Buchanan, C.M. , Reuman, D., Flanagan, C., & Mac Iver, D. (1993). Development during adolescence: The impact of stage-environment fit on young adolescents' experiences in schools and families. *American Psychologist,* 48(2), 90-101.

Elliott, J., Nembhard, M., Giannone, V., Surko, M., Medeiros, D., & Peake, K. (2004). Clinical uses of an adolescent intake questionnaire: Adquest as a bridge to engagement. *Social Work in Mental Health,* 3(1/2), 83-102.

Freud, A. (1998). Adolescence. In M. Perret-Catipovic., & F. Ladame (Eds.) Translated by Pierre Slotkin. *Adolescence and Psychoanalysis: The story and history.* London: Karnac Books, pp. 43-65.

Garcia Preto, N. (1989). Transformation of the family system in adolescence. In B. Carter, & M. McGoldrick (Eds.), *The changing family life cycle: A framework for family therapy. 2nd Edition.* Boston, MA: Allyn & Bacon, pp. 256- 285.

Greenspan, S.T. (1997). The growth of the mind. Reading, MA: Addison-Wesley Publishing Company, Inc.

Hauser, S.T., & Bowlds, M.K. (1990). Stress, coping and adaptation. In S. Feldman & G. Elliot (Eds.), *At the threshold: The developing adolescent.* Cambridge, MA: Harvard University Press, pp. 388-413.

Jessor, R.M. (1991). Risk behavior in adolescence: A framework for understanding and action. *Journal of Adolescent Health,* 12(8), 597-605.

Keating, D. (1990). Adolescent thinking. In S. Feldman, & G. Elliot (Eds.), *At the threshold: The developing adolescent.* Cambridge, MA: Harvard University Press, pp. 54- 90.

Medeiros, D., Kramnick, L., Diaz-Cruz, E., Surko, M., & Diaz, A., (2004). Adolescents seeking mental health services: Self-reported health risks and the need to talk. *Social Work in Mental Health,* 3(1/2), 121-133.

Medeiros, D., Carlson, E., Surko, M., Munoz, N., Castillo, M., & Epstein, I. (2004). Adolescents' self-reported substance risks and their need to talk about them in mental health counseling. *Social Work in Mental Health, 3*(1/2), 171-189.

Mirabito, D. (2001). Mining treatment termination data in an adolescent mental health service: A quantitative study. *Social Work in Health Care*, 33 (3/4), 71-90.

National Research Council. (1993). *Losing generations: Adolescents in high risk settings*. Washington, DC: National Academy Press/American Psychological Association.

Peake, K., & Epstein, I. (2004). Theoretical and practical imperatives for reflective social work organizations in health and mental health: The place of practice-based research. *Social Work in Mental Health, 3*(1/2), 23-37.

Peake, K., Epstein, I., Mirabito, D., & Surko, M. (2004) Development and utilization of a practice based, adolescent intake questionnaire (Adquest): Surveying which risks, worries, and concerns urban youth want to talk about. *Social Work in Mental Health, 3*(1/2), 55-82.

Powers, S.I., Hauser, S.T., & Kilner, L.A. (1989). Adolescent mental health. *American Psychologist, 44* (2), 200-208.

Savin-Williams, R.C., & Berndt, T.J. (1990). Friendship and peer relations. In S. Feldman, & G. Elliot (Eds.). *At the threshold: The developing adolescent*. Cambridge, MA: Harvard University Press, pp. 277-307.

Steinberg, L. (1990). Autonomy, conflict, and harmony in the family relationship. In S. Feldman & G. Elliot (Eds.), *At the threshold: The developing adolescent*. Cambridge, MA: Harvard University Press, pp. 255-276.

Sullivan, H.S. (1953). *The interpersonal theory of psychiatry*. New York, NY: Norton & Co.

Surko, M., Ciro, D., Carlson, E., Labor, N., Giannone, V., Diaz-Cruz, E., Peake, K., & Epstein, I. (2004). Which adolescents need to talk about safety and violence? *Social Work in Mental Health, 3*(1/2), 103-119.

Weisz, J.R., & Hawley, K.M. (2002). Developmental factors in the treatment of adolescents. *Journal of Clinical & Consulting Psychology, 70*(1) 21-43.

PART II

PART 1

Lesbian, Gay, Bisexual, Sexual-Orientation Questioning Adolescents Seeking Mental Health Services: Risk Factors, Worries, and Desire to Talk About Them

Dianne Ciro
Michael Surko
Kalpana Bhandarkar
Nora Helfgott
Ken Peake
Irwin Epstein

SUMMARY. Lesbian, gay, bisexual, and sexual-orientation questioning (LGBQ) adolescents have many of the same health needs as straight ado-

Dianne Ciro, MS, is Clinical Social Worker, Mount Sinai Adolescent Health Center (AHC) 320 East 94th Street, New York, NY 10128 (E-mail: Dianne.Ciro@msnyuhealth.org). Michael Surko, PhD, is Coordinator, AHC Center for Excellence. Kalpana Bhandarkar, BA, is Program Assistant, AHC Center for Excellence. Nora Helfgott, MSW, is Clinical Social Worker, AHC. Ken Peake, DSW, is Assistant Director, AHC. Irwin Epstein, PhD, is Helen Rehr Professor of Applied Social Work Research in Health, Hunter College School of Social Work, 129 East 79th Street, New York, NY 10021 (E-mail: iepstein@hunter.cuny.edu).

The authors would like to acknowledge the contributions made by Jenny DeBower, MSW.

[Haworth co-indexing entry note]: "Lesbian, Gay, Bisexual, and Sexual-Orientation Questioning Adolescents Seeking Mental Health Services: Risk Factors, Worries, and Desire to Talk About Them." Ciro, Dianne et al. Co-published simultaneously in *Social Work in Mental Health* (The Haworth Social Work Practice Press, an imprint of The Haworth Press, Inc.) Vol. 3, No. 3, 2005, pp. 213-234; and: *Clinical and Research Uses of an Adolescent Mental Health Intake Questionnaire: What Kids Need to Talk About* (ed: Ken Peake, Irwin Epstein, and Daniel Medeiros) The Haworth Social Work Practice Press, an imprint of The Haworth Press, Inc., 2005, pp. 213-234. Single or multiple copies of this article are available for a fee from The Haworth Document Delivery Service [1-800-HAWORTH, 9:00 a.m. - 5:00 p.m. (EST). E-mail address: docdelivery@haworthpress.com].

http://www.haworthpress.com/web/SWMH
© 2005 by The Haworth Press, Inc. All rights reserved.
Digital Object Identifier: 10.1300/J200v03n03_01

lescents. In addition, they must learn to manage a stigmatized identity that may create confusion, anxiety, and emotional turbulence for them. Beyond stigma, LGBQ youth are often found to be at higher risk for substance abuse, violence, depression, suicide, and sexual health problems. Based on responses given by urban adolescents seeking mental health services to a clinical self-assessment questionnaire (Adquest), this article examines the relationship between sexual identity and risk factors related to safety, health, sex, substance use, family and friends, worries, and their desire to talk about these in counseling. Findings indicate that LGBQ youth are at higher risk than straights, and express greater desire to talk about substance use, health, their personal lives, and their friends. Mental health practitioners working with these young persons must properly assess and address their risks by creating a sense of community and safe environment for open discussion. *[Article copies available for a fee from The Haworth Document Delivery Service: 1-800-HAWORTH. E-mail address: <docdelivery@haworthpress.com> Website: <http://www.HaworthPress.com> © 2005 by The Haworth Press, Inc. All rights reserved.]*

KEYWORDS. Adolescent, sexual identity, sexual orientation, mental health, help-seeking, risk, lesbian, gay, bisexual, questioning

The American Psychological Association defines sexual orientation as "rang[ing] from exclusive homosexuality to exclusive heterosexuality and includ[ing] various forms of bisexuality" (American Psychological Association [APA], 2003). Although studies show that sexual orientation is most likely set during childhood, realizations of sexual orientation and formation of sexual identity most often occurs during adolescence (Hershberger & D'Augelli, 2000; Ryan & Futterman, 1998).

Many lesbian, gay, bisexual adolescents, as well as those who are questioning their sexual orientations (LGBQ) may not know about or have access to health care providers that are sensitive to their unique mental health needs. This is an added burden for young people exploring their sexual identities, since they often lack adults with whom to talk about this topic. The normative developmental changes and experimentation that occur during adolescence, coupled with the confusion of acknowledging an LGBQ identity, only compounds the difficulties for mental health clinicians who are trying to engage and treat these youth.

Coming out, or recognizing one's gay, lesbian, bisexual, or questioning identity, is a complex, ongoing process (Ryan & Futterman, 1998). For adults, it can be an anxiety-ridden, emotional experience filled with fears and stresses. For adolescents, who are concurrently experiencing concomitant physical, cognitive, and emotional changes, exploring and coming to terms with a marginalized sexual orientation is a major challenge. Essentially, young people who are coming out are "learn[ing] to manage a stigmatized identity" (Ryan & Futterman, 1998, p. 9), most often with few or no positive adult role models, little access to reliable information, and lack of access to health and mental health care providers to help them during this stressful period in their lives (Hershberger & D'Augelli, 2000).

Risks of coming out for young people can be social isolation, rejection by peers, humiliation, discrimination, victimization, and abandonment by family and caregivers (Hershberger & D'Augelli, 2000; Mallon, 1997). As a result, LGBQ youth are considered to be at higher risk for self-isolation, substance abuse, violence, depression, suicide ideation and attempts, and sexual health problems (Hershberger & D'Augelli, 2000; Kulkin, Chauvin & Percle, 2000; Medeiros, Unpublished Manuscript; Ryan & Futterman, 1998; Sullivan & Wodarsky, 2002).

So, while LGBQ youth have the same risk factors as any other adolescent, they face unique challenges related to managing an LGBQ identity (Elze, 2002). Rosario, Schrimshaw, Hunter, and Gwadz (2002), in analysis of data from the National Longitudinal Study of Adolescent Health [Add Health], report that gay, lesbian, and bisexual youth are at higher risk than heterosexual youth for emotional distress including depression, anxiety, and suicidality. Further, high school students who reported same-sex contact were twice as likely to be threatened or injured with a weapon than students who reported only heterosexual activity. Young people who were romantically attracted to the same sex or to both sexes were more likely to be in a fight that required medical attention and to have witnessed violence than youth exclusively attracted to the opposite sex.

In a separate study, homosexual males were found to present with eating disorders and dissatisfaction with body image, more often then heterosexual men, women, and lesbian women (Ryan & Futterman, 1998).

Issues concerning sexual identity often arise in therapy with LGBQ adolescents. However, they are often manifested in, or masked by, different presenting problems such as isolation, impaired school performance, and family issues (Cooley, 1998). It is rare that a young person is entirely sure about his or her sexual orientation *and* clear about wishing to develop a gay, lesbian, or bisexual identity. More likely, an adolescent seen in treatment is unsure about her or his sexual orientation and sexual identity (Ryan & Futterman, 1998).

Ginsburg and colleagues (Ginsberg et al., 2002) identify several basic practice principles for clinicians to keep in mind when engaging and treating

LGBQ youth. First, LGBQ youth have the same primary care needs as hetero-sexual youth and these must be treated with equal and immediate attention. Second, LGBQ youth have many of the same mental health concerns as other adolescents. Third, LGBQ youth may present at health care centers for issues other than exploration of sexual identity and associated concerns. Fourth, these adolescents may not disclose either their sexual identity or related con-cerns to health care providers unless and until they are certain of confidential-ity and feel staff are not judgmental or discriminatory toward LGBQ youth.

This article considers the findings from an adolescent self-report question-naire (Adquest) gathered at intake at the Mount Sinai Adolescent Health Cen-ter (AHC). AHC is a comprehensive health and mental health center serving inner-city adolescents in New York City. An overview of the health risks, risk behaviors, and concerns of lesbian, gay, bisexual, and questioning youth is presented and compared with youth who identify themselves as heterosexual. From these empirical findings the authors derived a set of evidence-based, clinical implications for differentially engaging the LGBQ population in men-tal health treatment.

It should be noted that the study employs a clinical data-mining approach (Epstein, 2000) in that Adquest was not originally designed as a research in-strument. Nor were the needs of LGBQ adolescents identified as an issue for research exploration when the AHC staff began the Adquest data-mining pro-cess. However, interest in a study of LGBQ youth emerged during the process of three other Adquest studies concerning health (Medeiros, Kramnick, Diaz-Cruz, Surko, & Diaz, 2004), safety (Surko, Ciro, Carlson et al., 2004) and sexuality (Labor, Medeiros, Carlson et al., 2004) of the overall AHC client population. In conducting those studies practitioner-researchers recognized that LGBQ youth had unique mental health concerns and behavioral risks, jus-tifying their own exploratory study. This article is the result.

METHOD

Practice Context and Population Served

AHC is a comprehensive health center for inner city youth who make more than 20,000 mental health visits annually in a confidential setting, where cli-ents are seen regardless of their health insurance status or ability to pay. Rang-ing in age from 10 through 21, these urban adolescent applicants for mental health services come largely from low-income, minority households in New York City (Diaz, Peake, Surko, & Bhandarkar, 2004).

The study sample consisted of 758 adolescents presenting for mental health intake between 4/27/99 and 4/9/02. Of these, 36.4% were male and 63.6% were female; 5.3% of males identified as lesbian, gay, bisexual, or questioning (i.e., LGBQ), whereas 13.3% of females identified themselves as such. Of those who identified as LGBQ, 13.8% were between the ages of 17 and 21, 10.3% were between the ages of 15 and 16, and 7.5% were between the ages of 11 and 14.

Adquest

Adquest is an indigenous, context-specific instrument designed by practitioners for practitioners. The 80-item adolescent self-report asks about life areas such as school and education, work, safety, health, sexuality, substance abuse, personal, and family/home life. Its primary purpose was to promote adolescent engagement in psychotherapy by asking young people who are requesting mental health services to reflect on their own lives, problems, needs, worries, and reasons for seeking counseling, and what they want to talk about (Peake, Epstein, Mirabito, & Surko, 2004).

Conceptualization of Adquest Risk and Behavior Items and Plan for Analysis

On Adquest, the item regarding sexual identity asks respondents to choose from among six possible responses: "straight," "lesbian," "gay," "bisexual," "transgender," or "not sure." The latter category is referred to in this article as "questioning." (Only one respondent identified as transgender, and is excluded from the population studied in this article. Since Adquest lists "transgender" as a choice under sexual orientation, this respondent's sexual orientation vis-à-vis attraction to one or both sexes is not known.) Further, for analytic purposes, it was necessary to collapse responses from adolescents who identified as lesbian or gay because the sample size was too small to meaningfully study lesbians and gays separately. Moreover, one male described himself as lesbian and six females described themselves as gay. Consequently, the paper does not differentiate gay males or lesbian females. Instead, lesbian and gay adolescents are treated as a single category. Nonetheless, within this group gender differences are noted in the subsequent analysis.

In this article, self-reported sexual identity is treated as the independent variable; gender as an intervening variable; and risk and behavior items as well as desire to talk as dependent variables. An acknowledged limitation of Adquest with regard to sexual identity is that it does not ask adolescents what stage they are at in exploring their sexual identity, nor does it ask whether they have come out to peers or family. Further, it does not measure *directly* how much adolescents want to talk to clinicians about sexual identity, *per se* though AHC clinicians do engage many adolescents specifically on this topic.

In presenting the findings, we first present a *snapshot* of respondent self-identification with one of the sexual orientation categories, and cross-tabulate sexual orientation by age and gender. Second, exposure to risk, risk behaviors, and experience with family and peer relations is looked at across all four sexual identity categories used in our sample, e.g., what percentage of those reporting a particular sexual orientation has experienced "forced sex?" Third, we considered the gender and sexual identity differences associated with these risks and experiences (e.g., what percentages of LGBQ males report binging and purging, as compared with LGBQ females and straight males and females?). Fourth, we report on LGBQ youth's desire to talk to a counselor about multiple problems. The clinical and program implications of these findings conclude the article.

FINDINGS

Of 758 respondents, 723 gave a response on the sexual identity question. Of these, 89.7% identified themselves as straight, 5.1% responded they were "not sure" about their sexual identity, 3.4% identified themselves as bisexual, and 1.8% identified themselves as gay or lesbian (see Table 1).

Gender, Stage of Adolescent Development and Sexual Identity

Sexual identity was significantly associated with gender (see Table 2). Hence, more males than females identified themselves as straight (94.7% versus 86.7%). However, comparable proportions identified themselves as gay or lesbian (1.9% for males, 1.7% for females).

More females than males identified themselves as bisexual (5.2% versus 0.4%, respectively) and as questioning (6.3% versus 3.0%, respectively). Finally, there was no significant association between stage of adolescence and sexual identity.

TABLE 1. Sexual Identity (N = 723 Number of Valid Responses)

Sexual identity	%(n)
Straight	89.7% (650)
Not Sure	5.1% (37)
Bisexual	3.4% (25)
Lesbian/gay	1.8% (13)

TABLE 2. Reported Sexual Identity by Gender (N = 723)

	Straight %(n)	Not Sure %(n)	Bisexual %(n)	Lesbian/gay %(n)	χ^2
Gender					16.004**
Male	94.7 (249)	3.0 (8)	.4 (1)	1.9 (5)	
Female	86.7 (399)	6.3 (29)	5.2 (24)	1.7 (8)	

*$p < .05$, **$p < .01$, ***$p < .001$

Sexual Identity and Risk

Significant associations were observed between sexual identity and several indicators of risk, worry, and well-being. Among items asking about school and work, for example, self-report of failing one or more classes was significantly associated with sexual identity (see Table 3); 58.8% of questioning adolescents reporting failing classes, as compared to 49.2%, 46.2%, and 45.5% for straight, lesbian/gay, and bisexual adolescents, respectively. This would suggest that adolescents who are in the process of questioning their own sexual identities are less capable of focusing on their schoolwork.

Seven items assessing safety were significantly associated with sexual identity: having witnessed violence, feeling unsafe, having been a victim of violence, having been touched uncomfortably, having been forced to have sex, worry about hurting self or others, and being able to get a gun. For all but one item (feeling unsafe), bisexual adolescents had the highest levels of safety risk and exposure.

Thus, bisexual adolescents were most likely to have witnessed violence (92.0%), followed by lesbian/gay and straight adolescents (75.0% and 74.9% respectively), and questioning adolescents (50.0%). Bisexual adolescents were most likely to report being victims of violence (80.0%), followed by straight adolescents (44.1%), then by questioning and lesbian/gay adolescents (32.4% and 30.8% respectively). Bisexual adolescents were most likely to have been touched in a way that made them uncomfortable (60.0%); followed by questioning adolescents (50%), lesbian/gay adolescents (38.5%) and straight adolescents (24.1%). A similar pattern was observed in reports of forced sex: bisexual adolescents had the highest proportion of reports (30.4%), followed by questioning adolescents (21.6%), lesbian/gay adolescents (15.4%), and straight adolescents (9.7%). With regard to reported ability to get a gun, bisexuals were again highest (54.5%), followed by lesbian/gay adolescents (30.8%), straight adolescents (25.5%), and questioning adoles-

TABLE 3. Risk, Developmental, and Well-Being Indicators; by Sexual Identity (N = 723)

[S = Straight (n = 648); LG = Lesbian/Gay (n = 13); B = Bisexual (n = 25); NS = Not Sure (n = 37)]

	Highest	<---	--->	Lowest	χ^2
Work/School					
Failing classes	NS 58.8	S 49.2	LG 46.2	B 45.5	17.150*
Safety					
Witnessed violence	B 92.0	LG 75.0	S 74.9	NS 50.0	15.322**
Feel unsafe	LG 61.5	NS 59.5	B 56.0	S 39.3	10.463*
Victim of violence	B 80.0	S 44.1	NS 32.4	LG 30.8	15.977*
Touched uncomfortably	B 60.0	NS 50.0	LG 38.5	S 24.1	27.221***
Forced sex	B 30.4	NS 21.6	LG 15.4	S 9.7	14.375**
Worry hurt self/others	B 76.0	LG 53.8	NS 50.0	S 47.6	7.940*
Get gun	B 54.5	LG 30.8	S 25.6	NS 18.9	10.406*
Health					
Binge/purge	LG 23.1	NS 18.9	B 8.3	S 6.4	12.891**
How doing/health (poor/very poor)	NS 38.7	LG 33.3	S 13.7	B 13.6	17.347**
Sexuality					
Ever had sex	B 88.0	S 51.1	LG 46.2	NS 37.1	16.414**
Taught/re: body and sex (yes)	B 96.0	S 83.8	NS 63.9	LG 61.5	16.610**
Thought about HIV testing	B 84.0	S 35.0	NS 32.4	LG 30.8	25.371***
Used drugs to make sex better	B 32.0	LG 15.4	S 8.9	NS 5.4	15.929**
Worry/re: sex	B 80.0	LG 46.2	NS 43.2	S 38.2	17.833***
Substance abuse risk					
Offered drugs	B 84.0	LG 69.2	NS 56.8	S 51.6	11.732**
Time with user	B 84.0	LG 61.5	NS 52.8	S 48.8	12.718*

	Highest	<---	--->	Lowest	χ^2
Tried tobacco	B 91.3	LG 63.6	NS 62.1	S 52.1	14.756**
Tried alcohol	B 91.7	LG 83.3	NS 64.5	S 64.3	9.304*
Tried marijuana	B 78.3	LG 63.6	NS 55.2	S 45.9	10.969*
Tried other drugs	B 36.8	LG 18.2	NS 14.3	S 4.4	39.239*
Worry own drug use	B 56.0	NS 23.5	S 16.7	LG 0	28.503***
Worry others' drug use	B 64.0	NS 62.9	LG 38.5	S 33.3	21.527***
How doing/drugs (poor)	B 20.0	LG 15.4	NS 11.1	S 5.8	10.459*
Family/Friends					
How doing/friends (poor)	LG 41.7	NS 33.3	B 24.0	S 10.7	27.598***
Worry family/home life	B 84.0	NS 74.3	S 60.2	LG 50.0	8.918*
How doing family/home life (poor/very poor)	B 48.0	LG 46.2	NS 37.1	S 26.6	9.052*
How doing personal life (poor/very poor)	NS 41.2	LG 40.0	B 30.4	S 18.9	13.381**

$*p < .05$, $**p < .01$, $***p < .001$

cents (18.9%). With regard to feeling unsafe, however, lesbian and gay youth ranked highest (61.5%), followed by questioning youth (59.5%), bisexuals (56.0%) and straight adolescents (39.3%).

When asked to give an overall assessment of how they were doing with regard to health issues, questioning adolescents were most likely to report not doing well (38.7%), followed by lesbian/gay (33.3%), straight (23.7%) and bisexual adolescents (23.6%). Also, lesbian/gay adolescents were highest in reporting having binged or purged (23.1%), followed by questioning youth (18.9%), bisexuals (8.3%), and straights (6.4%).

However, bisexual adolescents appeared to be the most sexually active group and were most likely to express sexual health concerns, with mixed patterns for the other groups. So, for example, bisexual adolescents were most likely to report having had sex (88.0%), followed by straight (51.1%), lesbian/gay (46.2%), and questioning adolescents (37.1%). Likewise, bisexual adolescents were more than twice as likely than any other group to have thought about HIV testing (84.0%), followed by straights (35.0%), questioning (32.4%) and lesbian/gay (30.8%). In addition, bisexual youth were at least twice as likely than any other group to report having "used drugs to make sex easier, longer, or more fun" (32.0%) versus lesbian/gay (15.4%), straight (8.9%), and questioning (5.4%). Similarly, bisexual adolescents were almost twice as likely to express worry about sex, body, and birth control than other identity groups (80.0%), versus lesbian/gay (46.2%), questioning (43.2%), and straight (38.2%). Surprisingly, however, bisexual adolescents were most likely to report having been taught about their bodies and sex (96%), followed by straights (83.8%), questioning (63.9%), and lesbian/gay adolescents (61.5%).

Bisexual adolescents scored highest on all indicators of substance use and substance abuse risk exposure, with lesbian/gay and questioning adolescents generally reporting levels of use and risk exposure that were somewhat higher than straight adolescents. So, for example, bisexuals were most likely to say they had been offered drugs (84%), followed by lesbian/gay (69.2%), questioning (56.8%), and straight (51.6%) adolescents. Likewise, bisexual youth were most likely to have spent time with a drug user (84%), compared to lesbian/gay (61.5%), questioning (52.8%), and straight adolescents (48.8%). Bisexuals as well were most likely to report having tried tobacco (91.3%), versus lesbian/gay (63.6%), questioning (62.1%), and straight (52.1%) adolescents. The same pattern is noted for trying alcohol with (91.7%) of the bisexuals reporting doing so, compared to lesbian/gay (83.3%), questioning (64.5%), and straight (64.3%) adolescents. Bisexuals were as well most likely to report having tried marijuana (78.3%), compared to lesbian/gay (63.6%), questioning (55.2%), and straight (45.9%) youth. Finally, over one-third of the bisexuals reported having tried other drugs (36.8%), versus lesbian/gay (18.2%), questioning (14.3%), and straight (4.4%) adolescents.

Fifty-six percent of bisexual adolescents said they worried about their own drug use, compared to 23.5% of questioning adolescents, 16.7% of straight adolescents, and none of the lesbian/gay adolescents. Although bisexual youth scored even higher in their reported worry about the drug use of another person (64.0%), they were closely followed by questioning youth (62.9%). On this measure, lesbian/gay and straight adolescents shared lower but similar degrees of concern (38.5% and 33.3%, respectively). Finally, bisexual and lesbian/gay adolescents had the highest proportions reporting they were doing poorly when it came to drugs and alcohol (20.0% and 15.4% respectively), versus questioning (11.1%), and straight (5.8%) adolescents.

In contrast to the substance use findings, lesbian/gay and questioning adolescents had the highest proportion of respondents saying that they were doing poorly with friends (41.7% and 33.3%, respectively), as contrasted with bisexual (24.0%), and straight (10.7%) adolescents. Similarly, questioning and lesbian/gay adolescents had the highest proportion reporting that they did poorly with their personal lives. And while a high proportion of all adolescents in the sample reported worry about their family and home lives, bisexual and questioning adolescents had the highest proportions reporting such worry (84.0% and 74.3%, respectively), followed by straight (60.2%), and lesbian/gay (50%) adolescents. Similarly, nearly half of the bisexual (48.0%) and questioning youth (46.2%) said they were doing poorly at home with their families compared to slightly more than a third of the questioning youth (37.1%) and a quarter of the straight youth (26.6%).

Gender, Sexual Identity, and Risk

The relatively small number of LGBQ males in the sample (N = 14), precluded a comprehensive analysis of the relationship between gender, sexual identity and the foregoing risk factors. However, when gay and bisexual males are combined, sexual identity was found to be significantly related to two risk indicators: often feeling unsafe (questioning 75.0%; LGB 66.7%; straight 36.2%) and ever having binged or purged (LGB 33.3%; questioning 12.5%; straight 2.4%).

By contrast with the males, there were adequate numbers of females self-identifying as other than straight to allow a more comprehensive analysis (see Table 4). Here again, however, the most productive analysis was derived by combining lesbian/gay and bisexual (LGB) females into one sexual identity status category. As with the males, questioning females were treated as a separate group because their risk profiles appeared quite distinct from lesbian/gay and bisexual females. As this analysis will show (see Table 4) LGB and questioning females HAD similar rates of ever having "been touched uncomfortably" (59.4% and 57.1%, respectively) as well as "feeling unsafe" (56.3% and 55.2%, respectively). However, in most risk exposure categories questioning females reported considerably lower rates than LGB females–either being midway between LGB and straights or very similar to straights. In fact, on a number of risk indicators, questioning females scored lower than straight females.

More specifically, among females, most safety items were significantly associated with sexual identity. For example, LGB females were most likely to have witnessed violence (87.5%), followed by straights (68.1%) and then by those who are questioning their sexual identities (46.4%). Similarly, LGB females were most likely to have been victims of violence (68.8%), followed by straights (40%), and questioning (31%) females. LGB females were as well most likely to have been touched uncomfortably (59.4%) and to have experienced forced sex (30%). On these external risk factors, however, questioning

TABLE 4. Risk, Developmental, and Well-Being Indicators; by Sexual Identity, Among Females (N = 460)

	Highest <---	--->	Lowest	χ^2
Safety				
Witnessed violence	LGB 87.5	S 68.1	NS 46.4	11.605**
Victim of violence	LGB 68.8	S 40.0	NS 31.0	11.466**
Touched uncomfortably	LGB 59.4	NS 57.1	S 32.6	15.043**
Forced sex	LGB 30.0	NS 24.1	S 13.6	7.655*
Could get a gun	LGB 51.7	NS 20.7	S 18.7	17.738***
Often feel unsafe	LGB 56.3	NS 55.2	S 41.3	4.517
Health				
Binge/purge	NS 20.7	LGB 9.7	S 8.9	4.302
Sexuality				
Ever had sex	LGB 81.3	S 50.5	NS 42.9	12.255**
Thought about HIV testing	LGB 68.8	S 39.8	NS 37.9	10.352**
Used drugs to make sex better	LGB 25.0	S 7.3	NS 6.9	12.055**
Worry about sex, body, or birth control	LGB 75.0	NS 48.3	S 45.3	10.476**
Substance Abuse Risk				
Ever offered drugs	LGB 84.4	NS 62.1	S 50.6	14.403**
Spent time with drug user	LGB 81.3	NS 60.7	S 48.2	13.978**
Used tobacco ever	LGB 86.7	NS 60.9	S 55.5	10.980**
Used alcohol ever	LGB 90.6	NS 68.0	S 67.1	7.593*
Used marijuana ever	LGB 76.7	NS 58.3	S 45.3	11.722**
Worry about own drug use	LGB 43.8	NS 26.9	S 13.2	22.719***
Worry about others who use drugs	NS 70.4	LGB 56.3	S 34.5	18.544***
Doing poorly/very poorly with drugs in general	LGB 19.7	NS 14.4	S 4.1	15.542***

*$p < .05$, **$p < .01$, ***$p < .001$

females ranked second with 57.1% reporting that they had been touched uncomfortably and 24.1% having had sex forced upon them. By contrast, rates of being touched uncomfortably were lowest among straight adolescents (32.6%) as well as for forced sex (13.6%). LGB females were most likely to report that they could get a gun if they wanted to (51.7%), followed by questioning (20.7), and straight (18.7%) females. However, for females, neither feeling unsafe nor health concerns were significantly associated with sexual identity.

Despite this, sexual identity was significantly associated with sexual risks and worries in females. In general, LGB females reported higher rates of sexual experience and risks than straight or questioning females. More specifically, 81.3% of LGB females said that they had "ever had sex" compared to 50.5% of straights and 42.9% of females who were questioning their sexual identities. Likewise, 25% of LGB females reported using drugs to make sex feel better contrasted with 7.3% of straights and 6.9% of those who had questions about their sexual identities. Sexual identity was also significantly associated with being "worried about sex, your body, or birth control." Hence, LGB females were most likely to express worry (75%) compared to about half of the straight females (48.3%) and slightly less of those questioning (45.3%) females.

Sexual identity was also significantly associated with exposure to "someone who uses drugs," use of tobacco, alcohol and drugs, worries about one's "own drug use," as well as worries about "others drug use." Among LGB females for example, 81.3% had spent time with a drug user, compared to 60.7% of questioning, and 48.2% of straights. The vast majority of LGB females (90.6%) reported having used alcohol, followed by questioning females (68%), who in turn are followed closely by straights (67.1%). Furthermore, 43.8% of LGB females worried about their own drug use, compared to 26.9% of questioning females, and 13.2% of straights. Sexual identity among females was as well associated with "doing poorly/very poorly with drugs in general": 19.7% of LGB females said so, compared to 14.4% of questioning and 4.1% of straights.

Sexual Identity and Desire to Talk About Personal Problems and Risks

As shown in Table 5, the final area of analysis conducted was of the impact of sexual identity on the desire to talk about ten life areas covered in Adquest, i.e., race and racism, education, work, safety, health, substance abuse, sex, family or home life, friends, and personal life. In this analysis, lesbian, gay, bisexual, and questioning (LGBQ) as a group were compared with straight adolescents. This heuristic decision was based on three considerations.

TABLE 5. Desire to Talk with a Counselor About Adquest Life Areas by Sexual Identity (N = 723)

Life Area	Sexual Identity Status		
	Lesbian, Gay, Bisexual, or Not Sure	Straight	x^2
Race	53.3	49.5	.404
Education	88.0	81.0	2.190
Work	76.1	76.1	.000
Safety	79.7	69.9	3.113
Health	86.7	72.9	6.674*
Substance use	74.7	60.8	5.509*
Sex, body, or birth control	74.7	67.2	1.727
Family or home life	86.3	79.3	2.005
Friends	86.5	74.2	5.426*
Personal life	90.4	81.2	3.798*

*$p < .05$

First, theoretical reasons influenced this decision. Although questioning adolescents displayed greater *empirical* variability in the way they responded to the prior risk questions in comparison with lesbian, gay, and bisexual adolescents, they cannot be viewed *phenomenologically* as similar to straight adolescents. Instead, by questioning their own sexual identities and possibly owning the stigma associated with not being straight, they approximate a *clinical constituency* along with those who have identified themselves with being either gay, lesbian, or bisexual.

Second, in subsequent empirical analysis when desire to talk about problems in each of Adquest's ten areas of concern were compared for adolescents in each of the four identity categories, questioning adolescents scored most like bisexual youth (in seven areas), like lesbian/gay adolescents (in two areas), and were closest to straights in only one.

Third, the limits imposed by the relatively small sample of sexual minority youth meant that creating an LGBQ category generated the most flexibility and yielded the clearest results concerning desire to talk.

In general, it should be noted that adolescents in the study reported high levels of wanting to talk about most of these life concerns. After all, most are voluntarily seeking mental health counseling. However, LGBQ status was significantly associated with the desire to talk about four life areas: health, substance use, friends, and personal life. More specifically, among LGBQ adolescents 86.7% wanted to discuss health concerns as compared to 72.9% of straights; 74.7% wanted to talk about substance use, as compared to 60.8% of straights; and 86.5% wanted to talk about friends as compared to 79.3% of straights. Finally, 90.4% of LGBQ adolescents wanted to talk about their personal lives as compared to 81.2% of straights.

In this context however, *statistical significance* should not be equated with *clinical significance*. Because the desire to talk is as high as it is for the entire sample, differences between LGBQ and straight adolescents are not always statistically significant. Thus, despite LGBQ youth reporting high levels of exposure to safety risks, there was no significant association between sexual identity and wanting to talk about safety. More specifically, of LGBQ youth, 80% wanted to talk about safety as compared with 70% of straight adolescents. This difference was not statistically significant. Nonetheless, given the multiple safety risks reported earlier by LGBQ youth, clinicians might have reason to be concerned. This combination of findings suggests that practitioners should pay careful attention to adolescent safety risks, particularly among those LGBQ adolescents who do not seem eager to talk about them, *especially* with bisexual adolescents who are at highest risk.

DISCUSSION

The findings presented in this paper strongly suggest that LGBQ adolescents offer many serious clinical challenges to mental health practitioners. LGBQ adolescents appear to be at much higher risk on multiple dimensions than youth who identify themselves as straight. Indeed, bisexual adolescents seem to be doing most poorly across several indicators of risk, worry, and well-being. However, there is no consistent pattern for any one of the sexual identity categories across all risk indicators, and each appears to have its own particular vulnerabilities. Therefore, the findings will be summarized for each category, before going on to discuss issues that apply to LGBQ youth in general.

Bisexual Adolescents

Self-reported bisexual adolescents indicated that they were engaging in, and being exposed to, higher rates of risk in several areas: these included having had sex, having spent time with a drug user, having tried marijuana, alcohol, cigarettes, and other drugs, and having used drugs to improve sex. Cognizant of their sexual and substance abuse risk, they appeared to be most worried about sex, their body, and birth control. Similarly, they report the highest levels of feeling worried about their own drug use and that of friends and associates.

Bisexual adolescents have many safety risks and clinicians need to be particularly concerned about this when working with them. They are at higher risk for violence and report high rates for being touched uncomfortably and having forced sex. They have extremely high rates of worrying about hurting themselves or others, and report greatest access to guns. This should be of particular concern, given the high suicide and homicide rates among adolescents in general (Kulkin, Chauvin, & Percle, 2000).

Discovering that bisexual adolescents report *lower* rates of feeling unsafe than lesbian/gay and questioning adolescents despite their *higher* safety risks is of particular concern. A questionnaire such as Adquest does not allow us to explore *why* bisexual adolescents who are at risk do not feel unsafe. This is a matter for clinical exploration. However, this contradiction does present a particular problem for clinicians while assessing for safety during the early stages of treatment. During this period of engagement and trust-building, it is essential that practitioners be comfortable in keeping issues of safety on the table, while remaining open to understanding the nature of the bisexual adolescent's experience as she or he defines it. This is an especially complex task when clients, themselves, do not acknowledge feeling unsafe.

Bisexual adolescents report doing poorly with friends but to a lesser degree than do lesbian/gay and questioning adolescents. However, bisexual adolescents reported doing poorer than other sexual identity groups in their family/home-lives and are most worried about this. Perhaps this is because they are most sexually active but have no defined cultural support group the way lesbian or gay youth have. Clinicians may need to help them negotiate peer and familial relationships. Also, clinical experience suggests that adolescents need to feel connected to others like themselves. For those whose relationships with family and peers are especially problematic, clinical programs may need to provide a sense of belonging, self-acceptance and self-care through alternative support groups. This might involve some form of *coming-out* process as well.

As indicated earlier, Adquest does not allow exploration of why bisexual adolescents appear at highest risk across so many life areas. It may be symptomatic of a personal struggle associated with managing an identity that is not as clearly defined as being gay, lesbian, or straight. Identity-development theory (Ryan & Futterman, 1998) suggests that a bisexual identity is more difficult to assimilate than a lesbian or gay identity because it develops only *after* a straight identity has first been assimilated. Bisexual adolescents may find that, unlike those who identify with the *clearer* categories of lesbian and gay, it is particularly difficult to identify with a more *fluid* label. Consequently, clinicians need to help these adolescents process the unique internal challenges they face as well as their experiences with others' negative reactions to bisexuality.

Lesbian and Gay Adolescents

Feeling unsafe appears to be a particular problem for lesbian and gay adolescents. They report the highest levels of feeling unsafe despite having the lowest levels of victimization by violence, and having witnessed violence at the same rates as straight adolescents. They report lower levels of forced sex and being touched uncomfortably than bisexual or questioning youth, though they have higher levels than straight adolescents. This suggests that practitioners working with gay or lesbian youth need to make a point of exploring feelings of being unsafe to determine specific areas of vulnerability and fear.

This heightened feeling of being unsafe might result from concerns about disclosure of their sexual identity in a new, clinical setting, or about negative consequences of disclosure (intentional or otherwise) that have already occurred elsewhere. The intake questionnaire format of Adquest does not allow for further exploration of this issue. We wonder, however, whether more needs to be done at AHC to reassure gay and lesbian clients that the setting is a safe one for disclosure, that practitioners are open, accepting, and competent enough to help and that there is programming specifically designed for these young persons.

Interestingly, lesbian and gay adolescents were least likely to report being taught about sex and their bodies. Possibly, this reflects the heterosexist bias in institutionally sanctioned sex education and a failure to address the sexual health questions that lesbian and gay adolescents may have. Combined with the fact that lesbian and gay youth also report the highest levels of binging and purging and second highest concerns about their health in general, emphasizes the need for programming that is tailored to their specific health information, mental health counseling and social support needs.

Questioning Adolescents

Questioning adolescents report the highest rates of school failure. They also report high rates of being touched uncomfortably and having experienced forced sex. On several other indicators of worry, risk, and absence of well-being they score most closely to lesbian and gay adolescents (e.g., feeling unsafe, experiencing forced sex, worry about hurting self or others, binging and purging, etc.). At the same time, they are less likely than all other groups to have had sex, witnessed violence, or have access to a gun. Their alcohol use and drug exposure is lower than bisexual, gay and lesbian adolescents. Nonetheless, many questioning adolescents appear to worry: They report second highest level of worry about safety, their own drug use, and the drug use of others.

Questioning adolescents may be struggling with sexual identity, peer acceptance, security, and as a result, unable to concentrate or perform fully in school. It may be that questioning youth are in some ways more risk averse than LGB adolescents. Perhaps they are resisting acknowledging and *coming out* as lesbian, gay, or bisexual youth. Perhaps they are similar to these other sexual minority youth but at an earlier stage of identity formation. Perhaps they are a group unto themselves. Adquest information does not allow further empirical exploration of these possibilities. What Adquest does tell us is that each of these groups has its own unique risk profile to which effective clinicians and clinical programming must be responsive.

Gender and LGBQ Status

Though the sample size did not allow for an analysis that controlled for gender, some findings do relate to LGBQ status and gender. Female LGB adolescents appear to be exceptionally vulnerable when compared to straight females. They are at very high risk in almost all areas of risk exposure explored by Adquest, i.e., safety, sexual activity, worries about friends and family, and most indicators of substance abuse risk. They also report the highest rates of feeling unsafe, worry about substance abuse, and worry about sex, their bodies, and birth control. Though questioning females, *per se*, have greater variability in their exposure to risk, they appear to be as worried as LGB females.

LGBQ males also seem to be vulnerable to feeling unsafe, and though Adquest data could not go further than saying this, clinicians should pay careful attention to this vulnerability. In addition, the finding that LGBQ males report such high rates of binging and purging is surprising and disturbing. Although this has been noted in other studies (Bradford et al., 1994), we are concerned that many clinicians may not be aware of this problem, and think of binging and purging as an entirely female mental health symptom.

LGBQ Adolescents' Desire to Talk

Most of the adolescents in our sample want to talk about some aspects of their lives. LGBQ adolescents are especially desirous of talking about their health, substance abuse, friends, and personal lives. However, given the multiple safety risks reported by LGBQ youth, practitioners should pay particular attention to this area, particularly among those LGBQ adolescents who do not seem eager to talk about them. Here again, it must be remembered that bisexual adolescents are at highest risk and most likely to deny feeling at risk. For them as a group the gap between *wanting* to talk about safety and *needing* to talk about it is perhaps greatest.

Substance abuse risk is very high for LGBQ adolescents. Fortunately, a very large proportion of them are open to discussing their risk exposure and behaviors, as well as other concerns about drugs. This profile of risk and openness presents practitioners with opportunities for initial engagement. Likewise, LGBQ adolescents' greater desire to talk about friends and personal life than their straight peers suggests a need that LGBQ have to work out issues of identity, coming out, and negotiating peer relationships.

At AHC and at many other mental health programs, LGBQ youth appear to be at greater risk than straight adolescents. Consequently, it is incumbent upon mental health program planners and managers to ensure that practitioners are competent to assess and address the particular needs of LGBQ youth and the subgroups represented within this broad category. Mental health agencies that serve these adolescents need to create a community for young persons who may not feel they fit in anywhere by offering and providing access to programs specifically designed to work with LGBQ youth.

At AHC adolescents attending LGBQ support groups have helped in creating just such a community. They have made sure that a gay pride flag hangs prominently in the facility and that posters, created by LGBQ adolescents who have received services, advertise those services and provide testimony to AHC being a safe place for LGBQ youth to seek help.

Access to services must be made easier for LGBQ adolescents. Ironically, analyzing Adquest-generated data has alerted us to the possibility that feelings of being unsafe might be intensified when adolescents applying for mental health services must complete an extensive mental health intake (particularly one that is problem focused) in order to obtain services. This means that AHC staff along with client representatives will need to examine the pros and cons of present intake practices.

One lesson learned through this data-mining process might be that adolescent services should not pathologize the need for connection among LGBQ adolescents, no matter how high their risk status may appear. It may well be that provision of a sense of community might in itself support other treatment interventions in reducing risky behaviors such as alcohol and drug use.

Programs must also show that they are *safe* places where adolescents will be seen confidentially. At AHC services are mainstreamed–rather than being compartmentalized into separate clinics for different types of adolescents. Moreover, strenuous efforts are made to ensure that confidentiality of LGBQ clients will not be compromised by appointment time, waiting area or primary therapist.

We suggest, however, that organizational competencies in serving these youth should be embedded in all mental health and in all comprehensive health services such as AHC where a full range of health and reproductive health services are available to adolescents. Having been embedded in these programs, services can be tailored to the specific concerns, mental health and health needs of this differentially vulnerable group of young people.

As was described earlier, this article originated from observations made by practitioners conducting analyses of the health and safety concerns of AHC's general client population, and the discovery of concerns and patterns that seemed particular to, and variegated within, LGBQ youth. One consequence of this study has been the recognition that Adquest does not allow *in depth* exploration of the needs of LGBQ adolescents and that more organizational development needs to take place to ensure that this happens.

Consequently, a new version of Adquest needs to allow for more complete but less threatening exploration of the issues faced by LGBQ youth, particularly where a particular LGBQ adolescent may be in the process of coming out. Although a challenging, complex, and potentially controversial task, it can help us understand how services can facilitate this process. For example, Adquest is presently given to adolescents only at time of intake and, as such, the way adolescents self-identify represents only a snapshot in time. Since sexual identity formation is an evolving project of adolescence, more needs to be understood about how that evolution occurs over time. This could be achieved through repeated administration and analysis of a modified version of Adquest that puts less emphasis on risk factors and more on strengths. Alternatively, it could be achieved through sensitive exploration by clinicians who are alert to the unique as well as common needs of this population.

On the other hand, it should be noted that until AHC accumulated a sample of sufficient size and analyzed existing Adquest data, none of this would have been known. Finally, this practice-based research experience has led us to revisit and refine a commonly held assumption that, where possible, mental health programs should not aspire to match each individual adolescent client with a therapist who mirrors her or his racial, ethnic, or sexual identity. Instead, it is AHC's philosophy that adolescents should experience the organizational staffing, competencies, and culture that *as a whole* reflects the range of identities of the population served. In such an environment, competent programming for LGBQ is easier to develop because staffing is diverse and includes lesbian, gay, and bisexual professionals.

CONCLUSION

LGBQ adolescents seeking mental health services have, in most respects, many of the same concerns and needs as other young people. Furthermore, to feel comfortable in sharing their concerns they need to feel welcomed and understood. The fact that LGBQ adolescents are more vulnerable than straight adolescents for some specific safety, health, and substance use risks means that clinicians working with these adolescents need to be aware of how these vulnerabilities might impact initial and ongoing engagement. In addition, practitioners should attend to how these vulnerabilities may be heightened for adolescents struggling with an evolving identity and the coming-out process.

LGBQ youth present at generally higher risk than straight adolescents, particularly in the area of safety. To effectively engage these adolescents, services must address how issues of feeling unsafe might interfere with engagement, and design outreach and interventions accordingly. It is encouraging that LGBQ adolescents particularly want to talk about their health, substance abuse, friends, and personal lives. However, their multiple safety risks mean that practitioners should pay particular attention to this, especially among those LGBQ adolescents who do not seem eager to talk about safety.

At AHC, more needs to be done to identify specific cultural competencies that will enable us to better serve these young people. Those who work with LGBQ adolescents must be aware of the special challenges these young people face and must be equipped to address these challenges. Above all, they must be comfortable addressing issues pertinent to LGBQ adolescents and must be willing to develop interventions to address their special needs. When providing mental health services to LGBQ youth, providers need to ensure appropriate, nonjudgmental counseling and support.

REFERENCES

American Psychological Association [APA]. (2003). Answers to your questions about sexual orientation and homosexuality. Retrieved from the Internet at *http://www. apa.org/pubinfo/answers.html*

Bradford, J., Ryan, C., & Rothblum. E. (1994). National lesbian health care survey: Implications for mental health care. *Journal of Consulting & Clinical Psychology, 62* (2), 228-242.

Cooley, J. J. (1998). Gay and lesbian adolescents: Presenting problems and the counselor's role. *Professional School Counseling, 1*(3), 30-34.

Diaz, A., Peake, K., Surko, M., & Bhandarkar, K. (2004). Including "at risk" adolescents in their own health and mental health care: A youth development in perspective. *Social Work in Mental Health*, 3(1/2), 3-22.

Elze, D. (2002). Risk factors for internalizing and externalizing problems among gay, lesbian, and bisexual adolescents. *Social Work Research, 26*(2), 65-128.

Ginsburg, K., Winn, R., Rudy, B., Crawford, J., Zhao, H., & Schwarz. D. (2002). How to reach sexual minority youth in the health care setting: The teens offer guidance. *Journal of Adolescent Health, 31*, 401-416.

Hershberger, S., & D'Augelli, A. (2000). Issues in counseling lesbian, gay, and bisexual adolescents. In R. Perez, K. DeBord, & K. Bieschke (Eds.), *Handbook of Counseling and Psychotherapy with Lesbian, Gay, and Bisexual Clients.* Washington, DC: American Psychological Association.

Kulkin, H. S., Chauvin, E. A., & Percle, G. A. (2000). Suicide among gay and lesbian adolescents and young adults: A review of the literature. *Journal of Homosexuality, 40*(10), 1-29.

Labor, N., Medeiros, D., Carlson, E., Pullo, N., Seehaus, M., Peake, K., & Epstein, I. (2004). Adolescents' need to talk about sex and sexuality in an urban mental health setting. *Social Work in Mental Health, 3*(1/2), 133-151.

Mallon, G. (1997). Basic premises, guiding principles, and competent practices for a positive youth development approach to working with gay, lesbian, and bisexual youths in out-of-home care. *Child Welfare, 76*(5), September/October, 591-608.

Medeiros, D. (2003) Adolescent self-report of sexual orientation: Comparisons based on gender, age, and racial/ethnic identity. Unpublished Manuscript.

Medeiros, D., Kramnick, L., Diaz-Cruz, E., Surko, M., & Diaz, A. (2004). Adolescents seeking mental health services: Self-reported health risks and the need to talk. *Social Work in Mental Health, 3*(1/2), 121-134.

Peake, K., Epstein, I., Mirabito, D., & Surko, M. (2004). Development and utilization of a practice-based adolescent intake questionnaire (Adquest): Surveying which risks, worries, and concerns urban youth want to talk about. *Social Work in Mental Health, 3*(1/2), 55-82.

Rosario, M., Schrimshaw, E., Hunter, J., & Gwadz. M. (2002). Gay-related stress and emotional distress among gay, lesbian, and bisexual youths: A longitudinal examination. *Journal of Consulting & Clinical Psychology, 70*(4), 967-975.

Ryan, C., & Futterman, D. (1998). *Lesbian & Gay Youth: Care & Counseling.* Columbia University Press: New York, NY.

Sullivan M., & Wodarski, J. S. (2002). Social alienation in gay youth. *Journal of Human Behavior in the Social Environment, 5*(1), 1-17.

Surko, M., Ciro, D., Carlson, E., Labor, N., Giannone, V., Diaz-Cruz, E., Peake, K., & Epstein, I. (2004). Which adolescents need to talk about safety and violence? *Social Work in Mental Health, 3*(1/2), 103-120.

Experience of Racism as a Correlate of Developmental and Health Outcomes Among Urban Adolescent Mental Health Clients

Michael Surko
Dianne Ciro
Caryl Blackwood
Michael Nembhard
Ken Peake

SUMMARY. Correlates of race/ethnicity and perceived racism among 760 urban, predominantly Hispanic/Latino and African-American, adolescent mental health clients were investigated using an exploratory, clinical data-mining approach. All racial/ethnic groups reported substantial rates of racism, ranging from 80.0% for Asian/Pacific Islanders to 32.4% for Hispanic/Latinos. Racism was associated with significantly elevated environmental risk (e.g., violence, sexual abuse or assault, exposure to drug use), behavioral risk (e.g., drug use) and worry (e.g., worry about hurting self or others, worry about doing dangerous

Michael Surko, PhD, is Coordinator of the Center for Excellence at Mount Sinai Adolescent Health Center (AHC). Dianne Ciro, MS, Caryl Blackwood, CSW, and Michael Nembhard, CSW, are Clinical Social Workers at AHC. Ken Peake, DSW, is Assistant Director of AHC, 320 East 94th Street, New York, NY 10128.

[Haworth co-indexing entry note]: "Experience of Racism as a Correlate of Developmental and Health Outcomes Among Urban Adolescent Mental Health Clients." Surko, Michael et al. Co-published simultaneously in *Social Work in Mental Health* (The Haworth Social Work Practice Press, an imprint of The Haworth Press, Inc.) Vol. 3, No. 3, 2005, pp. 235-260; and: *Clinical and Research Uses of an Adolescent Mental Health Intake Questionnaire: What Kids Need to Talk About* (ed: Ken Peake, Irwin Epstein, and Daniel Medeiros) The Haworth Social Work Practice Press, an imprint of The Haworth Press, Inc., 2005, pp. 235-260. Single or multiple copies of this article are available for a fee from The Haworth Document Delivery Service [1-800-HAWORTH, 9:00 a.m. - 5:00 p.m. (EST). E-mail address: docdelivery@haworthpress.com].

http://www.haworthpress.com/web/SWMH
© 2005 by The Haworth Press, Inc. All rights reserved.
Digital Object Identifier: 10.1300/J200v03n03_02

things). Overall, racism *was significantly associated with* more negative health and well-being outcomes than ability to get a gun, sexual orientation, and being enrolled in school. The authors conclude that *experience of racism should* be routinely assessed at intake to mental health services along *with traumatic* experiences such as physical or sexual abuse. *[Article copies available for a fee from The Haworth Document Delivery Service: 1-800-HAWORTH. E-mail address: <docdelivery@haworthpress.com> Website: <http://www.HaworthPress.com> © 2005 by The Haworth Press, Inc. All rights reserved.]*

KEYWORDS. Adolescent, racism, mental health, race/ethnicity, trauma, help-seeking, risk factors

In clinical mental health work with urban adolescents, the authors hear varied behavioral, emotional, educational, and other problems that represent responses to, and attempts at coping with, the developmental challenges of adolescence. Despite a racially and ethnically diverse population, however, and despite the wide range of issues with which adolescents present for mental health services, we rarely see adolescents who raise issues of race, ethnicity, or racism, as presenting problems. With adolescents in a racially and culturally diverse society, we believe it is vital to not overlook these complex and developmentally important issues. Clinicians, therefore, need a means for routinely exploring issues of ethnic identity, and assessing and addressing the impact of racism on the adolescent's functioning, in psychotherapy.

In order to understand these issues better relative to our own clinical work, we conducted an exploratory data-mining study on data collected from an adolescent self-report questionnaire at a health center in New York City primarily serving inner-city adolescents. Although the data were collected primarily for the purposes of clinical assessment and treatment planning, an aggregate analysis affords the opportunity for evidence-based, clinical, and programmatic reflection (Peake & Epstein, 2004). In employing such a *practice-based research* (PBR) approach (Epstein, 2001), practitioners can address questions derived from practice concerns and dilemmas using research methodologies most suited to the practice context. The ultimate aim of conducting a PBR study is reflection on existing methods of practice and generation and refinement of practice knowledge, both at the individual and organizational levels.

This study focuses on correlates of perceived racism, ethnic pride, and race and ethnicity; and the implications for culturally competent mental health care. The literature review examines bodies of theory relevant for understanding these adolescents' experiences of ethnic identity and racism. Finally, in the discussion, we share developmental and clinical implications of the findings for contextually appropriate clinical assessment and for forming therapeutic relationships with adolescents.

ETHNIC IDENTITY

Achieving a positive self-identity is a critical psychological component of adolescence (Meeus, 1996; Erickson, 1968) and may present particular challenges to adolescents who are from racial and ethnic minority groups (Utsey, Chae, Brown, & Kelly, 2002; Zayas, 2001). Ethnic identity has been conceptualized in many ways, including as an analog of *ego identity* (Meeus, 1996) and as the ethnic component of *social identity theory* (Blascovich, Wyer, Swart, & Kibler, 1997). In addition, for many adolescents, issues of *acculturation* (Ryder, Aldenor, & Palhus, 2000) constitute a crucial backdrop against which ethnic identity development plays out. These literatures provide useful conceptual frameworks for understanding ethnic identity formation, clinical and developmental impacts of racism, and the clinical implications that need to be accounted for in our work with adolescents.

Erikson (1968) posited that adolescence is a developmental period characterized by identity crisis, and that *ego identity* is achieved, generally during this time, after a normal period of experimentation and exploration. This process culminates in social and occupational commitments and decisions about occupation, sex roles, religion, and political ideology. Marcia (1966, 1980) articulated the idea of a *commitment* to one of four identity statuses, arranged hierarchically: (1) *Identity diffusion* (no active exploration or commitment); (2) *Identity foreclosure* (commitment has been reached without exploration, e.g., an adolescent simply takes on parental beliefs); (3) *Moratorium* (the individual is exploring but has not yet committed to an identity); and (4) *Achieved identity* (commitment is made to an identity after exploration). Others (Cote & Levine, 1988) viewed identity formation as a more fluid process, in which a person could rethink his or her commitment and return to earlier statuses. In this alternate view, then, an achieved identity status does not necessarily signal the end of the identity formation process.

Yoder (2000) expanded on this model by including social and environmental barriers to ego identity formation such as racism, gender bias, and sociocultural limitation in addition to the purely internal processes posited by Marcia and others. So, for example, an adolescent's experiences of racism may lead to more limited choices in exploring career opportunities and in committing to social and occupational goals and aspirations.

From the perspective of *social identity theory* (Tajfel, 1981; Phinney, 1990), ethnic identity is the part of an individual's self-worth that derives from self-identification with a social group [or groups] together with the values and emotional significance attached to that membership. In this process a positive social identity can be achieved simply through self-identification with a group, or groups, held in high regard. Conversely, being a member of an ethnic group that is different from the dominant group and held in low esteem may contribute to a negative social identity (Phinney, 1990). Possible paths for achieving a positive social identity in the face of prejudice include developing pride in one's own group, reinterpreting characteristics that have been deemed inferior by the dominant culture so that they do not appear inferior, and stressing the distinctiveness of one's own group (Utsey et al., 2002). Some have hypothesized that, given evidence to suggest that prejudice is pervasive, recognizing the existence of racial and ethnic prejudice can also help lead to a positive self-identity and a stronger connection with the group held in low esteem (Branscombe, 1999; Utsey et al., 2002).

Acculturation theory concerns how ethnic minority individuals from a culture different from the dominant one adapt to the new culture and its associated beliefs, values, and prescribed behaviors. In the linear model of acculturation (Andujo, 1988; Triandis, Kashima, Shimada, & Villareal, 1988), acculturating individuals progressively surrender the attitudes, values, and behaviors of their natal culture over the course of time while simultaneously adopting those of the mainstream society. In the bipolar model (Berry, 1997), acculturation is understood as an interaction between inherited and mainstream cultural identities, which are seen as relatively independent of one another. Thus, individuals may adopt many of the values and behaviors of the mainstream culture without giving up facets of self-identity developed from their natal culture.

In the bipolar perspective, acculturating individuals can relate to the host culture in one of four ways: *integrate* (i.e., maintain their cultural heritage while also maintaining relations with the mainstream; *assimilate* (i.e., relinquish their particular cultural heritage and adopt the beliefs and behaviors of the new culture); *separate* (i.e., maintain their heritage culture without intergroup relations); or *marginalize* (i.e., reject both natal and host cultures). Using these categories, Rotheram-Borus (1990) found that integrated individuals reported less acculturative stress and manifested fewer psychological problems than those who were marginalized, separated or assimilated, and concluded that integration was the most psychologically adaptive pattern.

The acculturative status of adolescent's caregivers may have implications for the adjustment of adolescents as well. According to a model proposed by Knight, Bernal, Cota, Garza, and Ocampo (1993) for example, parents indirectly model and reinforce ethnic behaviors in addition to directly teaching their children about the traditions, beliefs, and values associated with their cultural background. In a study examining the impact of parents' acculturative status on children, Roer-Strier and Rosenthal (2001) found that adolescents with immigrant parents maintaining a separate status toward the host culture had more psychological problems than adolescents whose parents were integrated.

Finally, the environment beyond the family may have important implications for identity development. Many ethnic minority adolescents living in the United States grow up in contrasting, yet parallel, cultures. At home, they may be expected to maintain traditional values and beliefs, whereas at school they may want to fit in with their peers. As a result, in the struggle to balance these conflicting allegiances and establish a distinct self-identity, as well as an ethnic identity that is compatible with both their natal culture and the American mainstream, adolescents may experience increased family conflict, heightened anxiety, low self-esteem, and poor school functioning (Roer-Strier & Rosenthal, 2001).

IMPACTS OF RACISM

Racism can be conceptualized as occurring at three levels: individual, institutional, and cultural (Jones, 1997). *Individual racism* refers to racial prejudice that occurs in the context of face to face interactions. *Institutional racism* refers to racial prejudice embedded within social institutions that manifest in social policies, norms, and practices. *Cultural racism* refers to a patterned way of thinking or a worldview that perpetuates the belief that the cultural values, traditions, and beliefs of the dominant group are superior to those of the other cultures. At each of these levels, racism, discrimination, and marginalization can tax individual and collective resources and threaten individual well-being, in turn impairing an individual's ethnic identity formation (Utsey et al., 2002; Zayas, 2001).

At the psychological level, perceptions of a racially stressful situation that taxes one's ability to cope may result in feelings of anger, anxiety, paranoia, helplessness, frustration, resentment, and fear (Utsey et al., 2002). Perceived racism or prejudice can be internalized and be manifested through anxiety, depression, and low self-esteem (Branscombe, 1990), and somatization, obsessive-compulsive symptoms, interpersonal sensitivity, depression, and subjective distress (Utsey et al., 2002). Physiological stress responses to racism can include changes in immune, neuroendocrine, and cardiovascular system functioning (Clark, Anderson, Clark, & Williams, 1999; Harrell, 2000).

The psychological and physiological symptoms associated with racism have been hypothesized to result from excessively burdened stress-responses accompanied by inadequate coping skills (Utsey et al., 2002; Clark et al., 1999). These responses can then activate coping skills that may or may not be adaptive. In time, overextended stress responses and coping skills may fall short in protecting the adolescent's self-worth and positive identity formation (Zayas, 2001) and may result in psychological and physiological distress (Clark et al., 1999).

Culturally competent clinicians familiar with typical psychological and physical responses to chronic experiences of discrimination and racism can be effective in identifying instances when these experiences are driving presenting problems (Zayas, 2001). This study seeks to identify ways that clinicians can best be attuned to these issues with the population we serve.

In this article, the data are analyzed in four steps. First, we examine the connections between race/ethnicity and the following: environmental and behavioral risk, desire to talk with a counselor about each of ten life areas (e.g., education, safety, sexuality, substance use), and worry about each life area. Second, we consider the connections between ethnic pride and: gender, stage of adolescence, and race/ethnicity. Third, we explore the connections between experienced racism and: race/ethnicity, gender, stage of adolescence, environmental and behavioral risk, worry in each of the life areas, and desire to talk about each of the life areas. Finally, we compare racism with other environmental risk factors on the number of significant correlates each has among indicators of behavioral risk, worry about each of the life areas, and coping in each of the life areas. We conclude with clinical and program implications.

METHOD

Practice Context and Population Served

Mount Sinai Adolescent Health Center (AHC) is a comprehensive health center for a diverse population of inner-city youth and offers medical, reproductive health, mental health, and health education services, as well as specialized clinical programs (e.g., programs focusing on eating disorders, special needs of HIV-infected or affected adolescents). Adolescent mental health clients make more than 20,000 mental health visits annually in a confidential setting, where they are seen regardless of their health insurance status or ability to pay. The study sample consisted of 759 adolescents presenting for intake to mental health services between 4/27/1999 and 4/9/2002. Of these, 36.0% were male and 64.0% were female. Ranging in age from 10 through 21, these urban adolescent applicants for mental health services come primarily from low-income, minority households in New York City (Diaz et al., 2004).

Adquest

Adquest is an indigenous, context-specific instrument designed by practitioners for practitioners. The 80-item adolescent self-report asks about life areas such as race/ethnicity and racism, school and education, work, safety, health, sexuality, substance abuse, and personal/family life. The instrument was intended to facilitate adolescent engagement in mental health services in a developmentally appropriate way by having young people seeking services to self-assess their own lives, problems, needs, worries, and reasons for seeking counseling, and what they want to talk about (Peake, Epstein, Mirabito, & Surko, 2004). This self-assessment, carried out before the adolescent meets a clinician for the first time, communicates AHC's philosophy of making adolescents partners in, and responsible consumers of, their own health care services.

Race/ethnicity categories for Adquest were developed by conducting focus groups in which AHC clients were asked how they identified themselves. AHC staff developed categories based on those responses, then piloted and discussed them with clients in order to assure they were consistent with how most clients self-identified. The resulting categories were Hispanic/Latino, African-American, White, West Indian/Caribbean, Asian/Pacific Islander, Other, and "Don't Know."

A question about racism was included as one of the first items on the survey in part because of clinician's experience that racism is an important environmental feature in the lives of AHC's population; it was also included to communicate to young people of color that clinicians at AHC are equipped to work with adolescents on issues of race, ethnicity, and racism; and regard these issues as important ones. Sample Adquest questions including those relating to race/ethnicity, ethnic pride, and perceived racism, and items regarding safety, are shown in the Appendix.

Adquest asks adolescents about their desire to talk about each of ten life areas: race/ethnicity, education, employment, safety, health, sex/body/birth control, drugs and alcohol, friends/associates, family/home life, and personal life. In analyzing desire-to-talk responses on Adquest, Peake, Epstein, Mirabito, and Surko (2004) grouped "don't know" responses with affirmative responses because the need to detect and address safety risks with this population makes de-

sirable a moderate bias toward over-inquiring rather than asking too little. Furthermore, adolescents responding "don't know" on questions regarding experiences of violence, sexual abuse, forced sex, etc., generally expressed a similar or greater level of wanting to talk about safety in comparison to those answering "yes" to having experienced these events (Peake et al., 2004). This analysis, therefore, follows the convention of grouping "don't know" responses on questions about desire to talk with affirmative answers.

FINDINGS

Of 759 adolescents completing Adquest in the sample, 748 gave a response on the item asking about their race/ethnicity. The majority identified as either Hispanic/Latino (44.7%) or African-American (29.8%; see Table 1). A substantial proportion (10.2%) gave multiple responses; other response categories included White (6.0%), West Indian/Caribbean (4.5%), Other (2.8%), and Asian/Pacific Islander (1.6%). A small proportion (.4%) answered "Don't Know." For the analyses presented in this article, adolescents giving multiple responses, and identifying as either "Other" or "Don't Know" were collapsed into a single category, and will be referred to as Multiethnic. This was done for two reasons. First, aggregating these groups simplified analysis by yielding a group comparable in size to the others. Second, in our clinical experience, adolescents with multiple ethnicities often self-identify in ways that are quite fluid, even to the extent of self-identifying one way in a predominantly White neighborhood, then later in the day, self-identifying differently in a predominantly Black and Latino neighborhood. Race/ethnicity was not significantly associated with either gender or with stage of adolescence, categorized into early (ages 11-14), middle (ages 15-16) and late (17-21) adolescence.

Ten indicators of environmental and behavioral risk were significantly associated with race/ethnicity (see Table 1). Asian/Pacific Islander and West Indian/Caribbean adolescents experienced environmental risk in the highest proportions, as seen in Table 1. For example, Asian/Pacific Islanders were most likely to have witnessed violence (91.7%) and been a victim of violence (75.0%) and were second most likely to report spending time with a drug user (66.7%). West Indian/Caribbean adolescents were most likely to report having been touched in a manner that made them uncomfortable (50.0%) and having experienced forced sex (20.6%), and relatively high proportions reported having witnessed violence (78.8%) and having been a victim of violence (52.9%). Whites, Hispanic/Latinos, and African-Americans reported lower levels of environmental risk than the other three racial/ethnic groups, although levels of risk remained substantial. For example, those three groups had the smallest

TABLE 1. Selected Environmental and Behavioral Risk Indicators by Race/ Ethnicity (%; N = 748)

	Higher	<----	----	----	---->	Lower	χ^2
Environmental Risk							
Witnessed violence	A/PI 91.7	Other 86.7	W. Ind. 78.8	Af-Am 75.8	Hisp/Lat 67.9	White 63.6	19.344**
Victim of violence	A/PI 75.0	W. Ind. 52.9	White 52.3	Other 50.0	Af-Am 42.0	Hisp/Lat 39.3	11.743*
Touched uncomfortably	W. Ind. 50.0	A/PI 45.5	Other 30.6	Hisp/Lat 25.7	Af-Am 22.7	White 17.8	16.039**
Forced sex	W. Ind. 20.6	Other 18.9	Af-Am 11.0	Hisp/Lat 8.8	A/PI 8.3	White 6.8	11.522*
Spent time with drug user	White 67.4	A/PI 66.7	Other 63.4	Hisp/Lat 49.8	W. Ind. 45.5	Af-Am 40.6	21.237**
Behavioral Risk							
Failing classes	A/PI 72.7	Hisp/Lat 68.5	Other 65.6	Af-Am 65.5	W. Ind. 56.7	White 37.2	17.317**
Ever had sex	Hisp/Lat 56.7	Af-Am 52.7	W. Ind. 51.5	Other 44.7	A/PI 41.7	White 26.7	16.896**
Tried alcohol	White 84.6	A/PI 81.8	Other 72.8	W. Ind. 69.0	Hisp/Lat 64.0	Af-Am 58.6	13.547*
Tried marijuana	White 72.2	Af-Am 52.6	A/PI 50.0	Other 44.9	Hisp/Lat 42.9	W. Ind. 41.7	13.347*
Tried other drugs	White 31.0	Other 13.9	W. Ind. 4.5	Hisp/Lat 4.1	Af-Am 2.0	A/PI 0	43.645***

*$p < .05$, **$p < .01$, ***$p < .001$

proportions reporting having witnessed violence (63.6%, 67.9%, and 75.8% respectively) and having been touched uncomfortably (17.8%, 25.7%, and 22.7% respectively) and also had generally lower proportions reporting being a victim of violence and having experienced forced sex than the other racial/ethnic groups.

Among the behavioral risk items significantly associated with race/ethnicity, whites had the highest proportions reporting having tried alcohol (84.6%), marijuana (72.2%), and other drugs (31.0%). Asian/Pacific Islanders had the highest proportion reporting failing classes (72.7%) and the lowest proportion reporting having tried drugs other than tobacco, alcohol, and marijuana (0.0%).

Desire to talk with a counselor was associated with race/ethnicity for only two of the ten possible life areas: education ($\chi^2 = 14.175$, $p < .05$) and work ($\chi^2 =$

24.118, $p < .001$). Differences among the six race/ethnicity groups were relatively modest. Proportions of adolescents wanting to talk about education were 91.7% for Asian/Pacific Islanders, 86.7% for Hispanic/Latinos, 80.0% for Whites, 78.2% for African-Americans, 76.5% for West Indian/Caribbeans, and 72.2% for Multiethnic adolescents. Proportions of adolescents wanting to talk about work were 80.8% for Hispanic/Latinos, 78.8% for West Indian/Caribbeans, 78.1% for African-Americans, 75.0% for Asian/Pacific Islanders, 66.3% for Multiethnic adolescents, and 51.2% for Whites. Desire to talk about race/ethnicity was not significantly associated with race/ethnicity itself.

Two of the fifteen items related to worry were significantly associated with race/ethnicity; worry about doing dangerous things ($\chi^2 = 12.165$, $p < .05$) and worries or concerns about health ($\chi^2 = 11.730$, $p < .05$). Multiethnic adolescents had the highest proportion worried that they did dangerous things (50.0%), followed by West Indian/Caribbeans (47.1%), Asian/Pacific Islanders (41.7%), Whites (38.6%), Hispanic/Latinos (35.3%), and African-Americans (31.2%). West Indian/Caribbeans had the highest proportion with health worries or concerns (64.7%), followed by Asian/Pacific Islanders (60.0%), Whites (56.8%), Multiethnic adolescents (50.5%), Hispanic/Latinos (45.1%), and African-Americans (40.0%).

A large majority of adolescents reported being proud of their race/ethnicity (90.5%); 2.5% reported being not proud and 6.9% responded "don't know." Ethnic pride was significantly associated with gender ($\chi^2 = 6.415$, $p < .05$). Most males (88.2%) and females (92.1%) were proud of their race or ethnicity and similar proportions of males and females were not proud (1.8% and 2.7%, respectively). However, more males than females said they didn't know whether they were proud (10.0% vs. 5.2%, respectively). There was no significant relationship between ethnic pride and stage of adolescence.

Ethnic pride also varied significantly by race/ethnicity ($\chi^2 = 70.307$, $p < .001$; see Table 2). West Indian/Caribbeans and Hispanic/Latinos had the highest proportions expressing pride (100.0% and 95.2% respectively) and the lowest proportions reporting not being proud (0.0% and 0.6% respectively). Asian/Pacific Islanders and Whites had the lowest proportions reporting pride (75.0% and 61.4%, respectively) and the highest proportion reporting not being proud (16.7% and 9.1%, respectively). Whites and Multiethnic adolescents had the highest proportion answering they didn't know whether they were proud of their race/ethnicity (29.5% and 11.0%, respectively), and Hispanic/Latinos and West Indian/Caribbeans had the lowest proportions responding "don't know" (4.2% and 0.0% respectively).

Perceived racism varied significantly by race/ethnicity ($\chi^2 = 27.196$, $p < .001$). Asian/Pacific Islanders had the highest proportion of adolescents reporting ex-

TABLE 2. Ethnic Pride by Race/Ethnicity (%; N = 748)

	Higher	<----	----	----	---->	Lower	χ^2
Proud of race/ethnicity							70.307***
Yes	W. Ind. 100.0	Hisp/Lat 95.2	Af-Am 91.0	Other 85.0	A/PI 75.0	White 61.4	
No	A/PI 16.7	White 9.1	Other 4.0	Af-Am 3.2	Hisp/La .6	W. Ind. 0	
Don't know	White 29.5	Other 11.0	A/PI 8.3	Af-Am 5.9	Hisp/Lat 4.2	W. Ind. 0	

*$p < .05$, **$p < .01$, ***$p < .001$

periences of racism, with 80.0%. Proportions among the other groups were as follows: 60.6% of West Indian/Caribbeans; 52.5% of Multiethnic adolescents; 45.5% of Whites; 40.1% of African-Americans; and 32.4% of Hispanic/Latinos. There was no significant relationship between gender and lifetime experience of perceived racism, but stage of adolescence was significantly related to lifetime experience of perceived racism ($\chi^2 = 26.640$, $p < .001$). Fewer than a third of early adolescents (29.2%) reported experiencing racism, 40.5% of middle adolescents reported experiencing racism, and 53.6% of late adolescents reported experiencing racism. There was no significant relationship between perceived racism and ethnic pride.

Racism was significantly associated with several indicators of environmental and behavioral risk (see Table 3). Because racism was associated with stage of adolescence, the association between racism and indicators of risk, worry, and well-being was broken down by age. With all indicators and age groups where a significant association existed, racism *was significantly associated with* higher risk. Early adolescents reporting racism were more likely to have witnessed violence (87.3% versus 54.4% for those not having experienced racism) and to have been a victim of violence (56.3% versus 30.0% for those not having experienced racism). Racism was significantly associated with the most risk indicators for middle adolescents, and it was associated with substantially higher risk in some cases; for example, having been threatened with a weapon (37.3% versus 14.0% for those reporting not having experienced racism), having been a victim of violence (55.1% versus 35.3%), having been touched uncomfortably (37.3% versus 22.5%), and having used drugs in the prior month (42.6% versus 26.0%). Late adolescents reporting racism also had higher proportions reporting environmental, but not behavioral, risk; for example, having been threatened with a weapon (47.1% versus 26.1% for late adolescents

TABLE 3. Selected Environmental and Behavioral Risk Indicators by Perceived Racism and Stage of Adolescence (%; N = 748)

	Experienced Racism?		
Item	YES	NO	χ^2
Environmental Risk			
Witnessed violence			
Early (10-14)	87.3	54.4	23.638***
Middle (15-16)	91.5	69.6	19.935***
Late (17-21)	92.2	69.0	16.736***
Threatened with weapon			
Early (10-14)	21.1	15.4	1.164
Middle (15-16)	37.3	14.0	21.230***
Late (17-21)	47.1	26.1	8.836**
Victim of violence			
Early (10-14)	56.3	30.0	14.783***
Middle (15-16)	55.1	35.3	11.230**
Late (17-21)	67.0	43.2	10.769**
Touched uncomfortably			
Early (10-14)	23.9	15.2	2.622
Middle (15-16)	37.3	22.5	7.481**
Late (17-21)	42.2	28.4	3.885*
Get gun			
Early (10-14)	17.9	16.7	.052
Middle (15-16)	39.7	22.5	9.794**
Late (17-21)	44.9	21.6	11.245**
Offered drugs			
Early (10-14)	43.3	33.7	1.878
Middle (15-16)	72.2	50.9	13.001***
Late (17-21)	75.0	55.7	7.780**
Spent time drug user			
Early (10-14)	37.3	33.9	.239
Middle (15-16)	68.7	49.4	10.458**
Late (17-21)	65.7	52.9	3.144
Behavioral Risk			
Tried tobacco			
Early (10-14)	41.3	35.3	.514
Middle (15-16)	66.7	52.6	4.745*
Late (17-21)	68.5	59.4	1.413

| | Experienced Racism? | | |
Item	YES	NO	χ^2
Tried other drugs			
Early (10-14)	4.7	0.9	2.192
Middle (15-16)	11.1	3.6	4.248*
Late (17-21)	15.2	5.0	3.678
Used drugs last month			
Early (10-14)	7.7	13.9	1.666
Middle (15-16)	42.6	26.0	8.655**
Late (17-21)	43.1	35.2	1.237

*$p < .05$, **$p < .01$, ***$p < .001$

not having experienced racism), having been a victim of violence (67.0% versus 43.2%), having been touched uncomfortably (42.4% versus 28.4%), and being able to get a gun (44.9% versus 21.6%). In contrast to racism, ethnic pride was generally not significantly associated with environmental and behavioral risk, worry, and desire to talk with a counselor; therefore, those results are not presented here.

For some environmental and behavioral risks, racism *was significantly associated with* higher risk for one gender but not the other. Females, but not males, who had experienced racism had a higher proportion who also had had their body touched in a way that made them uncomfortable (49.7% versus 26.7%, $\chi^2 = 25.820$, $p < .001$), who had been offered drugs (71.5% versus 43.5%, $\chi^2 = 33.529$, $p < .001$), and who had tried drugs other than tobacco, alcohol, and marijuana (13.3% among those who had experienced racism, versus 2.7% among those who had not; $\chi^2 = 12.851$, $p < .001$). Males, but not females, who had experienced racism were more likely to have had sex (58.6% versus 45.0%, $\chi^2 = 4.702$, $p < .05$) and to have used drugs in the prior month (39.4% versus 19.7%, $\chi^2 = 12.043$, $p < .01$).

Racism was significantly associated with worry among middle and late adolescents but not for early adolescents (see Table 4). Among middle adolescents, for example, having experienced racism was associated with higher proportions experiencing worry about hurting self or others (60.0% versus 44.0% for those not having experienced racism), getting enough sleep (64.1% versus 48.5%), and another person's drug use (47.0% versus 30.2%). Among late adolescents, racism was associated with higher proportions reporting worry about hurting self or others (65.7% versus 44.3%), one's own danger-

TABLE 4. Selected Worry Items by Perceived Racism and Stage of Adolescence (%; N = 748)

Worry Item	Experienced Racism?		
	YES	NO	χ^2
Often feel unsafe			
Early (10-14)	50.0	37.6	3.122
Middle (15-16)	35.6	36.2	.011
Late (17-21)	60.8	34.1	13.478***
Worry/hurt self/others			
Early (10-14)	42.9	40.0	.168
Middle (15-16)	60.0	44.0	7.107**
Late (17-21)	65.7	44.3	8.594**
Worry about friends or associates			
Early (10-14)	73.9	62.0	3.090
Middle (15-16)	68.1	58.6	2.668
Late (17-21)	67.3	48.3	6.988**
Worry/do dangerous things			
Early (10-14)	42.9	31.6	2.782
Middle (15-16)	43.2	35.4	1.806
Late (17-21)	46.1	29.5	5.458*
Health problems/worries			
Early (10-14)	46.4	33.5	3.466
Middle (15-16)	54.3	36.3	9.162**
Late (17-21)	64.1	58.4	.644
Worry about sleep			
Early (10-14)	43.7	32.4	2.791
Middle (15-16)	64.1	48.5	6.796**
Late (17-21)	72.5	53.9	7.139**
Worry about sex, body, birth control			
Early (10-14)	29.4	20.7	2.028
Middle (15-16)	49.1	39.3	2.735
Late (17-21)	64.0	44.9	6.910**
Worry about own drug use			
Early (10-14)	8.1	9.9	.173
Middle (15-16)	25.0	14.8	4.586*
Late (17-21)	31.7	24.1	1.314

	Experienced Racism?		
Worry Item	YES	NO	χ^2
Worry about another's drug use			
Early (10-14)	37.9	24.5	4.112*
Middle (15-16)	47.0	30.2	8.268**
Late (17-21)	46.0	36.8	1.626

*$p < .05$, **$p < .01$, ***$p < .001$

ous behavior (46.1% versus 29.5%), getting enough sleep (72.5% versus 53.9%), and worry about friends or associates (57.0% versus 49.4%). Among early adolescents, experienced racism was associated with higher proportions reporting worry on only two items: drug use of another person (37.9% versus 24.5%) and things not on the survey (23.9% versus 12.7%).

Experienced racism *was associated with* higher proportions of worry among females but not males on the following items (see Table 5): worry about hurting self or others (65.5% versus 46.1%), health worries or concerns (64.4% versus 44.3%), worry about another person's drug use (46.7% versus 30.4%), worry about friends or associates (64.9% versus 48.6%), worry about family and home life (75.3% versus 63.3%), and worry about things not mentioned on the survey (52.8% versus 25.1%). Experienced racism *was associated with* higher proportions of worry among males but not females on the following items: worry about doing dangerous things (53.6% versus 35.1%), worry about one's own drug use (30.2% versus 15.5%).

Racism was significantly associated with desire to talk with a counselor: middle and late adolescents having experienced racism wanted to talk about race and ethnicity more than those who had not experienced racism (61.5% versus 45.1% for middle; $\chi^2 = 7.549$, $p < .01$; 54.9% versus 39.3% for late, $\chi^2 = 4.623$, $p < .05$). Unexpectedly, a lower proportion of early adolescents having experienced racism wanted to talk about safety than those who had not experienced racism (58.6% versus 72.2%; $\chi^2 = 4.233$, $p < .05$). Finally, a higher proportion of middle adolescents having experienced racism wanted to talk about family and home life than those who had not experienced racism (92.1% versus 82.8%; $\chi^2 = 5.027$, $p < .05$).

As a means of determining the relative strength of racism as a *correlate* of health and well-being, chi-square analyses were conducted examining the number of health and well-being indicators significantly associated with environ-

TABLE 5. Proportion of Adolescents Expressing Worry, by Perceived Racism and Gender (%; N = 748)

Worry Item	Experienced Racism?		χ^2
	YES	NO	
Worry about hurting self/others			
Male	45.5	35.3	2.718
Female	65.5	46.1	16.310***
Worry about doing dangerous things			
Male	53.6	35.1	8.954**
Female	38.2	31.6	2.141
Health concerns or worries			
Male	42.3	30.9	3.642
Female	64.4	44.3	17.593***
Worry about own drug use			
Male	30.2	15.5	7.695**
Female	19.5	14.5	1.890
Worry about another's drug use			
Male	36.4	26.9	2.622
Female	49.7	30.4	16.659***
Worry about friends or associates			
Male	48.6	37.4	3.224
Female	64.9	48.6	11.581**
Worry about family and home life			
Male	57.3	46.6	2.865
Female	75.3	63.3	7.061**
Worry about things not on the survey			
Male	17.6	14.2	.538
Female	52.8	25.1	33.562***

$*p < .05, **p < .01, ***p < .001$

mental and demographic variables, shown in Table 6. *The assumption here was that the more widespread the influences of an environmental risk factor, the greater the number of health and well-being outcomes with which it would be significantly correlated.* Health and well-being indicators included 10 behavioral risk items, 17 worry items, and 10 perceived coping items. As seen in Table 6, racism *was significantly associated with* more health and well-being

TABLE 6. Environmental Risk Factors, Including Racism, Ranked by Number of Significant Correlates (*p* < .05) Among 37 Indicators of Behavioral Risk, Worry, and Coping

Adquest Item	Number of Significant Correlates
Touched uncomfortably	30
Ever offered drugs	28
Forced sex	27
Spend time with friends who use drugs	27
Victim of violence	26
Witnessed violence	25
Ever experienced racism	**24**
Could get a gun	21
Threatened with weapon	18
Currently working	17
In school	13
Taught about body/sexuality	12
How do you rate school	10
Anyone close died in last year	10
Race/Ethnicity	8
How often attend religious services	7

outcomes than about half of the other variables examined, including ability to get a gun, sexual orientation, having been threatened with a weapon, and being enrolled in school.

DISCUSSION

Risk Exposure and Race/Ethnicity

Although all adolescents in the sample seemed vulnerable for many risk factors across all life areas, within each racial/ethnic category there were widespread variations in frequencies of self-reported risks. Notable exceptions were related to safety and alcohol/substance risk. West Indian/Caribbean adolescents and Asian/Pacific Islanders were particularly vulnerable for environmental safety risks. West Indian/Caribbean adolescents had the highest reports for forced sex and having been touched uncomfortably, and were second highest with regard to witnessing violence and having been a victim of violence. Asian/Pacific Islanders reported the highest rates of being victims of violence and witnessing violence at extremely high rates. However, although West Indian/Caribbean adolescents and Asian/Pacific Islanders were consistently at highest safety risk, safety risks were disturbingly high for all groups, as from a developmental perspective all adolescents should be able to feel safe.

White adolescents reported the highest levels on all Adquest substance abuse risk items, including ever tried alcohol, marijuana, and other drugs as well as exposure to a drug user. Though there were considerable variations in substance abuse risk within all other racial/ethnic groups, rates of ever having tried alcohol were extremely high for all groups and the rate for Asian/Pacific Islanders was comparable to that for whites.

In presenting findings about patterns across racial and ethnic groups, we hope to support clinicians' culturally competent practice in conducting effective and efficient initial assessments. We of course also recognize a tension here; these findings are aggregated data, and each individual must be assessed separately. Culturally competent assessment requires being aware of, and making use of, group patterns without being blinded by them.

One way in which findings like these can be useful in a practice setting is for clinicians to reflect on their pattern of assessment and diagnosis in the aggregate. Knowing the aggregate pattern of self-reported problems can give clinicians a point of reference by which to assess their aggregate patterns of diagnosis across racial and ethnic groups. In some cases, disparities between rates of self-report and diagnosis may reflect culturally determined differences in style of self-reporting; in others, they may identify opportunities for individual clinicians to more effectively engage adolescents from particular ethnic or cultural groups.

Ethnic Pride

Ethnic pride, as measured by Adquest, did not appear to be either a risk or protective factor for adolescents in this sample, and level of ethnic pride did not seem to be affected by the experience of racism. Neither was ethnic pride associated with adolescents' self-reports of coping or desire to talk about Adquest life areas, including race/ethnicity. Ethnic pride was also not correlated with reports of having experienced racism. It may be that no connection exists; alternately, the statistical power to identify an association may have been attenuated by the low proportion of adolescents indicating lack of pride or uncertainty about pride.

That Asian/Pacific Islanders had the highest proportion not being proud of their race and ethnicity may call for particular attention to issues of self-concept in clinical work with these young people. This may be especially pertinent given that they had the highest proportion reporting racism: an alarming rate of eight in ten. These adolescents might have been struggling with acculturation issues. Male adolescents were less likely to report feeling proud of their race/ethnicity than females. While the format of Adquest does not allow further exploration as to why that might be, the authors wondered whether this might be a cause for concern with male clients.

The Experience of Racism

Racism is a common experience among the inner-city adolescents seeking mental health services at the AHC. Even among Latinos, who reported the lowest rates, more than three in ten adolescents reported the experience. This is disturbing. Furthermore, racism was *associated with* a wide range of risks, worries, and indicators of poor coping–almost as powerful as having experienced forced sex, having been a victim of violence, and witnessing violence (as seen in Table 6). This suggests that the *experience of racism should* be routinely assessed for when working with adolescent clients in diverse settings.

For females, the experience of racism was associated with having been touched uncomfortably, having been offered drugs, and having used substances other than alcohol and marijuana, i.e., harder drugs. For males, experience of racism was *associated with substance use and ever having* had sex. When looking at the impact of racism on worry, other gender differences were evident. Compared to peers who had not experienced racism, females who had were more likely to worry about hurting themselves or others, their health, another's drug use, friends and associates, and family and home life. Males who had experienced racism were more likely to worry about doing dangerous things and their own drug use than males who did not report the experience. These findings suggest that the *impacts of racism manifest themselves* differently for males and females.

Rates of reported racism increased with age, which was expected, given that older adolescents have had a longer time in which to accumulate such experiences. The older adolescents may also have been exposed to a wider assortment of social situations, and wider segments of society, which could have increased their exposure to racism. Finally, it is also possible that the older adolescents were better able to identify and articulate instances of racism in their relationships with others, due to their higher levels of cognitive and social functioning as compared to younger adolescents.

In contrast, the relationship between the experience of racism and *other* environmental risks seemed unlikely to be an artifact of their respective associations with age. When controlling for stage of adolescence, adolescents who reported having experienced racism were, generally, significantly more at risk than those who did not report the experience. Adolescents who experienced racism were particularly vulnerable around issues of safety, being more likely to be victims of violence, forced sex, and other forms of abuse. This suggests that practitioners need to be sensitive to the fact that racism co-occurs with other *environmental risks. Clinicians should assess for experiences of racism when other environmental risks are reported, and conversely, when adolescents report experiences of racism, clinicians should be sure to assess for other environmental risks.*

The findings also suggest that experience of racism affects adolescents differently based on their stage of development. In particular *early* adolescents who experienced racism reported far fewer worries than middle and late adolescents (see summary in Table 7). Furthermore, these adolescents wanted to talk about race and ethnicity *less* than their peers who reported not having experienced racism.

In contrast, for *middle and late* adolescents, having experienced racism was *associated with* greater risk exposure and increased worries across a wide spectrum of Adquest life areas (see Table 7). For middle adolescents, in particular, having experienced racism was associated with increased substance use. Both middle and late adolescents who had experienced racism were more likely to be able to get a gun and more likely to worry about hurting themselves or others. Consistent with the aforementioned literature, racism can interfere with healthy identity development (Jones, 1997). For some adolescents, racism may have a negative impact on their identity development and self-worth, and may lead to increased risk behaviors and poorer coping.

The finding that middle and late adolescents who had experienced racism had significantly greater desire to talk about race and racism than their peers who had not experienced racism was encouraging. However, it was disturbing that early adolescents who experienced racism had *less* desire to talk about race and ethnicity than those who did not report racism. This suggests that programs should actively include racism as a health issue to be addressed through health education and public service announcements, and that particular focus may need to be paid to children and early adolescents.

The experience of racism was generally not associated with an increased desire to talk about various life areas except, as reported earlier, the desire of middle and late adolescents to talk about issues of race and ethnicity. Overall, for adolescents in this sample, racism appears to have been associated with a

TABLE 7. Environmental and Behavioral Risk, Worry, and Coping Items Significantly Correlated with Perceived Racism; by Developmental Stage

Developmental Stage		
Early adolescence	Middle adolescence	Late adolescence
Witnessed violence	Witnessed violence	Witnessed violence
	Threatened with weapon	Threatened with weapon
Victim of violence	Victim of violence	Victim of violence
	Touched uncomfortably	Touched uncomfortably
	Able to get a gun	Able to get a gun
	Offered drugs	Offered drugs
	Spent time with drug user	
	Tried tobacco	
	Tried other drugs	
	Used drugs last month	
	Worry about hurting self or others	Worry about hurting self or others
		Feel unsafe
		Worry do dangerous things
	Worry about own drug use	
	Health concerns and worries	
		Worry about sex, body, birth control
	Worry about sleep amount	Worry about sleep amount
Worry about another's drug use	Worry about another's drug use	
		Worry about friends/ associates
Worry about things not on survey	Worry about things not on survey	

more generalized vulnerability across many life areas *rather than particular risk behaviors.*

Practice Implications

This study shows that experiences with racism, and their sequelae, must be considered in the assessment, engagement, and mental health treatment of urban adolescents of *all* ethnicities. While it is commonly accepted that practitioners need to understand their clients' cultures, that is not enough. These findings highlight the fact that valuing diversity in the organizational culture and recruiting a diverse staff cannot, in itself, adequately ensure cultural competence, nor can it ensure that client experiences of, or concerns about, racism are addressed.

Based on our clinical experience that adolescents can be idealistic about issues such as race and racism, we suggest that practitioners may need to carefully assess how experiences of racism affect the developing self-concept of adolescents in treatment. Given the fact that all groups reported high levels of perceived racism, we urge that this assessment be part of the ongoing work with adolescents from all racial and ethnic groups. In particular, these findings called our attention to racism reported by Asian/Pacific Islander and White adolescents. This moving beyond the prototype of racism as primarily a phenomenon with White perpetrators and African-American or other minority victims was an important, and potentially productive, finding for work with AHC's clinical population.

Adquest was not designed as a comprehensive assessment questionnaire but rather as a clinical tool intended to trigger discussion and thereby enhance engagement (Peake, Epstein, Mirabito, & Surko, 2004). When designing Adquest, AHC practitioners acknowledged the pernicious nature of racism and its destructive potential and thus included the question about the experience of racism. The findings illustrate the value that such questions can bring to a clinical instrument. Adquest illustrates that mental health intake practices should ensure that practitioners tap issues of culture, cultural and racial identity, and acculturation.

The authors suggest that racism should be first assessed *at intake* to allow the practitioner and client to recognize this as a legitimate area for discussion at any time in treatment. A further recommendation is that adolescents be asked about witnessing racism, and the impact of this experience. Similarly, a framework for exploration of ethnic identity and acculturation can be created at intake and returned to when pertinent. (Elsewhere in this volume this aspect of Adquest has been referred to as a framework for ensuring that clinical *conversations are kept open*) (Elliott et al., 2004). The authors suggest that it is difficult to have these discussions if permission is not given up front.

When parents are involved in their adolescent's treatment, the family's experiences should also be assessed. Similarly, assessment should include the family's ethnic identity framework and how this fits with that of the adolescent client. At times this may well be an issue to explore in family history through the genogram as experiences of earlier generations may well shape a family's identity (Carter & McGoldrick, 1999).

A revised Adquest might spark discussion of an adolescent's experiences in these areas, and their treatment needs. Similarly, the AHC intake questionnaire for parents (Peake, Epstein, Mirabito, & Surko, 2004) will be revised to ask about family experiences that might be relevant to an adolescent's cultural identity. A revised Adquest will also include "don't know" as an optional response when asking about experiences with racism. This option on other Adquest questions–such as "have you ever been forced to have sex?"–has proved itself highly productive (Surko, Ciro, Carlson et al., 2004). In that example, adolescents who responded "don't know" represented a population who may have been struggling to define a traumatic experience because empirically they were similar to those who acknowledged the trauma. These adolescents may need help making sense of their experience.

Practitioners should be equipped to help an adolescent describe and define his or her experiences and explore issues of cultural identity. The literature cited earlier can provide guidance to clinicians, and the authors suggest that practice competencies should be informed by it. For example Yoder's work underscores the fact that experiences of racism may limit life choices. For adolescents who are in the process of defining themselves and their future directions (Erikson, 1968) this is a particularly pertinent area that practitioners must keep in mind and–if they do not ask about racism–will overlook.

Jones (1997) typology of individual, institutional, and cultural racism, cited earlier, can provide clinicians with a framework to use when helping adolescents make sense of their experiences. This conceptual model can be helpful in working through the experience of racism, as one of many potentially negative experiences that have damaged an adolescent's self-esteem, as it offers a taxonomy for a cognitive reframing process or a narrative therapy approach (Cooper & Lesser, 2001).

Practice competencies could also include Berry's (1997) acculturation framework, described earlier; this could be useful in separately assessing adolescents and their families. Young people can feel a tension between the pull from their families to embrace and retain aspects of their families' natal cultures and the pull to adopt aspects of the dominant culture embraced by peers; this can lead to substantial conflict. Routinely assessing for such disjunctions is an important clinical competency in working with our population, which has a high proportion of immigrant families.

Cultural competency additionally means clinicians must be comfortable in asking clients about their experiences and views, be reflective on their own attitudes and experiences, be able to help an adolescent on his or her own path without imposing their own views, and be aware of power dynamics in the room. Adolescents like practitioners to be *genuine* and practitioners must be comfortable in learning from clients and not feel the need to be the expert at all times. These competencies can be encouraged and supported when the agency environment expects and promotes them, and at AHC they are incorporated in formal clinical competency protocols used in performance appraisal. Such competencies can also be reinforced through models of supervision that bring together diverse groups of clinicians who are able to learn from one another's experiences.

CONCLUSION

Actively assessing for experiences of racism has been a long-overlooked aspect of mental health treatment with adolescents. More needs to be done by practitioners to understand how racism impacts the development and identity of the young people they serve. Furthermore, the findings presented here strongly suggest that racism constitutes an *environmental risk* that should be routinely assessed at intake to mental health services along *with traumatic* experiences such as physical or sexual abuse.

REFERENCES

Andujo, E. (1988). Ethnic identity of transethnically adopted Hispanic adolescents. *Social Work*, *33*, 531-535.

Berry, J. W. (1997). Immigration, acculturation, and adaptation. *Applied Psychology: An International Review*, *46*, 5-68.

Blascovich, J., Wyer, N. A., Swart, L. A., & Kibler, J. L. (1997). Racism and racial categorization. *Journal of Personality and Social Psychology*, *72*, 1362-1372.

Branscombe, R. N., Schmitt, M. T., & Harvey, R. D. (1999). Perceiving pervasive discrimination among African Americans: Implications for group identification and well-being. *Journal of Personality and Social Psychology*, *77*, 135-149.

Carter, B., & McGoldrick, M. (1999). *The expanded family life cycle: Individual, family, and social perspectives, 3rd ed.* Needham Heights, MA: Allyn and Bacon.

Clark, R., Anderson, N. B., Clark, V. R., & Williams, D. R. (1999). Racism as a stressor for African Americans: A biopsychosocial model. *American Psychologist*, *54*, 805-816.

Cote, J. E., & Levine, C. (1988). A critical examination of the ego identity status paradigm. *Developmental Review*, *8*, 147-184.

Diaz, A., Peake, K., Surko, M., & Bhandarkar, K. (2004). Including at-risk adolescents in their own health and mental health care: A youth development perspective. *Social Work in Mental Health*, *3*(1/2), 3-22.

Epstein, I. (2001). Using available clinical information in practice-based research: Mining for silver while dreaming of gold. *Social Work in Health Care*, *33* (3), 15-32.

Erikson, E. (1968). *Identity: Youth and crisis.* New York: Norton.

Harrell, S. P. (2000). A multidimensional conceptualization of racism related stress: Implications for the well being of people of color. *American Journal of Orthopsychiatry*, *70*, 42-57.

Jackson, A. L., Sullivan, A. L., Harnish, R., & Hodge, N. C. (1996). Achieving positive social identity: Social mobility, social creativity, and permeability of group boundaries. *Journal of Personality and Social Psychology, 70,* 241-254.

Jones, J. M. (1997). *Prejudice and racism, 2nd ed.* New York: McGraw-Hill.

Knight, G. P., Bernal, M. E., Costa, M., Garza, C., & Ocampo, K. (1993). Ethnic identity: Formation and transmission among Hispanics and other minorities. Albany, NY: State University of New York Press.

Marcia, J. (1966). Development and validation of ego-identity status. *Journal of Personality and Social Psychology, 3,* 551-558.

Marcia, J. (1980). Identity in adolescence. In J. Adelson (Ed.), *Handbook of adolescent psychology* (pp. 159-187). New York: Wiley.

Meeus, W. (1996). Studies on identity development in adolescence: An overview of research and some new data. *Journal of Youth and Adolescence, 25,* 569-598.

Peake, K., & Epstein, I. (2004). Theoretical and practical imperatives for reflective social work organizations in health and mental health: The place of practice-based research. *Social Work in Mental Health, 3*(1/2), 23-38.

Peake, K., Epstein, I., Mirabito, D., & Surko, M. (2004). Development and utilization of a practice-based adolescent intake questionnaire (Adquest): Surveying which risks, worries, and concerns urban youth want to talk about. *Social Work in Mental Health, 3*(1/2), 55-82.

Phinney, J. S. (1990). Ethnic identity in adolescents and adults: Review of research. *Psychological Bulletin, 108*(3), 499-514.

Roer-Strier, D., & Rosenthal, M. K. (2001). Socialization in changing cultural contexts: A search for images of the "adaptive adult." *Social Work, 46*(3), 215-228.

Rotheram-Borus, M. J. (1990). Adolescents' reference-group choices, self-esteem, and adjustment. *Journal of Personality and Social Psychology, 59*(5), 1075-1081.

Ryder, A. G., Aldenor, L. E., & Palhus, D. L. (2000). Is acculturation unidimensional or bidimensional? A head to head comparison in the prediction of personality, self- identity, and adjustment. *Journal of Personality and Social Psychology, 79*(1), 49-65.

Surko, M., Ciro, D., Carlson, E., Labor, N., Giannone, V., Diaz-Cruz, E., Peake, K., & Epstein, I. (2004). Which adolescents need to talk about safety and violence? *Social Work in Mental Health, 3*(1/2), 103-120.

Triandis, H. C., Kashima, E., Shimada, E., & Villareal, M. (1988). Acculturation indices as a means of confirming cultural differences. *International Journal of Psychology, 21,* 43-70.

Utsey, S. O., Chae, M. H., Brown, C. F., & Kelly, D. (2002). Effect of ethnic group membership on ethnic identity, race-related stress, and quality of life. *Cultural Diversity and Ethnic Minority Psychology, 8,* 366-377.

Yoder, A. E. (2000). Barriers to ego identity status formation: A contextual qualification of Marcia's identity status paradigm. *Journal of Adolescence, 23*(1), 95-106.

Zaslow, M. J., & Takanishi, R. (1993). Priorities for research on adolescent development. *American Psychologist, 48*(2), 185-192.

Zayas, L. H. (2001). Incorporating struggles with racism and ethnic identity in therapy with adolescents. *Clinical Social Work Journal, 29,* 361-373.

APPENDIX

Adquest items assessing race/ethnicity, ethnic pride, perceived racism, and safety risk

- What is your race or ethnicity? [African-American/West Indian,Caribbean/Asian, or Pacific Islander/White(non-Hispanic)/Hispanic, Latino/Don't Know/Other (please write in)]
- Are you proud of your race and ethnicity? [Yes/No/Don't Know]
- Have you ever experienced racism? [Yes/No]
- Have you ever witnessed violence? [Yes/No]
- Do you ever feel unsafe? [Yes/No]
- Have you ever been threatened with a weapon? [Yes/No]
- Have you ever been a victim of violence? [Yes/No/Don't Know]
- Has anyone ever touched your body in a way that made you feel uncomfortable? [Yes/No/Don't Know]
- Do you and your boyfriend/girlfriend ever physically fight? [Yes/No/Don't Know]
- Have you ever been forced to have sex when you didn't want to? [Yes/No/Don't Know]
- Have you ever worried about hurting yourself or someone else in any way? [Yes/No/Don't Know]
- Do you ever worry about the friends or associates that you hang out with? [Yes/No]
- Do you ever worry that things you do are dangerous? [Yes/No]
- Do your friends or family members ever worry that things you do are dangerous? [Yes/No/Don't Know]
- Could you get a gun if you wanted to? [Yes/No]
- Do your friends or family members ever worry about your safety? [Yes/No/Don't Know]
- In general, when it comes to your own safety, how often do you feel unsafe? [Always/Often/Sometimes/Rarely/Never]
- How much do you want to talk to your counselor here about your safety? [Not At All/Somewhat/Very Much/Don't Know]

Multiple Risks, Multiple Worries, and Adolescent Coping: What Clinicians Need to Ask About

Michael Surko
Ken Peake
Irwin Epstein
Daniel Medeiros

SUMMARY. To describe the process that clinicians use to engage vulnerable urban adolescents in mental health counseling, the authors propose a tri-partite model of clinical engagement that takes into account: (1) *consumer preference*; (2) *risk and worry*; and (3) *youth development* (YD) perspectives. These conceptual lenses embody what adolescents want to talk about, their exposure to behavioral and environmental risks, and their coping and strengths. Based on responses given by urban adolescents seeking mental health services to a clinical self-assessment questionnaire (Adquest), this paper uses this tripartite model to summarize patterns of risk that service applicants experience, what they worry about, and how they cope. It explores the *substructure* of adolescent risk and vulnerability, through factor analysis of relevant items *across* a

---

Michael Surko, PhD, Ken Peake, DSW, Irwin Epstein, PhD, and Daniel Medeiros, MD, are affiliated with the Mount Sinai Adolescent Health Center, 320 East 94th Street, New York, NY 10128.

[Haworth co-indexing entry note]: "Multiple Risks, Multiple Worries, and Adolescent Coping: What Clinicians Need to Ask About." Surko, Michael et al. Co-published simultaneously in *Social Work in Mental Health* (The Haworth Social Work Practice Press, an imprint of The Haworth Press, Inc.) Vol. 3, No. 3, 2005, pp. 261-285; and: *Clinical and Research Uses of an Adolescent Mental Health Intake Questionnaire: What Kids Need to Talk About* (ed: Ken Peake, Irwin Epstein, and Daniel Medeiros) The Haworth Social Work Practice Press, an imprint of The Haworth Press, Inc., 2005, pp. 261-285. Single or multiple copies of this article are available for a fee from The Haworth Document Delivery Service [1-800-HAWORTH, 9:00 a.m. - 5:00 p.m. (EST). E-mail address: docdelivery@haworthpress.com].

http://www.haworthpress.com/web/SWMH
© 2005 by The Haworth Press, Inc. All rights reserved.
Digital Object Identifier: 10.1300/J200v03n03_03

broad range of Adquest life areas, to develop a typology of adolescents by *risk* and *worry*. Patterns of coping and desire to talk across a range of life areas within this typology are described, as are the practice implications. The authors conclude that even those adolescents who most concern clinicians–because they have high environmental and behavioral risk and low worry–present many different opportunities for engagement. *[Article copies available for a fee from The Haworth Document Delivery Service: 1-800-HAWORTH. E-mail address: <docdelivery@haworthpress.com> Website: <http://www.HaworthPress.com> © 2005 by The Haworth Press, Inc. All rights reserved.]*

KEYWORDS. Adolescent, risks, worries, coping, consumer, youth development, mental health, help-seeking

Urban adolescents from low-income communities face multiple health and mental health risks in their efforts at achieving healthy adulthood (Abernathy, Webster, & Vermeulen, 2002; Escarce, 2003). Some manage with their own personal, family and community resources. Others require help in the form of comprehensive community-based, health and mental health services. Too often, however, programs and/or professional efforts at helping take forms that are incompatible with what adolescents are seeking or with the ways they might define their concerns (Pittman, Irby, & Ferber, 2000; Carrera, 2003).

Too often, adolescents report that they leave their initial contacts with clinicians wishing they had been asked more about issues such as tobacco, alcohol, or drug use; sexual abuse, and other areas of risk (Schoen, Davis, Scott, & Collins et al., 1997; Klein & Wilson, 2002; Ackard & Neumark-Sztainer, 2001; Steiner & Gest, 1996). In other words, the majority of young people–including those engaging in risky behaviors–want to talk about their lives, their concerns, their behaviors and the potential consequences of these behaviors.

But to talk openly, they need to be asked about sensitive issues in ways that demonstrate that providers are competent to address adolescent concerns in a non-judgmental manner and that take into account client perspectives about what they want to talk about (Diaz, Peake, Surko, & Bhandarkar, 2004; Elliott, Nembhard, Giannone, Surko, Medeiros, & Peake, 2004). Unfortunately, however, the aforementioned studies suggest that practitioners are missing opportunities to engage young people, and that programs do not take into account what young people can contribute to programmatic knowledge about how to help them.

Seeking to avoid these engagement problems, Mount Sinai Adolescent Health Center (AHC) strives to ensure that its services are compatible with the needs and help-seeking patterns of urban adolescents. On the most direct level, AHC conducts peer-based street outreach to highest risk youth and welcomes any adolescent through its doors regardless of his or her insurance coverage and ability to pay. However, recognizing that these activities, in themselves, are not enough, AHC endeavors to learn from and about its clients in order to refine its services and tailor help to forms most compatible with client needs as they see them. To accomplish this the agency utilizes a number of information-gathering and processing strategies, including practice-based research (Peake, Mirabito, Epstein, & Giannone, 2004).

Employing a clinical "data-mining" approach (Epstein, 2001), the previous practice-based empirical studies in this collection (Peake & Epstein, 2004) exemplify one strategy. These studies analyze aggregate data drawn from an adolescent intake questionnaire (Adquest) completed by applicants for services before receiving their first clinical interview at AHC. Each of the preceding studies focused on a singular Adquest-explored domain in clients' lives. By contrast, this article attempts to summarize the patterns of risk that AHC mental health service applicants experience, what they worry about and how they cope. It places these informational components in a tri-partite model of clinical engagement that takes into account: (1) consumer preference; (2) risk and worry; and (3) youth development (YD) perspectives. Clinical implications are then discussed in the context of this expanded approach to the clinical engagement of adolescents.

As a practice tool, Adquest was originally intended by practitioners to enhance individual clinical engagement and provide practitioners with a profile of individual applicant risks, concerns, and needs. In so doing, Adquest asks each young person who is coming for mental health counseling to reflect on her or his own social environment, risk factors, worries, and coping across a range of life areas. It explores how these factors affect what individuals want and need to talk about in mental health counseling (Peake, Epstein, Mirabito, & Surko, 2004).

Practice experience suggests that Adquest itself enhances engagement by giving clients permission to talk about a range of life areas. Even when clients are initially reluctant to talk about these issues Adquest gets them on the table for discussion later in treatment (Elliot, Nembhard, Giannone, Surko, Medeiros, & Peake, 2004). By asking colloquially about a range of life concerns and risks even before a first meeting with a clinician, Adquest is intended to convey to service applicants that AHC is a place where highly charged issues such as racism, sexuality, substance use, abuse and violence, and other areas, are routinely explored and addressed.

Questions and response categories are intended as well to indirectly educate service applicants about behavioral and health issues before the first
in-person contact (e.g., questions related to sexual abuse are grouped with
other safety-related issues to indicate to patients that sexual violence and exploitation are not the client's fault, and should be considered differently than
the patient's own sexual behavior). Additionally, Adquest helps clinicians and
clinical trainees maintain a broad perspective on the intersections among a
wide range of behavioral and mental health issues in young persons' lives.

A secondary purpose of Adquest was to create a rich informational resource
in the form of an aggregate database for subsequent analysis that would contribute to staff reflectivity, clinical effectiveness, and program improvement
(Peake, Epstein, Mirabito, & Surko, 2004). This paper demonstrates how this
database was "mined" in order to create an overall picture of adolescent desire
to talk, their environmental and behavioral risks, their worries, and their
self-perceived coping.

A CONCEPTUAL MODEL
OF ADOLESCENT CLINICAL ENGAGEMENT

Based on the clinical experiences of AHC practitioners and prior analyses
of Adquest data, we suggest a tri-partite conceptual model of clinical engagement for adolescent mental health service providers. This approach combines
consumer, risk and youth development perspectives and is informed by
Adquest-generated findings as well as by AHC practitioners' experience. More
specifically, we suggest that clinical engagement must be viewed through three
different, but equally important lenses:

1. A *consumer* lens (i.e., how the client defines need);
2. A *vulnerability/risk/worries* lens (i.e., what client risks should the practitioner be concerned about); and,
3. A *youth development* lens (Pittman et al., 2000) (i.e., what contributions
   does the client bring and what are his/her strengths and coping capacities
   upon which treatment must build).

In this article, we contend that when working with adolescent clients, effective practitioners must *integrate* a view through all three lenses simultaneously
in order to get a complete clinical picture. However, we believe that it is useful
to conceptualize the clinical engagement process as one in which there is a *se-
quential shift in emphasis* from one lens to the other.

So, for example, to begin the engagement process a practitioner must understand that an adolescent who walks through the door physically has not yet crossed the self-perceived threshold as a client. To establish *clienthood* (i.e., to achieve trust and mutually define a problem to begin working on), the practitioner must understand which life domains the client wants to talk about and which–though important clinically–are at least initially off-limits. In other words, at the first point of contact, the effective practitioner must assess and validate what the client is initially seeking help with, and lend some assurances that this need will be addressed on the client's own terms. As AHC clinicians frequently comment: "Often the whole point of the first session is to secure a second session." With this precarious moment in mind, clinicians designed Adquest as a consumer-oriented intake instrument that asks service applicants what they want to talk about.

Once a client begins to talk openly and engagement begins, clinicians can then allow the "vulnerability/risk lens" to focus their assessment. As with low-income and minority youth in other large cities, AHC clients have considerable risk exposure, including poverty, racism, community violence, abuse, refugee-related dislocation, loss of caregivers, and–for many–high rates of behaviorally related health risks (Medeiros, Kramnick et al., 2004). And often they know it. Consequently, complete *risk* assessment involves not only what the practitioner determines places the client at-risk, but also the client's own worries and self-perceived vulnerability.

To competently proceed therapeutically, the practitioner must have a good sense of behavioral and environmental risk factors that contribute to the presenting problem and that s/he is not missing issues that may put the client at immediate risk. The vulnerability/risk lens distills these experiences while allowing the clinician and client to be comfortable with moving forward. Getting both sets of concerns on the table in a non-judgmental way also can serve to demonstrate the clinician's genuine interest in the client, as well as signal that therapy is a safe place to talk about loaded issues–if not now then later (Elliot et al., 2004). With risk and vulnerability in mind, Adquest surveys service applicants' environmental and behavioral risks as well as what they themselves worry about.

As therapeutic goals and strategies evolve, the YD lens–which takes into account client's strengths and resources–is applied. Successful therapy with adolescents requires the assessment and consideration of current and past coping patterns that serve as a foundation upon which to build. As a YD tool, Adquest asks adolescent clients to make a self-assessment of both coping and vulnerabilities. However, AHC's theory of help is that the most developmentally appropriate service model is one that recognizes and builds on adolescent clients' competencies by engaging them as partners in managing their own health and mental health care.

The empirical data analysis presented in this paper utilizes the foregoing conceptual framework to describe consumer desire to talk, a typology of risk and worry, and coping across various life areas of AHC service applicants. Additionally, the analysis considers the relationship between the risk/worry typology and desire to talk as well as age and gender differences in client wants, risks, worries, and coping patterns.

This analysis builds on the prior set of studies conducted by AHC practitioners examining client risk, coping, and need to talk about these to a counselor. Following the framework of previous studies, we begin our analysis by offering a broadly focused *snapshot* of desire to talk across multiple life areas. Second, we present the results of an exploratory factor analysis that examines the interrelationships among environmental and behavioral risks and adolescent worries across the life areas. Third, we show how these factors are related to stage of adolescence and gender. Fourth, we present a typology of adolescents by risk and worry—and the percentage of adolescents in each type. Fifth, we then present the percent in each risk/worry type by stage of adolescence and gender. Sixth, we present how well adolescents perceive themselves to be coping across the life areas. Finally, we discuss the implications of the findings for planning and delivery of mental health services.

METHOD

Practice Context and Population Served

AHC is a comprehensive health and mental health center serving inner-city youth (described in Diaz, Peake, Surko, & Bhandarkar, 2004). The study sample consisted of 759 adolescents presenting for intake to mental health services at AHC between 4/27/1999 and 4/9/2002. Of these, 36.0% were male and 64.0% were female. Ranging in age from 10 through 21, these urban adolescent applicants for mental health services come primarily from low-income, minority households in New York City.

Adquest

Adquest is an indigenous, context-specific instrument designed by practitioners for practitioners. The 80-item adolescent self-report asks about life areas such as race/ethnicity and racism, education, employment, safety, health, sex/body/birth control, substance abuse, friends/associates, family/home life, and personal life. The instrument asks young people seeking services to assess their own problems, needs, worries, and reasons for seeking counseling (Peake, Epstein et al., 2004). Thus Adquest embodies all three lenses.

The consumer perspective is represented in its focus on what each adolescent wants to talk about in counseling. Taking a risk/vulnerability perspective Adquest also queries adolescents about their behavioral and environmental risks as well as about their worries across a broad range of life areas. Finally, the YD perspective is embodied in questions that ask how well they see themselves coping with each life area.

A Clinical Data-Mining Approach

The questions posed in each of Adquest's life areas are more general than typical traditional research questionnaires. For example, a question from the safety section asks, "Have you ever been touched in a way that made you feel uncomfortable?" Affirmative responses to the question are likely to point to a broad range of issues relating to physical safety and sexual abuse or harassment. This reflects a strategy of using very broad trigger questions designed to alert clinicians to issues of concern that need further exploration.

For purposes of rapport and trust, adolescents Adquest intentionally does not ask for information that might lead to negative consequences for them (e.g., their own weapon-carrying, being in a fight, domestic violence within the home that could lead to involvement of child welfare authorities), as these issues are best addressed during the in-person interview where confidentiality can be negotiated. As a result, the data about risk are not highly specific. From a practice standpoint, however, this bias toward capturing a range of possibly problematic experiences is the most efficient clinically; the clinician uses affirmative answers to the trigger questions as starting points for a discussion about the young person's life and experiences.

Although its designers intended that one use of Adquest would be research, no analytic strategies were initially specified. In preparing for the data-mining process, a group of ten AHC practitioners and managers reviewed the 80 items and assigned items to one of five categories: Environmental risk, behavioral risk, worry, coping, and desire to talk with a counselor. These categories were used to analyze data pertaining to life areas based on the clinical organization of Adquest in psychosocial domains.

The previous Adquest studies built on *a priori* assumptions about discrete psychosocial domains in young persons' lives. Consequently, they focused on school and work (Diaz-Cruz, Medeiros, Surko, Hoffman, & Epstein, 2004) health (Medeiros, Kramnick, Diaz-Cruz, Surko, & Diaz, 2004), substance use (Medeiros, Carlson, Surko, Munoz, Castillo, & Epstein, 2004), family and friends (Giannone, Medeiros, Elliott, Perez, Carlson, & Epstein 2004), etc. Only two studies–one of lesbian, gay, bisexual, and questioning adolescents (Ciro, Surko, Bhandarkar, Helfgott, Peake, & Epstein, 2005), the second of racism and race/ethnicity (Surko, Ciro, Blackwood, Nembhard, & Peake, 2005)–were not limited to a single psychosocial area but explored issues across all life areas. Nonetheless, all of these studies focused on the desire to talk with a counselor about the different life areas as a dependent variable of primary interest.

This article extends previous analyses in a number of ways. First, it summarizes the other studies by presenting patterns of desire to talk *across* all ten life-areas. Second, it complements prior categorizations of the data by exploring the *substructure* of adolescent risk and vulnerability through factor analysis of relevant items *across* all of the life areas in Adquest. By creating and exploring the age and gender implications of a typology of risk and vulnerability, the article provides additional empirical support for the disjuncture between objective *risk* and *sense of vulnerability* in adolescents' lives. This further supports an earlier conceptual/empirical distinction made between client *wants* and *needs* (Peake, Epstein, Mirabito, & Surko, 2004). Finally, the paper presents patterns of coping across all life areas. In so doing, the analysis follows the clinically derived logic of engagement as a process of shifting emphasis from a consumer-oriented, to a risk/worry, to a YD strengths-based approach to clinical engagement and assessment.

FINDINGS

What Clients Want to Talk About?

To begin our analysis, Table 1 presents a broadly focused "snapshot" of adolescent desire to talk to a mental health counselor by life area, both in the full sample and broken down separately by stage of adolescence and by gender. Our findings indicate that at least initially, adolescents were most likely to want to talk about education (with 80.5% expressing a desire to talk), friends/associates (73.1%), health (73.0%), and employment (71.8%); and were least likely to want to talk about race/ethnicity (49.7%) and alcohol/drugs (59.0%).

Four areas reflected statistically significant differences by stage of adolescence: health, sex/body/birth control, family/home life, and personal life. More specifically, desire to talk about health increased across the stages of early, middle, and late adolescence, with 65.1% of early adolescents, 73.8% of middle adolescents, and 82.0% of late adolescents wanting to talk. Desire to talk about sex, body, or birth control showed the greatest difference between

TABLE 1. Proportion of Adolescents Wanting to Talk to a Counselor by Life Area, in Full Sample and Broken Down by Stage of Adolescence and Gender

Talk area	Full sample % (n)	Stage of adolescence				Gender		
		11-14 % (n)	15-16 % (n)	17-21 % (n)	χ^2	Male % (n)	Female % (n)	χ^2
Race/ethnicity	49.7 (377)	49.8 (127)	51.3 (155)	47.5 (95)	.704	48.9 (133)	50.2 (243)	.119
Education	80.5 (611)	76.1 (194)	84.1 (254)	81.0 (162)	5.724	76.1 (207)	83.1 (402)	5.378*
Employment	71.8 (545)	67.5 (172)	74.5 (225)	74.0 (148)	3.953	72.4 (197)	71.9 (348)	.024
Safety	69.4 (527)	67.1 (171)	70.2 (212)	71.5 (143)	1.163	62.1 (169)	73.6 (356)	10.705**
Health	73.0 (554)	65.1 (166)	73.8 (223)	82.0 (164)	16.425***	64.7 (176)	77.7 (376)	14.891***
Sex/body/birth control	66.1 (502)	50.6 (129)	71.5 (216)	78.5 (157)	17.708***	56.6 (154)	71.7 (347)	17.708***
Alcohol/drugs	59.0 (448)	53.7 (137)	63.6 (192)	59.0 (118)	5.548	55.5 (151)	61.0 (295)	2.127
Friends/associates	73.1 (555)	72.2 (184)	74.8 (226)	72.5 (145)	.599	66.2 (180)	77.3 (374)	10.950**
Family/home life	77.6 (589)	68.6 (175)	83.1 (251)	81.5 (163)	18.946***	68.4 (186)	83.1 (402)	21.699***
Personal life	78.4 (595)	66.7 (170)	82.5 (249)	88.0 (176)	34.756***	66.2 (180)	85.5 (414)	38.768***

early and middle adolescence; 50.6% of early adolescents wanted to talk, as opposed to 71.5% of middle adolescents and 78.5% of late adolescents. Similarly, larger proportions of middle and late adolescents expressed a desire to talk about family/home life and personal life: 83.1% of middle adolescents and 81.5% of late adolescents wanted to talk about family/home life, as opposed to 68.6% of early adolescents; and 82.5% of middle and 88.0% of late adolescents wanted to talk about their personal lives, as opposed to 66.7% of early adolescents.

When desire to talk was broken down by gender, seven of the ten life areas showed significant differences between males and females in proportion wanting to talk with a counselor: education, safety, health, sex/body/birth control, friends/associates, family/home life, and personal life. In each of these areas, females were more likely than males to express desire to talk with a counselor; proportions are shown in Table 1. These findings provide an overall picture through the "consumer lens," i.e., what AHC clients initially say they want to talk about.

Client Risks and Worries

Viewing Adquest data through a "risk/vulnerability lens" required looking at the substructure of risk and vulnerability items, in order to empirically identify clusters among the complete set of environmental and behavioral risk and worry responses. To do this, all self-reported behavioral and environmental risk items as well as worry items were subjected to factor analysis using the SPSS software package (SPSS Inc., 2003). Two factors, with eigenvalues of 5.773 and 2.697, were extracted and rotated using the varimax procedure. Items significantly loading (> .4) on these factors were identified as candidates for inclusion in scales measuring each factor. One item whose conceptual content diverged from the bulk of scale items was excluded (see below) from each scale. Items selected for inclusion in each of the scales are shown in Table 2.

Items loading on the first factor, which we designated the Environmental/Behavioral Risk factor, included: witnessed violence, threatened with a weapon, able to get a gun, ever offered drugs, ever spent time with a drug user, ever had sex, ever used drugs to make sex better, ever tried tobacco, ever tried alcohol, ever tried marijuana, and used alcohol or other drugs in the past month. Worry about own drug use also loaded significantly on the factor but was excluded from the risk scale because it was the lone worry item.

Items loading on the second factor, designated the Worry factor, included: ever worried about hurting self or others; worry about health issues; worry about weight; worry about sleep quantity; worry about sex, body, or birth control; worry about friends or associates; and worry about things not mentioned

TABLE 2. Environmental Risk, Behavioral Risk, and Worry Items Significantly Loading (> .4) onto Environmental/Behavioral Risk and Worry Factors

Type of variable	Environmental/Behavioral Risk factor[a] items	Worry factor[b] items
Environmental risk	Witnessed violence Threatened with weapon Able to get gun Offered drugs Spend time with drug user	
Behavioral risk	Ever had sex Used drugs to make sex better Tried tobacco Tried alcohol Tried marijuana Alcohol/drugs past month	
Worry		Worry hurt self/others Health worry Weight worry Sleep quantity worry Sex worry Worry friends/associates Things not on survey worry

[a]Eigenvalue = 5.773, [b]Eigenvalue = 2.697

on the survey. Having been touched in a way that made the client uncomfortable loaded significantly on this factor but was excluded because the content diverged from the other worry items and it was the lone environmental risk item among the remaining seven items. Furthermore, this item was significantly influenced by gender ($\chi^2 = 49.80$, $p < .001$), with far fewer males reporting this experience (11.0%) than females (34.5%).

Items loading on the Environmental/Behavioral Risk and Worry factors were separately summed to create two conceptually distinct scales, each measuring a single factor. Internal reliabilities of the scales, as measured with the Cronbach alpha statistic, were .82 for the 11-item Environmental/Behavioral Risk scale and .66 for the 7-item Worry scale. The resulting scales were modestly positively correlated with each other ($r = .37$, $p < .01$), supporting the assumption of independence. Both were split as close as possible to their respective medians (53.6 for Risk and 42.7 for Worry) to create "high" and "low" categories for each scale.

Proportions of adolescents scoring high and low on each of the factor scales were broken down by stage of adolescence and gender (see Table 3). Proportions of adolescents scoring high on each of the scales significantly increased

TABLE 3. Proportions of Adolescents with High Environmental/Behavioral Risk and Worry Scores, by Stage of Adolescence and Gender

	High Env/ Beh Risk % (n)	χ^2	High Worry % (n)	χ^2
Stage of adolescence		85.298***		53.245***
Early (11-14)	24.7 (63)		41.6 (106)	
Middle (15-16)	51.3 (155)		58.9 (178)	
Late (17-21)	67.0 (134)		75.5 (151)	
Gender		.012		39.765***
Male	46.7 (127)		42.3 (115)	
Female	46.3 (224)		65.9 (319)	

$*p < .05, **p < .01, ***p < .001$

across the three adolescent age groups. For example, for early adolescents, 24.7% had high Environmental/Behavioral Risk scale scores, as compared with 51.3% of middle adolescents, and 67.0% of late adolescents. Similarly, for the Worry scale, 41.6% of early adolescents had high scores, as compared with 58.9% of middle adolescents and 75.5% of late adolescents. Scores on the Environmental/Behavioral Risk scale were not significantly associated with gender, but females were significantly more likely than males to have a high score on the Worry scale (65.9% vs. 42.3%, respectively).

High and low scores on the Environmental/Behavioral Risk scale were significantly associated with high and low scores on the Worry scale (see Table 4). In other words, the higher the risk, the higher the worry. However, this was not always true. And, as we have seen before in our want/need to talk typology, at-risk adolescents do not always recognize their own vulnerability. Alternately, some adolescents who are relatively low-risk may consider themselves to be highly vulnerable.

With these potential disjunctures between objective risk and subjective sense of vulnerability in mind, each of the four possible combinations of low and high scores was designated as a "Risk-Worry type." Adolescent service applicants scoring low on both the Environmental/Behavioral Risk and Worry scales were designated Type I, those with low Environmental/Behavioral Risk and high Worry were designated Type II, those with high Environmental/Behavioral Risk and high Worry were designated Type III, and those with high

Environmental/Behavioral Risk and low Worry. Proportion of adolescents falling into each of the categories is shown in Table 4: 29.6% were Type I, 24.0% were Type II, 33.3% were Type III, and 13.0% were Type IV.

As shown in Table 5, stage of adolescence and gender were both significantly associated with Risk-Worry type as defined above (see Table 5). For example, the proportion of adolescents identified as Type I decreased across

TABLE 4. Distribution of Adolescents by Levels of Environmental/Behavioral Risk and Worry[a,b]

Level of Environmental/Behavioral Risk	Level of Worry	
	Low % (n)	High % (n)
Low	Type I 29.6 (225)	Type II 24.0 (182)
High	Type IV 13.0 (99)	Type III 33.3 (253)

[a]N = 759, [b]$\chi^2(1)$ = 56.902, $p < .001$

TABLE 5. Risk-Worry Type by Gender and Stage of Adolescence

	Risk-Worry Type			
	Type I (Low-Risk Low-Worry) % (n)	Type II (Low-Risk High-Worry) % (n)	Type III (High-Risk High-Worry) % (n)	Type IV (High-Risk Low-Worry) % (n)
Stage of Adolescence[a,b]				
Early (10-14)	49.4 (126)	25.9 (66)	15.7 (40)	9.0 (23)
Middle (15-16)	25.2 (76)	23.5 (71)	35.4 (107)	15.9 (48)
Late (17-21)	10.5 (21)	22.5 (45)	53.0 (106)	14.0 (28)
Gender[c,d]				
Male	38.6 (105)	14.7 (40)	27.6 (75)	19.1 (52)
Female	24.4 (118)	29.3 (142)	36.6 (177)	9.7 (47)

[a]N = 757, [b]χ^2 = 113.822, $p < .001$, [c]N = 756, [d]χ^2 = 43.426, $p < .001$

stages of adolescence (49.4%, 25.2%, and 10.5% for early, middle, and late, respectively), and proportion identified as Type III increased (15.7%, 35.4%, and 53.0%, respectively). More males than females were identified as Type I (38.5% for males versus 24.4% for females) and Type IV (19.1% for males versus 9.7% for females), and more females than males were identified as Type II (29.3% for females versus 14.7% for males) and Type III (36.6% for females versus 27.6% for males). Clearly then, AHC service applicants differ markedly in their risk/vulnerability profiles and these in turn, are significantly influenced by stage of adolescence as well as by gender.

Superimposing the "consumer lens" on the "risk/vulnerability lens" leads us to consideration of what each of the Risk-Worry types were interested in talking about and how they can best be clinically engaged. Accordingly, Table 6 indicates that adolescents in each of the Risk-Worry types were interested in talking about different life areas.

In general, higher proportions of adolescents in Types II and III wanted to talk about each of the life areas than did adolescents from Types I and IV. Second, the areas of education, family/home life, and personal life were among

TABLE 6. Desire to Talk About Life Areas by Risk-Worry Type

Life Area	Risk-Worry Type				x^2
	Type I	Type II	Type III	Type IV	
	(Low-Risk Low-Worry)	(Low-Risk High-Worry)	(High-Risk High-Worry)	(High-Risk Low-Worry)	
	% (n)	% (n)	% (n)	% (n)	
Race/ethnicity	44.4 (100)	54.9 (100)	55.3 (140)	37.4 (37)	13.720***
Education	73.3 (165)	86.8 (158)	87.7 (222)	66.7 (66)	32.517***
Employment	60.9 (137)	72.5 (132)	80.2 (203)	73.7 (73)	22.358***
Safety	60.9 (137)	81.3 (148)	76.3 (193)	49.5 (49)	43.993***
Health	53.3 (120)	84.1 (153)	90.5 (229)	52.5 (52)	115.864***
Sex/body/birth control	48.9 (110)	68.7 (125)	84.6 (214)	53.5 (53)	75.882***
Alcohol/drugs	44.4 (100)	55.5 (101)	73.9 (187)	60.6 (60)	44.005***
Friends/ associates	61.8 (139)	80.8 (147)	82.6 (209)	60.6 (60)	39.625***
Family/home life	63.6 (143)	83.5 (152)	89.7 (227)	67.7 (67)	56.201***
Personal life	64.9 (146)	87.9 (160)	90.1 (228)	61.6 (61)	70.946***

$p < .05$, **$p < .01$, ***$p < .001$

the ones adolescents wanted most to talk about across Risk-Worry types. Third, health was a life area that relatively high proportions of adolescents in Types II and III wanted to talk about (84.1% and 90.5%, respectively). Fourth, unlike adolescents from the other three Risk-Worry types, Type IV adolescents were most focused on talking about employment (73.7%).

Client Coping

The final component of this data analysis looks at adolescents from a YD perspective, namely patterns of positive coping in each life area and how these are influenced by stage of adolescence and by gender. Positive coping varied markedly by domain and was significantly related to stage of adolescence and gender for several of the life areas examined (see Table 7). Adolescents were most likely to report positive coping in the life areas of sex/body/birth control (95.0%) and alcohol/drugs (93.3%) and least likely to report positive coping with balancing school and work (60.6%; computed only for adolescents reporting working, n = 137) and employment (66.8%).

The proportion of clients reporting positive coping declined significantly across the stages of early, middle, and late adolescence (ages 11-14, 15-16, and 17-21) for four of the life areas and increased significantly in none. Thus, with regard to health, 90.4% of early adolescents reported positive coping, as opposed to 87.1% of middle adolescents and 75.8% of late adolescents. Similar patterns were noted with friendships (93.5%, 87.5%, and 79.0%), family/home life (85.0%, 69.4%, and 58.9%), and personal life (90.0%, 79.0%, and 67.4%). Significantly greater proportions of males than females reported positive coping in the life areas of health (92.2% of males vs. 80.9% of females) and personal life (85.2% of males vs. 76.6% of females).

DISCUSSION

Clinical Significance of Desire to Talk

Statistical significance is one thing; clinical significance is another. From a PBR perspective (Epstein, 2001), the former has value only if it informs the latter. Individual adolescents in this sample were asked about their various possible desires to talk via a self-report questionnaire administered prior to any encounter with a clinician. Though it is tempting to define the sample population as one that is *seeking* counseling in general, prior to our analysis we had no systematic data regarding variations in either help-seeking patterns or how these were influenced by developmental stage and gender. All we could counsel

TABLE 7. Proportions of Adolescents Reporting Positive Coping, in Full Sample and Broken Down by Stage of Adolescence and Gender

Life Area	Full Sample	Stage of Adolescence			x^2	Gender		x^2
		Early (11-14)	Middle (15-16)	Late (17-21)		Male	Female	
Education	78.8 (584)	79.8 (201)	76.5 (228)	81.1 (154)	1.651	74.2 (196)	81.3 (386)	4.999
Employment	66.8 (507)	62.0 (158)	68.2 (206)	71.0 (142)	4.557	65.8 (179)	67.4 (326)	.188
Balancing school/work[a]	60.6 (83)	68.2 (15)	68.0 (34)	51.6 (33)	3.850	63.0 (29)	58.9 (53)	.219
Health	85.0 (588)	90.4 (208)	87.1 (236)	75.8 (144)	18.897***	92.2 (236)	80.9 (351)	16.225***
Sex/body/birth control	95.0 (640)	96.2 (202)	94.9 (262)	93.6 (176)	1.372	95.9 (236)	94.4 (403)	.787
Alcohol/drugs	93.3 (653)	94.6 (212)	93.0 (264)	92.2 (177)	1.077	91.7 (232)	94.2 (420)	1.571
Friends/associates	87.3 (638)	93.5 (231)	87.5 (253)	79.0 (154)	20.801***	90.2 (238)	85.6 (399)	3.110
Family/home life	71.8 (525)	85.0 (209)	69.4 (200)	58.9 (116)	38.077***	77.4 (205)	68.8 (320)	6.098
Personal life	79.6 (546)	90.0 (206)	79.0 (218)	67.4 (122)	31.761***	85.2 (202)	76.6 (343)	7.165**

*p < .05, **p < .01, ***p < .001
[a]Computed for adolescents reporting working; N = 137

the counselors was to assume a positive and open stance toward providing adolescents with mental health treatment. At best, practice wisdom told us that the vast majority of prospective clients are initially ambivalent about being referred for mental health services, and usually enter services *under pressure* from parents, or from schools or other institutions (such as the criminal justice system).

Instead, our empirical findings suggest a picture of a population that is generally open to talking about many life issues and, thus, presents many opportunities for engagement. For example, even regarding drugs (the area perhaps most clearly defined as *problematic behavior* and one that adolescents were least desirous of talking about) more than half of all adolescents wanted to talk. This held true for all stages of adolescence and for males as well as females.

In other life areas–that are not, by definition, defined as problem-behaviors or *illegal*–particularly education, safety, friends, home life, personal life, large proportions of all groups wanted to talk. In fact, most adolescent service applicants are willing to talk about a range of subjects and the data suggest that almost all will have some life areas that open the door for clinical engagement.

Clearly, our findings reinforce the assumption that practitioners should be acutely aware of the consumer perspective when first meeting with adolescent clients. Furthermore, therapists must be extremely flexible when assessing where to begin and what issues should be put on the table for initial exploration. As a result, clinicians are challenged to think holistically about each client as a unique individual so that issues that the client is comfortable dis- cussing provide avenues into those life areas that are more loaded and less immediately available for exploration.

Interestingly, desire to talk about health, sex/body/birth control, family/home, and personal life increased with age. Although younger adolescents were less desirous of talking about these areas, they were equally as open as older adolescents to talking about race and racism, education and work, safety and friends. These findings can be understood in the context of two developmental trends. First, the areas which older adolescents were more interested in talking about are consistent with higher reported rates of sexual activity (Labor et al., 2004), higher reported rates of health concerns (Medeiros, Kramnick, Diaz-Cruz, Surko, & Diaz, 2004), and the developmental trend for some adolescents to experience conflict in family relationships as they begin to seek increasing autonomy (Smetana, 1995). Second, throughout adolescence, young people continue to gain cognitive skills and the ability to reflect on their own thinking and learning strategies (Zimmerman, 1989), although this may not necessarily make them better problem-solvers until they gain experience in mastering the application of these new cognitive abilities to concrete situations (Keating, 1990). It is therefore not surprising that issues in these areas are of more interest as a topic of discussion among older adolescents.

Although females were more likely to want to talk than males about education, safety, health, sex/body/birth control, friends/associates, family/home life, and personal life, more than half of males also wanted to talk about each of these topics. For instance, although significantly more females wanted to talk about safety than males, more than 62% of the males indicated a desire to talk about this issue before they had even met a practitioner. Clearly, the findings show that practitioners must avoid allowing gender stereotypes to determine what they view as pertinent issues for exploration during the engagement phase.

Nonetheless, the increase in desire to talk that occurs with age, coupled with the difference between males and females, suggests that, among the young people we serve, practitioners need to have a wide repertoire of clinical engagement approaches at their disposal. Furthermore, they must be able to be adaptable and creative in their use of these different therapeutic strategies. They must be comfortable with asking directly about issues–because the majority of adolescents are open to that approach. Simultaneously, they must also be comfortable shifting strategies and–with some younger adolescents–using more indirect engagement approaches, especially initially.

For most adolescents, however, we suggest that there is considerable benefit in having practitioners openly discuss what adolescents themselves want from treatment, up front. By taking this position, therapists can openly acknowledge that they cannot–and do not want to–control the clinical dialogue. Perhaps placing the discussion in a positive YD framework–one that takes into account the young person's perspective on what is relevant–best does this. This discussion should include a positive assessment of their social networks, especially their families and peers, recognizing that this discussion may be highly charged for the young person as well as for the therapist.

To manage the strains and ambiguities that a more consumer-oriented clinical stance generates, program managers, and supervisors need to provide practitioners with opportunities to share their experiences with one another, through group-based supervision, so that individual practitioners can support one another in this process.

Clinical Significance of Environmental/Behavioral Risk and Worry

The distinction made in prior Adquest analyses between what clients *want* to talk about and what they *need* to talk about is paralleled in the Risk/Worry typology developed in this paper. Both sets of analyses indicate that adolescents' service requests and clinical requisites are not simply a by-product of their exposures to risk but depend, importantly, on the meanings they attach to those experiences.

Programmatically, these findings validate the decision to independently assess adolescent risk as well as their perception of risk. Here again, however, the YD lens helps the clinician to place the discussion of risk and worry in a positive context. Hence, both the risk lens and the YD lens are essential to effective clinical engagement. This analysis suggests that the perspective provided by each lens needs to be synthesized in the context of the therapeutic dialogue.

Likewise, although it might seem clinically and conceptually logical to dichotomize adolescents as either *actively* being risk takers or *passively* being at-risk from socially toxic environments, a distinction between environmental and behavioral risk was not justified by our empirical analysis. Looking more closely at the items contained within the first factor generated in our factor analysis (i.e., Environmental/Behavioral Risk), we learned that exposure to environmental risks and involvements in risky behaviors were closely associated.

This suggests that clinicians should assess risk *holistically* and explore the possibility of behavioral risk-taking when discovering environmental risk exposure, and vice versa. Furthermore, it is important that definitions of *high-risk* among adolescents do not overemphasize one aspect of risk at the expense of the other.

Returning to our empirical analysis, we saw that scores on both the Environmental/Behavioral Risk and Worry scales increased steadily with age. This was anticipated for the Environmental/Behavioral Risk scale, because many Adquest items are posed in terms of lifetime prevalence (e.g., "Have you ever been a victim of violence?"). As young people get older, therefore, they have wider exposure to environmental risk and more opportunities for experimentation with risky behaviors.

However, a similar but unanticipated association was found between Worry scores and age. This is disturbing as well as surprising, because this scale is composed primarily of ratings of present worry in multiple life areas, and increase with age could not be dismissed as an artifact of the way questions were asked.

Not unexpectedly, females were more likely to score high on the Worry scale than males. However, scores on the Environmental/Behavioral Risk scale were not significantly associated with gender. This latter finding runs counter to the stereotype of males being more likely to engage in risk behaviors related to substance use and violence.

In part, our findings serve to remind us that females are also susceptible to both environmental risk exposure and involvement in high-risk behaviors. Consequently, assessment of risk for females, and planning services for them, should be predicated on an assumption that females are as at-risk as males—both behaviorally and environmentally–to ensure that high-risk females are identified.

Clinical Significance of the Risk/Worry Typology

The Risk/Worry typology findings suggest additional implications for clinical engagement. The proportion of adolescents in Type I (low risk-low worry) was almost five times smaller in late than in early adolescents. This is partially predictable because of the use of lifetime prevalence items in the Environmental/Behavioral Risk scale. And greater risk shows itself in part through a corresponding increase in worry in late adolescents. Thus, the proportion of adolescents falling into Type III (high risk-high worry) was more than three times greater for them than for early adolescents. The good news, however, such as it is, is that the majority of adolescents with high exposure to environmental and behavioral risks are worried about these risks and, thereby, likely to be available for clinical engagement and intervention.

From the standpoint of both engagement and risk, the young persons that seem most vulnerable, are of greatest concern, and who may require our most active clinical attention to engagement are those falling into Type IV (high risk-low worry). Across each age group, the proportion of these adolescents remained roughly constant, i.e., within the 10-15% range. Their low levels of worry or conversely high levels of denial about the issues facing them across life areas can be very misleading.

Paradoxically, the consumer lens is particularly important with this group as a tool for engagement, because they might well be harder to engage than other groups, and the stakes–in terms of negative consequences of risk–may be higher. Worry is less of what is driving them into therapy; therefore, attention to other means of engaging them needs to be explored. The challenge here is similar to that of clinicians seeking to help substance-abusing clients appreciate the problematic nature of their drug or alcohol use–there is often some work to be done before clients are interested in making changes. In substance abuse work, this challenge has been addressed with the stages of change model (Prochaska, DiClemente, & Norcross, 1992) and the development of techniques of motivational interviewing (Miller & Rollnick, 2002). In this approach, clinicians work to build clients' motivation to change by exploring, and helping clients resolve, their ambivalence. The approach has been found to be effective for helping clients change behavior related to alcohol and drugs, and also diet and exercise (Burke, Arkowitz, & Menchola, 2003). Similar strategies are indicated with Type IV adolescents.

The findings in this paper show that Type IV adolescents as a group were most interested in talking about education, employment, and family/home life.

This relatively external focus may need to be initially accepted by clinicians in order to promote client engagement. At the same time, the perspective from the risk/vulnerability lens should be employed in clinical assessment and tracking of environmental and behavioral risks over the course of treatment by the clinician. With these clients, practitioners need to make especially sound and comprehensive assessments based on what these applicants say they want from treatment, how at-risk they are and, ultimately how they cope.

Clinical Significance of Coping

Our final analysis indicated that positive coping scores were generally higher for early adolescents than for middle and late adolescents. More specifically, with increasing age, AHC treatment applicants declined in their self-assessed coping with health, friends/associates, family/home life, and personal life. This finding is particularly noteworthy and disturbing because it suggests that many within this clinical sample of adolescents are poorly prepared for adulthood. Consequently, the developmental needs of many–in regard to feeling competent–are easily overlooked if clinicians do not take coping into account in their assessments.

There were, however, exceptions to this age-related decline in coping. Adolescents' self-rated coping remained high (with over 90% reporting positive coping) across stages of adolescence with regard to the sex/body/birth control and alcohol/drugs domains. This would initially seem to be at odds with the view of many clinicians that adolescent experimentation in these areas is a substantial cause of concern, particularly in a clinical population. Practice-based research about the early engagement process may be needed in order to resolve this seeming contradiction.

Similarly, the increase in desire to talk about sex/body/birth control with increasing age may seem at odds with the finding that adolescents in all three groups reported coping well in that domain. However, this is true only if one assumes that counseling adolescents means talking only about dysfunctions and problem areas.

On the contrary, and consistent with a YD perspective, we view this finding as suggestive of the possibility that as adolescents get older, they are increasingly eager to gain mastery over sexuality as a developmental task and to achieve competence. Recognizing the need to talk about sex and sexuality is an important milestone in this process. As they get older, young persons often lack opportunities for discussion, information, and guidance offered in a developmentally appropriate way.

For example, while teachers, health educators, and parents might be comfortable offering sexuality education and counseling at levels that suit early adolescents, older adolescents may be seeking more sophisticated discussions of sex and sexuality. They may lack adult figures, professional or not, who feel comfortable or competent in addressing these needs.

This observation is consistent with a YD perspective that adolescent sexual behaviors are not merely a set of indicators of potential risk but an expression of a developmental need to master this aspect of approaching adulthood. Too often services have been designed only from a risk perspective (Labor et al., 2004).

On a different clinical tack, some AHC practitioners participating in this research hypothesized early on that a high proportion of adolescents would express a primary interest in talking about family and home life because it represented a *safe* starting point for testing a therapeutic relationship with a mental health counselor. However, although adolescents may well find this a relatively less threatening topic around which to initially frame problems, family and home life was also the area in which many indicated that they were coping least well. Certainly the reports on positive coping indicate that adolescents seeking counseling–especially older adolescents–identified their problems within the context of their personal lives and, especially, their family relationships. On multiple counts, therefore, our findings suggest that these are generally good starting points for therapists to begin to clinically engage adolescents.

A Limitation of the Study and Future Directions

This study used data collected from adolescents before they made their first face-to-face contact with a mental health clinician. Although it provided a rich picture of risk, worries, coping, and desire to talk about a variety of life areas, the conclusions drawn about engagement of adolescents must remain tentative as they were not tested, for example, against rates of second visits. One of the next steps in creating a picture of the early engagement process among our clients will be to examine Adquest data in conjunction with data about patterns of early engagement.

CONCLUSION: PRACTICE IMPLICATIONS

The foregoing findings and the lenses through which they have been interpreted suggest that adolescents present many different opportunities for engagement and possible intervention. The vast majority of AHC mental health counseling applicants want to talk about some life area, and most are willing to talk about multiple aspects of their lives. More report coping well than otherwise but they appear to be coping less well as they age. Generally, they want to talk most about those areas in which they experience themselves as doing poorly. A notable exception is the area of sex and sexuality, which with increasing age, they want to talk about more regardless of their self-perceived coping. Almost all want to talk about their families, and this is a realm in which they report the lowest level of coping.

The discovery of a "core" group of high risk/low worry adolescents, 10% to 15% of every age group, is cause for particular concern. These highest-risk adolescents require the most creative approach to engagement and the most careful application of the multiple lenses. Nevertheless, Adquest data analysis reveals that even among these adolescents high proportions are willing to talk about many issues.

Viewed through the *consumer* lens, the issues that they most want to talk about may seem surprising–employment, family, education, and substance abuse. And because employment and education ranked so high among issues adolescents wanted to discuss, a *Youth Development* lens is essential when considering how to engage *these* adolescents and how to build on their positive coping capacities. At the same time, a *risk/vulnerability* lens needs to be employed in clinically assessing and tracking these young persons.

Irrespective of their risk/vulnerability profiles, adolescent service applicants have something to tell us and practitioners must be prepared to listen. In order to be effective listeners we must be able to recognize the strengths of our clients, and cannot focus on risks to the exclusion of strengths. For some, the initial focus of talking may have to be on their strengths. Nonetheless, strengths should be recognized and mobilized for all.

To accomplish this we must be able to explore our clients' own perceptions of their self-perceived service requirements, risks, worries, and coping capacities. Furthermore, we must show that we value these perceptions even when they do not fit neatly with our own. Integrating the consumer, risk and YD perspectives necessitates that as practitioners we are able to see the big picture, even when concerned about particular risks and vulnerabilities.

In turn, this requires that we remain flexible, agile, and adept in shifting focus, at times leading the discussion into areas that represent our concerns and at others falling back and letting the client take the lead. We must be able to think strategically so that, over the course of establishing a mutually agreed upon treatment contract, we are able to bring conflicting perspectives together into focus. In the short run this demands that we are able to keep what may seem like mutually incompatible viewpoints and perspectives in our heads.

Lastly, practitioners must be competent in working with adolescents in developmentally appropriate ways and should take into account how well their clients' families, social environment, programs and services, and communities provide opportunities for meaningful participation in developmentally relevant ways. Discovering that older adolescents report the highest level of worry and poorest coping suggests that they require, and lack, more sophisticated opportunities for discussion and reflection about their life concerns. Community structures and services that offer opportunities that match their changing developmental needs are desperately needed by low-income adolescents. Mining Adquest information and interpreting it through multiple lenses has significantly sharpened our clinical picture of this need.

REFERENCES

Abernathy, T.J., Webster, G., & Vermeulen, M. (2002). Relationship between poverty and health among adolescents. *Adolescence, 37*(145), 55-67.

Ackard, D., & Neumark-Sztainer, D. (2001). Health care information sources for adolescents: Age and gender differences on use, concerns, and needs. *Journal of Adolescent Health, 29*, 170-6.

Burke, B., Arkowitz, H., & Menchola, M. (2003). The efficacy of motivational interviewing: A meta-analysis of controlled clinical trials. *Journal of Consulting and Clinical Psychology, 71*(5), 843-861.

Carrera, M. (2003). Getting your youth development message to stick. New York State Department of Health: Youth development Symposium, November 14, 2003, Albany NY.

Ciro, D., Surko, M., Bhandarkar, K., Helfgott, N., Peake, K., & Epstein, I. (2005). Lesbian, gay, bisexual, and sexual-orientation questioning adolescents seeking mental health services: Risk factors, worries, and desire to talk about them. *Social Work in Mental Health, 3* (3), 213-234.

Diaz-Cruz, E., Mederios, D., Surko, M., Hoffman, R., & Epstein, I. (2004). Adolescents need to talk about school and work in mental health treatment. *Social Work in Mental Health, 3*(1/2), 155-171.

Diaz, A., Peake, K., Surko, M., & Bhandarkar, K. (2004). Including at risk adolescents in their own health and mental health care: A Youth Development perspective. *Social Work in Mental Health, 3*(1/2), 3-22.

Elliott, J., Nembhard, M., Giannone, V., Surko, M., Medeiros, D., & Peake, K. (2004). Clinical uses of an adolescent intake questionnaire: Adquest as a bridge to engagement. *Social Work in Mental Health, 3*(1/2),83-102.

Epstein, I. (2001). Using available clinical information in practice-based research: Mining for silver while dreaming of gold. *Social Work in Health Care, 33*(3/4), 15-32.

Escarce, J.J. (2003). Socioeconomic status and the fates of adolescents. *Health Services Research, 38*(5), 1229-34.

Giannone, V., Medeiros, D., Elliott, J., Perez, C., Carlson, E., & Epstein, I. (2004). Adolescents' self-reported risk factors and desire to talk about family and friends: Implications for practice and research. *Social Work in Mental Health, 3*(1/2), 191-208.

Keating, D.P. (1990). Adolescent thinking. In S.S. Feldman, and G.R. Elliott (Eds.), *At the threshold: The developing adolescent*, Cambridge, MA: Harvard University Press.

Klein, J., & Wilson, K. (2002). Delivering quality care: Adolescents' discussion of health risks with their providers. *Journal of Adolescent Health, 30*, 190-195.

Labor, N., Medeiros, D., Carlson, E., Pullo, N., Seehaus, M., Peake, K., & Epstein, I. (2004). Adolescents' need to talk about sex and sexuality in an urban mental health setting. *Social Work in Mental Health, 3*(1/2), 135-154.

Medeiros, D., Carlson, E., Surko, M., Munoz, N., Castillo, M., & Epstein, I. (2004). Adolescent self-reported substance risks and their need to talk about them in mental health counseling. *Social Work in Mental Health 3*(1/2), 171-190.

Medeiros, D., Kramnick, L., Diaz-Cruz, E., Surko, M., & Diaz, A. (2004). Adolescents seeking mental health services: Self-reported health risks and the need to talk. *Social Work in Mental Health, 3*(1/2), 121-134.

Miller, W. R., & Rollnick, S. (2002). *Motivational interviewing: Preparing people for change* (2nd ed.). New York: Guilford Press.

Peake, K., & Epstein, I. (2004). Theoretical and practical imperatives for reflective social work organizations in health and mental health: The place of practice-based research. *Social Work in Mental Health, 3*(1/2), 23-38.

Peake, K., Epstein, I., Mirabito, D., & Surko, M. (2004). Development and utilization of a practice-based, adolescent intake questionnaire (Adquest): Surveying which risks, worries, and concerns urban youth want to talk about. *Social Work in Mental Health, 3*(1/2), 55-82.

Peake, K., Mirabito, D., Epstein, I., & Giannone, V. (2004). Creating and sustaining a practice-based research group in an urban adolescent mental health program. *Social Work in Mental Health, 3*(1/2), 39-54.

Pittman, K., Irby, M., & Ferber, T. (2000). Unfinished business: Further reflections on a decade of promoting youth development. In *Youth development: Issues, challenges, and directions.* Philadelphia, PA: Public/Private Ventures.

Prochaska, J.O., DiClemente, C.C., & Norcross, J.C. (1992). In search of how people change: Applications to addictive behaviors. *American Psychologist, 47,* 1102-1114.

Schoen, C., Davis, K., Scott Collins, K., Greenberg, L., Des Roches, C., & Abrams, M. (1997). *The Commonwealth Fund Survey of the Health of Adolescent Girls.* New York: The Commonwealth Fund. Retrieved on August 18, 2002 from http://www.cmwf.org/programs/women/adoleshl.asp#GIRLS

Smetana, J.G. (1995). Parenting styles and conceptions of parental authority during adolescence. *Child Development, 66,* 299-316.

SPSS Inc. (2003). Statistical Package for the Social Sciences (Version 11.5) [Computer software]. Chicago IL: SPSS Inc.

Steiner, B.D., & Gest, K.L. (1996). Do adolescents want to hear preventive counseling messages in outpatient settings? *Journal of Family Practice, 43*(4), 375-81.

Surko, M., Ciro, D., Blackwood, C., Nembhard, M., & Peake, K. (2005). Experience of racism as a correlate of developmental and health outcomes among urban adolescent mental health clients. *Social Work in Mental Health, 3*(3) 235-260.

Zimmerman, B. J. (1989). A social cognitive view of self-regulated academic learning. *Journal of Educational Psychology, 81*(3), 329-339.

Data-Mining Client Concerns
in Adolescent Mental Health Services:
Clinical and Program Implications

Ken Peake
Michael Surko
Irwin Epstein
Daniel Medeiros

SUMMARY. Via a practice-based research collaboration, clinicians, supervisors, and managers in an urban adolescent mental health program studied previously collected intake information concerning adolescent risk exposures, behaviors, worries, and self-assessed coping. In addition, desire to talk with a mental health counselor about specific risks and worries was systematically analyzed with the aim of generating practice insights into the *clinical challenge* of engaging urban adolescents in mental health services. Though provided with research consultation, practitioners were full participants in all aspects of the research

Ken Peake, DSW, is Assistant Director, Mount Sinai Adolescent Health Center (AHC), 320 East 94th Street, New York, NY 10128. Michael Surko, PhD, is Coordinator of the ACT for Youth Downstate Center for Excellence at AHC. Irwin Epstein, PhD, is Helen Rehr Professor of Applied Social Work Research in Health, Hunter College School of Social Work, 129 East 79th Street, New York, NY 10021 (E-mail: iepstein@ hunter.cuny.edu). Daniel Medeiros, MD, is AHC's Director of Mental Health Services.

[Haworth co-indexing entry note]: "Data-Mining Client Concerns in Adolescent Mental Health Services: Clinical and Program Implications." Peake, Ken et al. Co-published simultaneously in *Social Work in Mental Health* (The Haworth Social Work Practice Press, an imprint of The Haworth Press, Inc.) Vol. 3, No. 3, 2005, pp. 287-304; and: *Clinical and Research Uses of an Adolescent Mental Health Intake Questionnaire: What Kids Need to Talk About* (ed: Ken Peake, Irwin Epstein, and Daniel Medeiros) The Haworth Social Work Practice Press, an imprint of The Haworth Press, Inc., 2005, pp. 287-304. Single or multiple copies of this article are available for a fee from The Haworth Document Delivery Service [1-800-HAWORTH, 9:00 a.m. - 5:00 p.m. (EST). E-mail address: docdelivery@haworthpress.com].

http://www.haworthpress.com/web/SWMH
© 2005 by The Haworth Press, Inc. All rights reserved.
Digital Object Identifier: 10.1300/J200v03n03_04

process. This organizational development process placed strains on the participants and organization, but many benefits were derived from it. One significant benefit was that *mining* the expressed concerns of clients gave participants a powerful vehicle for reshaping services. The organization came to see its clients as more than mere service recipients, resulting in a recommitment to Youth Development principles and a renewed effort to increase *direct* client participation in organizational life. *[Article copies available for a fee from The Haworth Document Delivery Service: 1-800-HAWORTH. E-mail address: <docdelivery@haworthpress.com> Website: <http://www.HaworthPress.com> © 2005 by The Haworth Press, Inc. All rights reserved.]*

KEYWORDS. Data-mining, practice-based research, practitioner research, organizational reflection, organizational learning, adolescent, youth development

INTRODUCTION

This article describes an adolescent mental health clinic's experience in involving clinicians, supervisors and program managers in utilizing clinical data-mining (CDM) for practice-based research (PBR) purposes (Epstein, 2001). The data that were *mined* was information generated by an adolescent self-assessment questionnaire (Adquest) administered at intake.

Originally, practitioners designed Adquest in collaboration with a client advisory group to better understand the service requests and needs of *individual* service applicants as they presented themselves to the clinic and to more effectively engage them in long-term mental health treatment (Peake, Epstein, Mirabito, & Surko, 2004). Adquest's eighty items explored adolescents' self-described behaviors, risk exposures, concerns, desire to talk in counseling and levels of coping across a number of clinically derived psychosocial domains–school and work, safety, health, sexuality, substance use, and family and home life.

By retrieving, aggregating and analyzing intake information from a one-year cohort of adolescent mental health service applicants, staff could consider its *programmatic* implications. The project took place within the mental health component of the Mount Sinai Adolescent Health Center (AHC) a freestanding adolescent-specific health center (described in Diaz, Peake, Surko, & Bhandarkar, 2004). Although it had multiple goals, the two primary purposes were to improve services by: (1) promoting reflectivity among staff and; (2) providing insights about the *clinical challenge* of what adolescents want to and need to talk about.[1]

This article describes the how the CDM process helped meet these goals, the organizational experience of doing it, and lessons learned from it. More specifically, the article addresses the organizational and programmatic impact from the standpoint of program administration. A separate article will describe the experience from the standpoint of clinician participants (Ciro & Nembhard, 2005). Ultimately, however, this CDM project gives expression to the service wants and needs of AHC clients and the article concludes with a discussion of its implications for social workers and organizations elsewhere.

WHY SHOULD HIGHLY STRESSED SERVICE SETTINGS BOTHER WITH PRACTICE-BASED RESEARCH?

Describing the recent *corporatization* of health care with its emphasis on competition and drastic cost-control, Rosenberg and his colleagues (Rosenberg, Blumenfield, & Rehr, 1998; Rosenberg & Weissman, 1995) describe the impact on social workers in health care. For better and for worse, they are now compelled to create a well-articulated relationship between social work services and the larger organizational mission, especially as these services relate to the financial bottom-line.

Elsewhere, Peake and Epstein (2004) describe why this health care industry change challenges practitioners and administrators to develop strategies for organizational reflection to increase effectiveness and efficiency of social work services. Although engagement in organizational reflection is now a professional imperative, they acknowledge the paradox that increased administrative scrutiny and pressure to increase social work's *value-added* contribution to the organization commonly results in less time for reflection. However, pointing out that scarcity demands innovation, they recommend organizational learning strategies that: (1) bring together line and management to redefine and expand social workers' competencies; (2) introduce program innovation to benefit the organization and its clients; and (3) create new opportunities for professional growth. Practice-based research (PBR) (Epstein, 2001) is offered as one means of achieving these ends. These three organizational strategies and the PBR approach provided the foundation for the data-mining project described in this article.

PRACTICE-BASED INQUIRY BUILDS
ON PRACTITIONERS' SKILLS

The Adquest, CDM project was intended to improve programming for adolescents. An AHC senior manager initiated it, collaborating with senior program staff and an external research consultant. Together, they provided overall leadership, coordination, and CDM consultation. However, from start to finish, practitioner participation was vital to it. As experts in direct clinical work with clients, practitioners' perspectives would shape every aspect of the inquiry. After all, they would be the ones to carry into practice any clinical or program innovations that emerged from the project.

The knowledge and apprehensions that social work health practitioners bring to PBR have been described elsewhere (Hutson & Lichtiger, 2001), as have the skills and concerns that AHC practitioners brought to this initiative (Ciro & Nembhard, 2005). Briefly stated, these skills include: expert knowledge of the client, the ability to reflect on practice issues, case management skills, and collaborative skills. Their concerns involved questioning their own capacity to engage in research and the impact of that engagement on their commitment to clients.

Despite their initial apprehensions, AHC practitioners' client expertise, combined with their willingness to reflect on practice dilemmas that emerge in working with adolescents, shaped the research questions and analyses that drove this collective process of inquiry in a manner that was perceived as most compatible with practice and relevant to it. Interestingly, the same case management and collaborative skills that are central to their clinical practice proved to be essential in managing the workings of ten simultaneous PBR project groups. Furthermore, they provided necessary survival skills in the face of the inevitable stresses and strains of an ambitious project, conducted over and above their heavy clinical caseloads. Naturally, the latter commitment had to remain their top priority throughout the project.

SHAPING AN APPROACH: RESOURCES AND CONSTRAINTS

The implementation approach to the project was determined by its goals and limited by organizational constraints. Chief among constraints were scarce resources, particularly a lack of organizationally sanctioned time, beyond supervision, for practitioners to engage in PBR. It was recognized up front that, apart from coordination meetings, project work was to be done on participants' *own* time. This naturally meant participation by only those clinicians who were highly motivated to study practice and programs, and/or those who saw some professional development benefit from participating.

As a result, the project's organizers were able to rely on participating practitioners as a major intellectual resource, in the form of the previously described knowledge and skills they would contribute. The experience that some participants had previously gained in earlier PBR activities at the agency (Peake, Mirabito et al., 2004), and the organizational lessons learned about conducting program-wide PBR, were extremely helpful in shaping implementation.

Administration contracted with a PBR consultant who made himself available to work groups on an as needed basis each month. The participation of two staff from the agency's technical assistance and evaluation unit–whose work had previously been focused on constituents external to AHC–added basic skills in data management and analysis. However, the project was to rely chiefly on the abilities and work of clinical and program staff, some of whom already had basic skills in research and/or evaluation. One assumption, however, which later proved correct, was that a well-coordinated, collaborative effort would promote skill-building by further developing conceptual, literature review, data analytic, and writing skills among all project participants.

A proposal was developed and contract obtained for this volume with the anticipation that an opportunity to publish might be a further incentive for practitioner participation. Ten direct service social workers–about half of AHC's social work staff–participated in the project and authored papers, despite the fact that they were largely committing their personal time. One AHC psychologist, a psychiatrist, a supervisor, and a physician participated as well, along with five other AHC program staff.

DERIVATION OF A PRACTITIONER/MANAGER COLLABORATIVE MODEL

In response to this PBR initiative, a self-selected *core* group of eight practitioners and managers was formed and joined by the external research consultant. As stated earlier, five of the core's members had previously engaged in PBR at AHC and had been involved in the creation of Adquest. Its strategy was to follow the clinically derived organization of Adquest by forming separate practitioner-based work groups to study and write about each of its psychosocial risk and coping domains. Finally, a work group would complete the data-analytic component of the project by studying multiple risk factors across all of Adquest's domains, thus integrating the separate studies (Surko, Peake, Epstein, & Medeiros, 2005).

The first core group began by data-mining one of Adquest's psychosocial domains–*safety* (see: Surko, Ciro, Carlson, Labor, & Giannone et al., 2005)–so as to develop a conceptual framework or map to guide the other project workgroups. This strategy was chosen not to rigidly assure consistency for consistency's sake but for three very practical reasons.

First, given tight time lines *efficiency* was essential and therefore each workgroup would require a rough data-analytic guide or roadmap to get started. Again, the intention was not to create a prescription for each workgroup. Instead, the objective was to create a conceptual foundation on which each work group could build its unique discovery process, as it became more at ease with the CDM process.

Second, some practitioner *anxiety* about how to approach and organize this ambitious project with all its necessary multitasking was anticipated. In addition, images of quantitative research, statistical analysis and a sample of more than 700 clients were daunting to clinicians who were used to working with individual clients based on qualitative observations. Some had additional concerns about their skills in writing for publication. Providing a general road map reassured participants that each work group would have a similar destination and freedom to decide how to get there.

Third and last, a road map would enable each group to anticipate and plan for the multiple tasks that it needed to complete and to develop a division of labor. Finally, consultation, training, and technical assistance would be available to each group as needed.

Acknowledging each of the foregoing anxieties and responding to them throughout the project proved helpful in eliminating and/or containing participants' anxieties about what they should expect and what was expected of them. As a result, participants were each able to identify and augment their own unique profiles of competency. Thus, reflective exploration was not completely unconstrained. However, by choosing a practical approach, designed to allay practitioners' apprehensions, the process of reflection remained focused clearly on the intersection between practitioner interests and organizational ends.

Principles derived from prior experience of using PBR for organizational development at AHC (Peake, Mirabito et al., 2004) further informed the initiative. They were as follows:

- The widest practitioner participation possible was wanted for maximum program effect;
- Project work would be conducted largely on non-paid time so not all practitioners would participate, nor should they be expected to;

- Collaborators would be *equals in the inquiry process*: it would not be run by a specialist staff of researchers and, in contrast to an academic research model, practitioners would take the lead in all other aspects of the work;
- Clinical interest would drive participation by practitioners and small workgroups, each focusing on a particular Adquest psychosocial domain (e.g., health, sexuality, substance use, etc.) would most effectively encourage participation;
- Ambitious time lines were necessary as this was a broad-based, *in-vivo* project, led by non-researchers, with the ever-present risk of it being eclipsed by competing priorities;
- Each workgroup would evolve its own division of labor based on its unique skills mix;
- Practitioners would acquire new skills that would build on their practice skills;
- The research skills of some practitioners would provide a valuable resource and foundation and would be supplemented by the core group and PBR consultant;
- The primary audience for the project's intellectual products would be direct service practitioners, both at AHC and elsewhere.

Elsewhere, Ciro and Nembhard (2005) describe the project's impact on the clinicians who participated in it. This section will focus on lessons learned about Adquest itself, about the organization as a whole and the services it provides, and finally what was achieved in terms of the ultimate goal of supporting and encouraging organizational reflection.

Given its scope, originality and reliance on voluntary participation, the project progressed extremely efficiently. First steps were (1) formation of a core leadership group of practitioners and managers, (2) development of a conceptual map for proceeding, (3) *marketing* the project to practitioners and recruiting them as participants, and (4) creation of workgroups.

Workgroups were asked to develop and stick to a time line. Tasks of each workgroup included literature review, data analysis and interpretation, interpretation of findings, reflecting on their practice and program implications, and writing according to a peer-review publication format. Because several practitioners wanted to be involved in multiple workgroups, not all started simultaneously. However, once a topic was undertaken, each group operated within a four-month time frame. Moreover, each developed its own, unique division of labor. For example, some assigned a discrete task (literature review, data-analysis, writing, etc.) to a different member based on interest and/or competency. In others, members shared every task, taking collective responsibility for actively participating in each section of the final article.

The number of data-mining components to be studied and the even higher number of articles to be completed dictated a formalized and highly focused effort. Eight data-mining workgroups, plus one workgroup focusing on the clinical uses of Adquest, were initiated within a five-month period. A ninth CDM project that emerged from questions that surfaced in an earlier paper was identified and later developed. In addition, articles that were written to address the agency context, the theoretical underpinnings of the project, and Adquest's development, required four additional workgroups. All of this resulted in an ambitious time line, reinforced by a contract for publication one year after the work began.

THE EXPERIENCE

Overall, the convergence of each workgroup's analysis on what clients were saying about their concerns, behaviors, risk exposure, and desire to talk in counseling produced a focused organizational reflection on the intersection between services available and clients' needs. From the project's inception in June 2002, sixteen articles were completed and sent for peer review by November of 2003.

In the process, the PBR effort required and enhanced collaboration between organizational subsystems whose previous interactions had been tightly circumscribed or defined by more bureaucratic roles. For example, staff employed at different levels of the agency hierarchy worked together as equals in the discovery process. In some cases practitioners led and organized projects in which supervisors and managers were subordinate workgroup members. Thus, in this CDM project the usual hierarchical order of roles and responsibilities was on occasion suspended or reversed. Outside the project itself, however, formal organizational roles continued as previously.

Collaboration also routinely occurred between previously *separate* specialty areas of the agency. For example, AHC managers and clinicians worked together with staff from AHC's technical assistance and evaluation unit who had previously collaborated only with *outside* agencies. Similarly, clinicians and supervisors from different clinical program areas shared their findings and practice implications with one another, enhancing communication across specialized program areas.

Organizational Costs

Before discussing the organizational insights gained from the project, it is important to describe some of the inevitable strains that the project placed on the organization. One consequence of its unusual focus on identifiable *products* within tight time lines was that considerable attention had to be paid to proj- ect management. This was in stark contrast to clinical practice at AHC and as well to the looser, more individualized, PBR efforts previously undertaken by practitioners. Though the work was intellectually exciting and challenging, it was undeniably stressful to some.

More challenging, however, was the fact that the PBR approach to knowledge generation represented a relatively new paradigm for practitioners, which required a culture shift for those used to the more intuitively based reflection on clinical practice. Furthermore, the egalitarian approach to project management occasionally generated role ambiguity and confusion for both practitioners and managers. Practitioners in leadership roles in workgroups were suddenly in the uncomfortable position of having to push peers and/or superiors to meet deadlines. This required monitoring, attention, and support from managers. On other occasions, workgroup leaders were unable to anticipate or identify when help might be needed until after a problem arose. And problems did arise, usually manifested as a failure of a group member to complete an assigned task. Often, however, this was the result of an unanticipated need for assistance in understanding and managing work processes.

Similarly, hierarchical decision-making processes did not fit comfortably in this newly created collaborative environment, at best appearing heavy-handed. Because, managers were acutely aware that practitioner participation was voluntary, they had to step lightly when intervening to remove workgroup roadblocks or to identify learning needs. Just as practitioners needed help managing the work of colleagues, at times supervisors felt wrongly held accountable by senior managers for projects in which they had no formal supervisory/leadership role. Overall, these strains required constant monitoring and dialogue, and demanded that all participants be able to recheck and revise their assumptions about one another's multiple roles.

Another stress resulted from the perception by some project non-participants that participants' time was being diverted from other programmatic priorities. Although participants had a greatly increased workload, some non-participating staff members did not distinguish between project work done off the clock and other work. As a result, senior managers were occasionally called upon to manage these tensions and clarify perceptions of project and non-project role-responsibilities for participants as well as non-participants.

Amplifying the Voice of Practitioners and Clients

As individual studies were completed, it became harder for practitioners to view their adolescent clients as *mere consumers* of services. The reflection that occurred as findings were presented and discussed drew attention to needs for systems of care that were better tailored to the users, their risk profiles and their definitions of need. This was reinforced by the fact that many project participants were participating in more than one project, carrying the lessons from one project into their work with others. While Adquest had amplified each client's individual voice during the intake process (Elliott et al., 2004), *mining aggregate data from Adquest allowed the expressed concerns of a client population as a whole, and client subgroups, to emerge.* In other words, CDM gave clients an indirect but powerful voice in a reflective process of redesigning existing AHC services and planning new ones. Hence, many lessons for AHC's practice were derived from findings generated by each project group. A few examples follow.

So, for example, findings related to ethnicity, race, and racism (Surko, Ciro, Blackwood et al., 2005) suggested that ethnic and racial identity were insufficiently assessed at intake although likely to have a significant impact on client well being. Moreover, the perceived experience of racism was discovered to be a powerful predictor of other risk exposures, and a major safety risk. This led the agency to conclude that it should do more to understand and address the traumatic effects of this common and aversive client experience and more to comprehend how ethnic and racial identity affect our client population. As a result, a group of practitioners has begun development of a framework for routine and systematic assessment of implications of ethnic and racial identity at intake, as well as protocols for ensuring that experiences of racism and discrimination are taken into account and addressed.

Findings related to sex and sexuality (Labor, Medeiros, Carlson, Pullo, Seehaus, Peake,& Epstein, 2004) demonstrated that with AHC's client population, sexual behavior must be considered from both a risk and a competency perspective. Although many adolescent clients engage in risky sexual activity that puts them at risk for serious negative sequellae, sexuality also is an area of human behavior that requires their mastery and competence by adulthood. As a clinical engagement tool Adquest may well enable clinicians to more fully explore sexuality and sexual behavior during the engagement process (Elliott et al., 2004) in this dualistic manner. Clearly, however, as a research tool Adquest focused on sexuality from a risk perspective. More broadly, reflection on the programmatic implications of our findings suggested a *programmatic paradigm bias toward sexual risk to the neglect of sexual competence.* Currently, a group of AHC practitioners has taken on the task of revising Adquest and is working to ensure that it reflects a more holistic view of sexuality. It is also developing adolescent focus groups to inform the process.

Other organizational lessons learned and questions raised by reflecting on the plurality of client responses to Adquest emerged from the finding that lesbian, gay, bisexual, and sexual identity questioning youth felt particularly vulnerable and unsafe and that agency practices at intake might inadvertently compound these feelings (Ciro, Surko, Bhandarkar, Helfgott, Peake, & Epstein, 2005). As a result, streamlining mental health intake, to reduce perceived barriers to care, is now an organizational priority.

In another example, CDM contravened prior AHC "practice wisdom" that dating violence is a phenomenon that did not affect early-adolescent clients. As a result of this incorrect assumption, programming regarding this issue was previously offered only to older adolescents. AHC is now retargeting dating-violence protective techniques to younger clients.

Safety and violence proved to be a huge problem for AHC's clients in general (Surko, Ciro, Carlson et al., 2004)–as did exposure to other trauma. This led to the conclusion that more must be done to assess for safety and to explicitly communicate to clients that AHC is a safe environment in which to talk about trauma. These findings highlighted the need to have *all* practitioners specifically trained to comfortably address safety and trauma. However, a more significant realization has been the identification of the need to develop a broader organizational strategy–called a "toolbox"–that will include specific measures that AHC might take to signal that the agency environment is one in which clients feel comfortable discussing victimization, violence, and abuse, as well as other worries and fears.

While training clinical staff is one obvious component, currently, a number of other toolbox elements have been identified and some implemented. One AHC staff group is currently developing guidelines for a brief but focused orientation for all new clients to address safety and trauma. Another group has obtained one-year grant support to develop an extensive training curriculum for non-clinicians and will utilize this not only at AHC but also disseminate it for training youth workers in non-clinical settings. This will be achieved through newly developed collaborations with other regional organizations that serve adolescents.

Other toolbox components will focus on AHC's physical environment. First steps include development of a mural of photographs inside the agency's entrances, consisting of pictures of each of AHC's staff members and a brief description of the special skills of each. In addition, specific written messages about AHC being a safe place to talk will now be explicitly stated–on posters and in artwork throughout the facility.

These are just some examples. Many more programmatic implications were drawn from mining and aggregating information regarding school and work (Diaz-Cruz, Medeiros, Surko, Hoffman, & Epstein, 2004), health (Medeiros, Kramnick, Diaz-Cruz, Surko, & Diaz, 2004), cigarettes, alcohol and drugs

(Medeiros, Carlson, Surko, Munoz, Castillo, & Epstein, 2004), and family and friends (Giannone, Medeiros, Elliott, Perez, Carlson, & Epstein, 2004).

Most important are the broader awareness and implications of these findings and the reflections they generated. One was the managerial articulation of an uneasy feeling that AHC services had perhaps become too settled. This suggested that a more active approach to service design was needed to specifically address how the broad social contexts of our clients' lives influenced service utilization and the effort to address need, and that services needed to be more accessible.

Promoting More Effective and Efficient Services

Earlier, the authors asserted that social workers face an imperative to articulate the relationship between social work services and the organizational mission, as well as to improve the effectiveness and efficiency of services. Although not specifically designed with all of these broad challenges in mind, this project had the more modest goal of improving services by promoting reflectivity among staff. More specifically, it was intended to inform practitioner understanding of the *clinical challenge* of engaging urban adolescents in mental health treatment.

We do not know whether the introduction of Adquest effectively increased client retention during the intake phase because the original project evolved *organically* and incrementally, and was not initially conceptualized as an organizational intervention to be systematically evaluated (Peake, Epstein et al., 2004). Although hindsight suggests that this evaluative approach might be applied to future programmatic innovations, this article is concerned, more narrowly, with the impact of the Adquest CDM project. Despite this limited focus, there is considerable evidence that the CDM project improved *organizational efficiency* and had other programmatic and clinical benefits.

First and foremost, findings concerning multiple risks, generated by the process of cross-fertilization between project workgroups, provided powerful reminders that relationships between the organization's different subspecialty programs needed to be revisited. Accordingly, program managers and clinicians became aware that services had become overly fragmented over time–perhaps because of AHC reliance on grant funds. (Such funds are usually highly categorical, i.e., aimed at addressing specific risks such as HIV, substance abuse, or pregnancy.) By contrast, this project powerfully illustrated that in the lives of our clients complex interactions take place between risk factors (Surko, Peake, Epstein, & Medeiros, 2005.) In other words, their lives are not categorical. Consequently, practitioners saw a need to re-emphasize the fact that our clients are more alike than they are different–despite each of their individual risk profiles–a reminder that *programmatically* clients should be viewed as whole and services should be delivered holistically. While agency divisions based on clinical specialty might appear to be convenient programmatically, adolescents are not easily pushed into bureaucratic niches.

Because AHC's clients have multiple, inter-related problems and/or risk factors, divisions between specialty services appeared to result in considerable inefficiency in the work of client recruitment, service delivery and client retention. One striking example identified by the CDM project was AHC's grant-funded services for treating substance abuse in adolescents. Initially organized as its own specialty program within AHC, with its staff dedicated solely to drug treatment services, this service had struggled with extremely low recruitment despite the plethora of referrals in other AHC service areas. The Adquest-CDM project underscored the fact that many eligible adolescents were to be found within the general client population, and that the problem of recruitment was really one of poor service integration and poor case-finding methods.

In addition, the CDM project demonstrated that, in the initial stages of engagement, many adolescents often do not want to talk about their own substance use (Surko, Peake, Epstein, & Medeiros, 2005). Hence, while they are *not* easily enrolled in substance abuse counseling *per se*, they *are* willing to talk about other concerns. Accordingly, a first step to engagement must be based on what they want to engage about. Moreover, experience has also taught us that once a problem such as substance abuse is identified, neither the clients nor their therapists are generally desirous of a transfer to another practitioner. As a result the four social workers funded to provide substance abuse services had considerable difficulty in building caseloads and services such as groups.

As a result, a decision was made to disband the substance abuse program as a *stand-alone* division within AHC, and integrate this service into the general mental health work. Substance abuse funding would be spread across more staff and across all other program areas. In this way substance-abusing adolescents could be more readily and comfortably identified, and when that happened they could continue with the same primary therapist, with the treatment plan amended to address the newly emerging concerns. During the two months in which this redesign was initiated, recruitment rates improved by 25%, demonstrating that CDM had improved efficiency and effectiveness.

Despite AHC's avowed focus on holistic and integrated care (Diaz et al., 2004), internal barriers had incrementally evolved, barely noticed, over a prior decade of broad service expansion. One consequence of this was that AHC was not very *effectively* identifying and reporting the risk profiles of adolescents being served to the funders who financially support AHC services. Underreporting was a serious problem. As a consequence of the CDM project, senior managers made a decision that more regular attention to organizational redesign was necessary to reduce external and internal barriers to holistic care and more efficiently generate reports on service activity that more effectively capture work accomplished. Somewhat ironically, the metaphors that came from this dialogue referred to "organizational chiropractic" and the need for "a periodic readjustment." Metaphors aside, these discussions are more *data-driven* than ever before.

This insight was combined with the clear demonstration that context-specific tools such as Adquest provide a capacity for evidence-informed reflection and, thus, increase the potential for clinical, managerial and client voices in shaping program. Without specifically intending it, in Youth Development terms (YD) (Pittman, Irby, & Ferber, 2000; Diaz et al., 2004), *youth voice*– i.e., client participation in shaping services–was carried into program design.

As a result of data-based organizational reflection, AHC has initiated a process perhaps best characterized as a *recommitment to mission*. In particular, it has recommitted to YD principles such as meaningful youth involvement, ensuring that agency services are respectful of youth, and addressing barriers to long-term service involvement.

Another lesson was that new client self-assessment tools needed to be developed for more efficient *case finding* within AHC's primary care medical health services, thus extending the focus of Adquest to the many adolescents who come to AHC each year seeking health care alone but whose need for mental health services might otherwise go unnoticed. This became a new priority because Adquest had been developed and utilized only within AHC's mental health services. Improved identification and engagement in mental health services of vulnerable adolescents within AHC's primary care medical services would help integration between AHC's service divisions. Moreover, it would better take into account the relationships between health and mental health in the lives of adolescent clients.

At the same time, a refocus on YD principles underscored the realization that the current Adquest format was overly risk focused and should instead include greater exploration of client competencies. A newly formed PBR group of practitioners has begun refining Adquest by creating additional client self-assessment questions and integrating YD principles into them–such as exploring what opportunities are available to the client for positive social involvement, development of client strengths, etc.

Finally, practitioners and managers alike have seen the value of having available client information for subsequent data-mining studies. Developing additional tools based on the Adquest experience will not only provide new opportunities for practitioners to improve the practice dialogue but also provide a more complete database for future inquiry. Though such projects may perhaps be undertaken in a more routine and less demanding effort than that which was described in this article, they should continue to improve program development and service integration.

CONCLUSION

Clearly, valuable clinical and program lessons emerged from the ambitious PBR project. First and foremost was the re-emphasis of the YD perspective that adolescent services can be greatly enhanced when clients are not viewed as mere consumers but as participants. Although some young people were directly involved in designing Adquest (Peake, Epstein et al., 2004) and clients provided the data, the CDM research project, *per se*, did not *directly* involve young people as participants in the data-analysis and interpretation. However, it is spinning-off additional client involvement. Thus, a group of young people has begun to participate in a broad service redesign initiative, and other ways to involve adolescents as participants in services (rather than simply as recipients) are being developed. AHC is also developing a Youth Board as part of its Advisory Board and, to avoid mere token involvement, these young people will be trained and helped to conduct ongoing, youth-led evaluation.

Second, and equally important, the project powerfully demonstrated that practitioners can utilize PBR research methods to inform and enhance their own practice. Further, they should routinely be encouraged to reflect on both intervention approaches and organization of services. When they do, insights emerge and values are re-energized. Previous researchers have criticized practitioners for not consuming research and not applying research findings to their practice (Peake & Epstein, 2004; Epstein, 2000). This project underscores the limitations of viewing clinicians as mere consumers of research. *Just as staff learned that AHC clients could be more than consumers of services, we learned that social workers could be more than just consumers of research.*

This organizational case example amply demonstrates that practitioners can conduct research in collaborative groups and can use their practice skills to develop research questions that are highly relevant to practice. Their findings are then more likely to be *owned* and applied in their practice. Not all clinicians are able do all the tasks involved, though some are. Nonetheless, a division of labor that identifies and utilizes participants' skills is a practical approach that requires a relatively small investment in consultation and technical assistance.

What does this mean for AHC's future? Certainly the PBR initiative described in this article demanded extraordinary efforts on behalf of those who participated. It was an intense, time-consuming project that required that participants take risks, particularly the risk of feeling exposed for lack of research and/or writing skills and for acknowledging the limits of their own practice wisdom. Managers also took risks as they relinquished some control. Both groups committed to do work over and above their everyday duties.

Given the positive organizational outcomes achieved, it seems reasonable to assume that managers would condone future PBR activities, as integral to the everyday work of practitioners. However, severe strains on resources continue to hinder this process. At AHC, modest projects integrated into the everyday work will continue based upon the Adquest foundation, until such a time as the acquisition of additional resources allows an expanded effort.

What are implications for other organizations? Universally, resources remain scarce and all remain alert to the financial bottom line. This inevitably results in a narrow focus on service productivity and makes it difficult to initiate large-scale organizational reflection such as was described here. For PBR to gain organizational support, managers are challenged to specify the links between reflection and efficiency, improved effectiveness, or increased productivity. Clearly where innovative initiatives serve well-defined organizational ends–e.g., *case finding tools that help enroll or retain clients in services*–they will garner organizational support. Unfortunately, when too sharp a distinction is drawn between what is the officially sanctioned work of practitioners as distinct from the role of managers, the value of involving practitioners can easily be overlooked.

Finally, the authors have had to reconsider and refine their own understanding of organizational reflection. In the CDM project described here there was a sharpening of the focus of reflection that resulted from the way the initiative was structured in order to get work done efficiently. This produced many programmatic innovations precisely because it organized the reflection toward clear practice and organizational ends–i.e., how to better engage and serve adolescents.

Realizing this, the authors revisited the question: *"What are the qualities of organizational reflection?"* If the type of broadly focused, slower-paced reflection that AHC undertook previously (Peake, Mirabito et al., 2004) was lost, much was gained. Instead, it was replaced with a focused, well-honed, fast- paced, *nose-to-the-grindstone*, data-informed, reflective process. Reflection, in this instance, did not mean groupthink or individual introspection but rather an action-oriented collaborative process tied to clear organizational ends, benefiting program, practice, and, ultimately, our clients. In other words, reflection resulted in more than new ideas in participants' heads, but innovations that have profoundly changed AHC's organizational landscape and programmatic future.

NOTE

1. The dilemma, common for clinicians who work with at-risk or vulnerable adolescents, occurs when an adolescent client's explicit or implicit statements of what he or she wants to talk about are not congruent with reported experience and risk exposure and/or the clinician's assessment of risk, vulnerability, and coping (Peake, Mirabito, Epstein, & Giannone, 2004; Elliott, Nembhard, Giannone, Surko, Medeiros, & Peake, 2004).

REFERENCES

Ciro, D., & Nembhard, M. (2005). Collaborative Data-Mining in an Adolescent Mental Health Service: Clinicians Speak of Their Experience. *Social Work in Mental Health, 3*(3), 305-317.

Ciro, D., Surko, M., Bhandarkar, K., Helfgott, N., Peake, K., & Epstein, I. (2005). Lesbian, gay, bisexual, and sexual-orientation questioning adolescents seeking mental health services: Risk factors, worries, and desire to talk about them. *Social Work in Mental Health, 3*(3), 213-234.

Diaz, A., Peake, K. Surko, M., & Bhandarkar, K. (2004). Including at risk adolescents in their own health and mental health care: A Youth Development perspective. *Social Work in Mental Health, 3*(1/2), 3-22.

Diaz-Cruz, E., Medeiros, D., Surko, M., Hoffman, R., & Epstein, I. (2004). Adolescents, need to talk about school and work in mental health treatment. *Social Work in Mental Health, 3*(1/2), 155-171.

Elliott, J., Nembhard, M., Giannone, V., Surko, M., Medeiros, D., & Peake, K. (2004). Clinical uses of an adolescent intake questionnaire: Adquest as a bridge to engagement. *Social Work in Mental Health, 3*(1/2), 83-102.

Epstein, I. (2001). Using available clinical information in practice-based research: Mining for silver while dreaming of gold. *Social Work in Health Care, 33*(3/4), 15-32.

Epstein, I. (1995). Promoting reflective social work practice: Research strategies and consulting principles. In E. J. Mullen, and J. L. Magnabosco (Eds.), *Practitioner-Researcher Partnerships: Building Knowledge From, In, and For Practice.* 83-102. Washington DC: NASW Press.

Epstein, I. (1996). In quest of a research-based model for social work practice: Or why can't a social worker be more like a researcher? *Social Work Research and Abstracts, 20* (2): 97-100.

Giannone, V., Medeiros, D., Elliott, J., Perez, C., Carlson, E., & Epstein, I. (2004). Adolescents' self-reported risk factors and desire to talk about family and friends: Implications for practice and research. *Social Work in Mental Health, 3*(1/2), 191-208.

Hutson, C., and Lichtiger, E. (2001). Mining clinical information in the utilization of social services: Practitioners inform themselves. *Social Work in Health Care, 33* (3/4), 153-161.

Labor, N., Medeiros, D., Carlson, E., Pullo N., Seehaus, M., Peake, K., & Epstein, I. (2004). Adolescents' need to talk about sex and sexuality in an urban mental health setting. *Social Work in Mental Health, 3*(1/2), 135-154.

Medeiros, D., Carlson. E., Surko, M., Munoz, N., Castillo, M., & Epstein, I. (2004). Adolescents' self-reported substance risks and their need to talk about them in a mental health counseling. *Social Work in Mental Health, 3*(1/2), 169-187.

Medeiros, D., Kramnick, L., Diaz-Cruz, E., Surko, M., & Diaz, A. (2004). Adolescents seeking mental health services: Self-reported health risks and the need to talk *Social Work in Mental Health, 3*(1/2), 121-134.

Peake, K., & Epstein, I. (2004). Theoretical and practical imperatives for reflective social work organizations in health and mental health: The place of practice-based research. *Social Work in Mental Health, 3*(1/2), 23-38.

Peake, K., Epstein, I., Mirabito, D., & Surko, M. (2004) Development and utilization of a practice-based, adolescent intake questionnaire (Adquest): Surveying which risks, worries, and concerns urban youth want to talk about. *Social Work in Mental Health, 3*(1/2), 55-82.

Peake, K., Mirabito, D., Epstein, I., & Giannone, V. (2004). Creating and sustaining a practice-based research group in an urban adolescent mental health program. *Social Work in Mental Health, 3*(1/2), 39-54.

Pittman, K., Irby, M., & Ferber, T. (2000). Unfinished business: Further reflections on a decade of promoting youth development. In *Youth development: Issues, challenges, and directions.* Philadelphia, PA: Public/Private Ventures.

Rosenberg, G., Blumenfield, S., & Rehr, H. (1998). Program development, organization and administrative directions. In *Creative Social Work in Health Care.* New York: Springer.

Rosenberg, G., & Weissman, A. (1995). Social work leadership in health care: Directors' perspectives. *Social Work in Health Care, 20* (4).

Surko, M., Ciro, D., Blackwood, C., Nembhard, M., & Peake, K. (2005). Experience of racism as a correlate of developmental and health outcomes among urban adolescent mental health clients. *Social Work in Mental Health, 3*(3), 235-260.

Surko, M., Ciro, D., Carlson, E., Labor, N., Giannone, V., Diaz-Cruz, E., Peake, K., & Epstein, I. (2005). Which adolescents need to talk about safety and violence? *Social Work in Mental Health, 3*(1/2), 103-120.

Surko, M., Peake, K., Epstein, I., & Medeiros, D. (2005) Multiple Risks, Multiple Worries, and Adolescent Coping: What Clinicians Need to Ask About. *Social Work in Mental Health, 3*(3), 261-285.

Collaborative Data-Mining in an Adolescent Mental Health Service: Clinicians Speak of Their Experience

Dianne Ciro
Michael Nembhard

SUMMARY. As full participants in a collaborative *clinical data-mining* project intended to promote staff reflection and to improve services, clinicians discovered just how valuable their practice expertise was in maintaining project relevance. In this paper, they describe challenges they faced as non-experienced researchers and writers and how their practice skills enabled them to overcome these challenges. Benefits derived include: enhanced skills (in both practice and research), sensitization to previously overlooked areas of practice, and an increased sense of professionalism. *[Article copies available for a fee from The Haworth Document Delivery Service: 1-800-HAWORTH. E-mail address: <docdelivery@haworthpress.com> Website: <http://www.HaworthPress.com> © 2005 by The Haworth Press, Inc. All rights reserved.]*

Dianne Ciro, MS, is Clinical Social Worker, Mount Sinai Adolescent Health Center (AHC), 320 East 94th Street, New York, NY 10128. (E-mail: Dianne.Ciro@msnyuhealth.org). Michael Nembhard, MSW, is Clinical Social Worker, AHC.

The authors would like to acknowledge the contributions of AHC social work clinicians.

[Haworth co-indexing entry note]: "Collaborative Data-Mining in an Adolescent Mental Health Service: Clinicians Speak of Their Experience." Ciro, Dianne, and Michael Nembhard. Co-published simultaneously in *Social Work in Mental Health* (The Haworth Social Work Practice Press, an imprint of The Haworth Press, Inc.) Vol. 3, No. 3, 2005, pp. 305-317; and: *Clinical and Research Uses of an Adolescent Mental Health Intake Questionnaire: What Kids Need to Talk About* (ed: Ken Peake, Irwin Epstein, and Daniel Medeiros) The Haworth Social Work Practice Press, an imprint of The Haworth Press, Inc., 2005, pp. 305-317. Single or multiple copies of this article are available for a fee from The Haworth Document Delivery Service [1-800-HAWORTH, 9:00 a.m. - 5:00 p.m. (EST). E-mail address: docdelivery@haworthpress.com].

http://www.haworthpress.com/web/SWMH
© 2005 by The Haworth Press, Inc. All rights reserved.
Digital Object Identifier: 10.1300/J200v03n03_05

KEYWORDS. Clinician, reflection, practice-based research, collaboration, adolescent, engagement, professionalism, publication

INTRODUCTION

Participation in social work research is often avoided by social work clinicians for a variety of reasons. Some clinicians are uncomfortable with research technology and think of themselves as incapable of doing it (Sidell, Barnhart, Bowman, Fitzpatrick, Fulk, Hallock, & Metoff, 1996), while others feel they do not have time to generate quality research material and still serve clients adequately (Reid, 1997). Many academic researchers believe that clinicians lack time, skills and incentives to participate in research (Kirk, 1999). Despite these widely shared and negative perceptions, clinicians at the Mount Sinai Adolescent Health Center (AHC) took on the challenge of combining direct practice and research in a Practice-Based Research (PBR) project, employing a *clinical data-mining* (Epstein, 2001; Epstein & Blumenfield, 2001) study of AHC service applicants. Drawing on their own expertise as clinicians, supplementing their research knowledge through collaboration with colleagues from allied professions and with the assistance of a PBR consultant, the social work staff at AHC adopted a group approach to conducting practice-relevant research.

This article, written by two heavily involved clinicians, depicts their own experience and that of ten fellow social work clinicians who participated in this ambitious and ground-breaking research project.

CLINICAL DATA-MINING IN AN ADOLESCENT MENTAL HEALTH PROGRAM

AHC, a comprehensive health center for inner-city youth (see: Diaz, Peake, Surko, & Bhandarkar, 2004), has long recognized that the provision of high quality care to young people requires an ongoing process of organizational self-examination and program innovation. In turn, innovation has been, and remains, essential to ensuring program relevance and *goodness of fit* with client needs.

At AHC, PBR has been a primary strategy for achieving this goal (Peake, Mirabito, Epstein, & Giannone, 2004). In this setting, PBR is not viewed as the sole purview of a select set of researchers, but is considered an essential element of direct practice. This shared commitment to reflection that unites practice and research considerations led AHC practitioners to develop an indigenous questionnaire–Adquest–that adolescent applicants for mental health services are asked to complete prior to their intake interview (Peake, Epstein, Mirabito, & Surko, 2004).

The intention of the practitioners who designed Adquest was to improve engagement by asking adolescents about their experiences across a range of life areas, what their worries are, how well they feel they are handling each life area, and what they want to talk about in psychotherapy. In addition, Adquest generated information was intended to serve as a database for practitioner-led studies.

The twelve AHC clinicians, whose experiences are described in this article, were integrally involved in conducting and writing a series of studies that "mined" the clinical information captured by Adquest. These studies focused on life areas such as *school and work* (Diaz-Cruz, Medeiros, Surko, Hoffman, & Epstein, 2004), *safety and violence* (Surko, Ciro, Carlson, Labor, & Giannone et al., 2004), *health* (Medeiros, Kramnick, Diaz-Cruz, Surko, & Diaz, 2004), *sex and sexuality* (Labor, Medeiros, Carlson, Pullo, Seehaus, Peake, & Epstein, 2004), *substance abuse* (Medeiros, Carlson, Surko, Munoz, Castillo, & Epstein, 2004), *family and friends* (Giannone, Medeiros, Elliott, Perez, Carlson, & Epstein, 2004), *lesbian, gay, bisexual, and questioning adolescents* (Ciro, Surko, Bhandarkar, Helfgott, Peake, & Epstein, 2005), *racism and race/ethnicity* (Surko, Ciro, Blackwood, Nembhard, & Peake, 2005) and the *practice utilization of Adquest* to engage adolescents (Elliott, Nembhard, Giannone, Surko, Medeiros, & Peake, 2004).

WHAT CLINICIANS BROUGHT
TO THE PRACTICE-BASED RESEARCH

Even in the planning stages of this labor-intensive, year-long project, AHC clinicians were aware of some of the challenges full participation would present. The most concrete of these was time constraints. Clinicians knew that multiple projects would be running simultaneously and were aware that much of the work was to be done on their own time. This had the potential for an overwhelming and exhausting experience. Other challenges identified upfront included clinicians' worries about their lack of research and/or writing skills.

Challenges that were not identified initially emerged as the project progressed and clinicians took on multiple roles, many of which were new to them. These included project management, overseeing the work of clinical peers, establishing reasonable expectations of one another with regard to deadlines, and identifying when and where help might be needed. In differen-

tiating roles and contributions of participants in project groups, some participants feared letting others down by being unable to deliver on tasks.

Despite initial fears, clinicians found that these challenges were offset by
skills they already had. Clinicians brought their expert knowledge of the client, particularly clients' presenting issues, background characteristics, and the
challenges faced in engaging adolescents in psychotherapy. They also brought
the ability to reflect on practice and its dilemmas and to manage ambiguity,
make sense of conflicting information, and talk together to make sense of their
experiences. Case management and collaboration skills were also integral to
managing the work of the research project and the exchange of ideas that resulted.

Although clinicians were intensely involved in every aspect of the project,
not every clinician was involved in all aspects. For most, involvement came at
different stages of the project. Some were involved in the creation of Adquest.
These clinicians saw their participation in the research project as a natural ex-
tension of their prior experience. For others, however, this data-mining project
was a first-time experience and, though it seemed threatening–i.e., to fill the
shoes of writer, lead author, or researcher–the project also was seen as an opportunity to give *voice* to and represent the work that clinicians do with AHC
clients.

Some who had not previously participated in PBR at AHC or elsewhere but
remembered enjoying their Master's level research classes saw this as an opportunity to carry out *real live* research in order to learn more about their clients.
Consequently, when presented with the option to participate in this research
project many clinicians felt excitement as well as apprehension.

When the overall project was first presented to staff, the prospect of specific research inquiries organized by Adquest's clinically derived life areas
(e.g., "safety and violence," "health," "sex and sexuality," "substance use,"
etc.) and its focus on engagement made it seem highly relevant to, and "in
sync" with clinicians' own interests and ways of structuring their practice concerns and experiences. This array of clinically relevant topics was developed
with the input of clinicians who were involved in a core group that initiated the
project. It provided an anchor for participants' interests and simultaneously
helped offset their concerns that research might be too abstract and unrelated
to their practice. Moreover, using available data assured them that the research
process would not be intrusive.

Clearly, those who joined the clinical data-mining project did so in hope
that project participation would inform their practice thinking and improve
their clinical work. In addition, several clinicians became excited about writing for publication. Three social work practitioners expressed their expectation that participation would be an opportunity to bring together and integrate

their interests in research and practice. One in particular asserted that, for her, these interests had felt dichotomized and incompatible because her past exposure to research had led her to see it as irrelevant to everyday work.

Most saw project participation as an opportunity for career advancement; for example, as future applicants to doctoral programs, as future researchers or teachers, and as influential members of the social work profession.

THE EXPERIENCE OF PARTICIPATION

As expected, participating clinicians described experiencing a range of feelings about their involvement as the project progressed. Some found enjoyment in the experience. Others felt frustrated by the pace and demands of the project and wished they had never taken part in it. All viewed lack of *time* as by far the biggest obstacle to participation and as the most stressful and limiting factor when they did participate. Because clinicians knew prior to agreeing to participate that most of the project work would occur on their own time, they understood that this meant committing to work extra hours, evenings, and weekends. This meant that some could not or would not participate. Nonetheless, by the time the project ended, most participating clinicians agreed this PBR initiative was a useful and constructive one for AHC clients, the agency, and for themselves as professionals.

Much of the social work literature about practice-research utilization–generally written by academicians–faults clinicians for neither conducting, reading, nor utilizing research in their practice (Rehr, 2001; Bloom, Fischer, & Orme, 1995; Blythe, Tripodi, & Briar, 1995; Subramian, Siegel, & Garcia, 1994; Pruett, Shea, Zimmerman, & Parish, 1991). This critical stance is troubling for practitioners and has resulted in a "tense dichotomy" between research and practice (Sidell et al., 1996, p. 100). In this practice-research effort, however, things were different. In other words, the project felt "personal" and professionally meaningful to participants. The project did not completely resolve and dissolve the, perhaps inevitable, tensions between practice and research, but overall this gap was reduced. Each practitioner who participated progressed along the spectrum of comfort with research and research skills, and all felt that their appreciation for how research can enhance practice and how practice can enhance research was magnified.

This did not occur magically, i.e., simply by including practitioners in the Adquest studies and was not simply an artifact of the fact that the project took place in an academic medical center. While the organizational culture values research participation, resources were scant and clinicians' everyday work environment was extremely fast-paced and focused on productive, high quality service provision (Peake, Mirabito et al., 2004). Obtaining clinician participation resulted from both past experience and from careful planning.

Some clinicians had prior experience with practice-based research at AHC, including designing Adquest as a clinical tool (Peake, Epstein et al., 2004). Similarly, managers who were involved in initiating the project had learned through these prior experiences that clinicians are a valuable intellectual resource. In the planning process, clinicians were full partners and helped determine the shape that the overall project would take (Peake, Surko et al., 2005). As component projects were developed and implemented, practitioners led many project workgroups. In addition, within each workgroup clinicians were valued participants and each workgroup developed a unique division of labor that identified and built on the skills of participants. As a result, not only did the research feel relevant and useful to practice, but clinicians viewed themselves as full contributors who brought valuable skills and knowledge to the research process.

A key *driver* that shaped the research focus was the in-depth knowledge clinicians had of AHC's urban, poor, adolescent client population and, in particular, the challenges these clients presented for assessment and clinical engage- ment. This knowledge was used to develop the research strategy–to have projects that explored each of Adquest's aforementioned life areas with each focusing on "what do adolescents *want* and *need* to talk about?" Clinician expertise continued to identify directions for research exploration that were most relevant to practice.

Although an initial but secondary aim of Adquest was research, its creators had not specified an analytic strategy. Clinicians participated in the development of that strategy (Surko, Peake, Epstein, & Medeiros, 2005) and later came to lead individual projects from initial analysis to the creation of published articles.

In so doing, clinicians engaged in systematic reflection. They reflected on what were the most practice-relevant research questions, identified relevant literature, carried out literature reviews, analyzed data, and interpreted findings. As they wrote for publication, they reflected on clinical and programmatic implications of the findings, and on future research directions.

Initially the focus on "what adolescents *want* to talk about"–derived from Adquest's questions of *desire to talk* about each life area–evolved and was expanded into a construct of *need to talk* (Peake, Epstein, Mirabito, & Surko, 2004). Need to talk included not only desire to talk, but also exposure to risk. Thus, from a clinical perspective, an adolescent with high risk-exposure in a life area but expressing no interest in talking about that life area was treated as needing to talk. The decision to develop a construct of need to talk as the overall focus of several articles reflected a core clinical challenge and practice problem in engaging adolescents. Engagement requires that clinicians respect adolescents' comfort levels with talking or not talking about issues while simultaneously assessing and responding to factors that might put them at risk. This is often a difficult balancing act.

There were many other ways in which clinicians' knowledge shaped the research process and resulted in articles that were not initially anticipated. Although Adquest included questions regarding race/ethnicity, the experience of racism, and racial/ethnic pride, there was no distinct race/racism life area, nor was a separate study on race and racism planned. Likewise, researchers might have included race simply as an independent or intervening variable in the analyses of each life area. Clinicians, however, came to the position that the experience of racism for clients of color as well as their Caucasian counterparts merited an exploration in and of itself. Similarly, clinicians' reflection on findings in regard to *safety and violence* and *health* led to a separate study of these issues for lesbian, gay, bisexual, and questioning adolescents (Ciro, Surko et al., 2005).

More predictably, there were challenges clinicians faced due to their unfamiliarity with research methodology. Although some were more familiar than others with analyzing data, many lacked sufficient research knowledge or confidence in their research skills to fully take charge of this aspect. While wanting to be intensely involved, they feared feeling exposed. For this reason it was important that guidance, support and technical help were available throughout.

Typically, clinicians are most familiar with reflecting on single cases or clinical clusters developed from experientially derived information rather than aggregate data. Initially some clinicians needed to have colleagues with some research experience *walk them through* the data before they could feel comfortable in interpreting it and reflecting on its implications. Despite this, in a short, three-month period several clinicians achieved a comfort level reading through stacks of data. A smaller number of clinicians even learned to run data with SPSS (Statistical Package for the Social Sciences, 2003) by themselves.

Nonetheless, peering at pages of aggregate data seemed abstract at times and required the assistance of a practice-based research consultant, or staff with more research experience, to help interpret the numbers. However, the discovery that clinicians' work experience was a valuable asset in the interpretation of findings and the consideration of possible explanations gave clinicians the confidence to master this task and helped offset their fears that research findings might result in a prescriptive and limiting approach to practice.

As interpersonal practice proceeds there are ongoing opportunities to clarify information, revise clinical hypotheses, and change direction. In some instances, this type of reflectivity, to which clinicians were accustomed, felt constrained by the limits of the database. Some questions simply could not be answered, and when this occurred it was frustrating.

Practitioners found writing research reports a challenging experience, as it required a different set of skills from those used in reflecting on and recording clinical work. While accustomed to writing in summary form about the experience clients bring into the room, clinicians were not as accustomed to the *impersonal* quality of academic writing. However, their collaborative, group work and case management skills helped address this. By working in small groups together, clinicians were able to negotiate a division of labor so that those most comfortable with writing took on this role. However, for some groups the writing was laborious and difficult, and the most time-consuming and challenging aspect of the project work.

In addition to heavy clinical caseloads, clinicians also had to learn how to manage their research time and the stress of a different kind of work. Some were concerned that their supervisors or other managers might believe that project work, such as literature review and writing, was taking time from their everyday clinical work. Accordingly, reassurances needed to be obtained from managers and supervisory staff.

Some clinicians became project managers and lead authors, as the two roles often went hand in hand. Managing the work of a study group often resulted in challenges, as it was difficult to assess what were reasonable time allowances for co-authors to complete tasks. It was also sometimes difficult to push colleagues to produce. Line staff clinicians who became lead authors found it as awkward and complicated to manage the work of managers and supervisors. Furthermore, for clinicians–who ordinarily work with undefined endings– deadlines presented a sharp contrast with their everyday experience.

LESSONS LEARNED

Participating in the practice-based research project impacted the work of clinicians with adolescents. Clinicians expressed feeling encouraged to reflect on their work and sharpen their assessment and engagement skills. For some, this included rethinking how they might use Adquest during the initial assessment. Although some clinicians feel they have always made good use of Adquest, others find themselves utilizing it more in their work than they had.

Some report that participating in this PBR project sensitized them to the need to explore issues–such as racism and sexuality–more directly and more immediately than they had in the past. Previously, they felt uncomfortable addressing such *personal* issues before they had established a relationship with the client, now they see that many clients are clearly concerned about such issues and are willing to talk about them.

Clinicians found that participating in studies changed their approaches to assessment by challenging them to think about "preconceptions" they brought into the initial encounter with clients. In particular, one discovered that he had previously been mainly focused on risk *behaviors*. He reported now thinking more holistically and described having developed a *new* view of the intake process as one of "reconstructing the client." *Reconstruction*, in his view, is a rapid process in which he seeks to develop as holistic a picture and history as possible (i.e., looking beyond risk behaviors), to help answer the question: "How did this adolescent end up here with me?"

Another clinician, who participated in a study of lesbian, gay, bisexual and questioning adolescents (Ciro, Surko et al., 2005) reported that this sensitized her to the need to assess issues of safety, sexual behavior, and substance–as well as the interaction between these factors–when meeting for the first time with an adolescent who identifies as being part of this sexual minority group.

Clinicians who worked on a study of "family and friends" (Elliot at al., 2004) said that they were challenged to set aside the somewhat simplistic idea that adolescence, as a stage of development, is all about separation and individuation from family of origin. They found that they had to acknowledge how much more they needed to understand about clients' family relationships and views of their families. In particular, they suggested that the complex ways in which family factors impact risk behavior are not yet understood. One clinician described that she now assesses family issues and concerns in far more depth than previously because of the overwhelming evidence, derived from the data-mining study, that adolescent clients were highly concerned about their families, reported high rates of poor coping with their families, and had such high rates of desire to talk about family issues.

We anticipate that many more examples like these will emerge in the ongoing process of in-house presentation and discussion of study findings.

The practice based research project also impacted the work done in clinical supervision and team meetings. Clinicians have used the research findings to contribute in team discussions when reviewing assessments of new clients and formulating treatment plans. This has also encouraged new avenues for exploration of ongoing cases.

IMPLICATIONS FOR PRACTICE

Clinicians' participation in this PBR project honed their skills, sensitized them to previously overlooked aspects of their practice, and fostered collaboration within the agency. For some, it reinforced the belief that social workers have an ethical imperative to rigorously examine and evaluate their practice.

Participation also created a sense of pride in clinicians who feel they have contributed in bringing prestige to the agency. Overall, this experience increased clinicians' contributions to the agency–beyond their direct practice–by tapping into their wealth of clinical knowledge to help reshape agency practices. Simultaneously, it created new opportunities for them. Clinicians who participated have been invited to present at conferences and many have expressed interest in continuing to take on future research projects at AHC. All who participated take pride that they are now co-authors of published articles. In these ways, collaborative data-mining has increased clinicians' sense of professionalism.

Some advocates of clinician participation in research have pointed out that, in most settings, practitioners lack officially sanctioned time for research activities. This was a limitation of the project reported in this article, and may remain an obstacle to future projects. However, this project has underscored the value to the practice setting of clinician-driven projects that evaluate services, or provide new tools for engaging and assessing adolescents. This has resulted in some new service improvement initiatives that use PBR approaches and allow clinicians allotted time for participation. These include clinician participation in the development of new client self-assessment tools, grant applications to fund research, and a review of AHC's systems of care to improve the integration of previously fragmented services. These current AHC initiatives to better integrate services and to improve client access would not have been developed without the feedback that this project produced.

Thus, participation in PBR enhanced interdisciplinary and intra-disciplinary collaboration within the agency, and has now increased exposure of line social workers to a wider segment of the organization than might have been possible previously. Clinicians also take pride in the impact that the various studies in which they participated have begun to have on the agency.

We believe that clinicians elsewhere might also find opportunities to engage in practice research and in turn increase their participation in the agencies within which they work. Although this PBR project was conducted in a service division of a large academic medical center, it has implications for social workers in other service settings. While we are not blind to the potential benefits to practitioner research provided by the setting (particularly an organizational culture and social work department that formally recognizes engagement in research as a desirable and valued activity), these benefits should not be overstated. On a concrete level the project benefited from some available PBR consultant time (about six hours a month), and some support and technical expertise from staff from an AHC's unit that conducts evaluation and technical assistance external to AHC.

However, as has been noted, many constraints faced by the social workers on this project are common to all practitioners–lack of time, concern about lack of skills and viable roles, and concerns that researchers will not value practice. Similarly, we have noted that this initiative also relied on skills that are common to social work clinicians. We conclude, therefore, by providing some pointers for practitioners who might be interested in utilizing research methods to enhance their services.

SOME POINTERS FOR FELLOW CLINICIANS INTERESTED IN PRACTICE RESEARCH: WHAT YOU MIGHT KEEP IN MIND

- Finding a way to engage in research activities may require persistence and creativity, but clinicians should not assume that they cannot engage in research, or that their practice skills are irrelevant.
- Adquest was developed so as to better engage adolescents in services: likewise, clinicians should seek to make a case for research by anchoring their research questions in real, everyday practice issues and service challenges.
- Clinicians should not assume that managers are hostile to practice-based research; many managers utilize data in their everyday work, most know the value of information and evaluative methodologies (Weinbach, 1985).
- Clinicians should seek allies among supervisors and managers who are most invested in improving services and who understand the practice dilemmas they are interested in addressing.
- Clinicians should not assume a lack of research skills in their agency settings, inventorying available skills and interest is a useful first step (Peake, Mirabito et al., 2004). Looking for external resources should be done only when there is some clarity about what is lacking.
- Many academic social workers are interested in collaborative efforts to pursue research and often seek greater access to agency practice; in this way research skills can be enhanced and necessary resources obtained (Young, 1986). Clinicians can use their professional skills, such as networking, to identify potential allies.
- When seeking collaborations with academic social workers, we suggest that clinicians (along with managers and supervisors) engage as full partners in the endeavor and, thus, help shape the research questions and approach. We suggest that practitioner research be aimed at informing practice (not evaluating whether it works), and that it be conducted in a manner most compatible with practice. Practice-based research (Epstein, 2001) is one such approach.

REFERENCES

Bloom, M., Fischer, J., & Orme, J. (1995). *Evaluating practice: Guidelines for the accountable professional* (2nd ed.). Englewood Cliffs, NJ: Prentice-Hall.

Blumenfield, S., & Epstein, I. (2001). Promoting and maintaining a reflective professional staff in a hospital-based social work department. *Social Work in Health Care, 33* (3/4), 1-13.

Blythe, B., Tripodi, T., & Briar, S. (1994). *Direct Practice Research in Human Service Agencies.* New York: Columbia University Press.

Ciro, D., Surko, M., Bhandarkar, K., Helfgott, N., Peake, K., & Epstein, I. (2005). Lesbian, gay, bisexual, and sexual-orientation questioning adolescents seeking mental health services: Risk factors, worries, and desire to talk about them. *Social Work in Mental Health, 3*(3), 213-234.

Diaz, A., Peake, K., Surko, M., & Bhandarkar, K. (2004). Including at-risk adolescents in their own health and mental health care: A Youth Development perspective. *Social Work in Mental Health, 3*(1/2), 1-20.

Diaz-Cruz, E., Mederios, D., Surko, M., Hoffman, R., & Epstein, I. (2004). Adolescents' need to talk about school and work in mental health treatment. *Social Work in Mental Health, 3*(1/2), 155-170.

Elliott, J., Nembhard, M., Giannone, V., Surko, M., Medeiros, D., & Peake, K. (2004). Clinical uses of an adolescent intake questionnaire: Adquest as a bridge to engagement. *Social Work in Mental Health, 3*(1/2), 83-102.

Epstein, I. (2001). Using available clinical information in practice-based research: Mining for silver while dreaming of gold. *Social Work in Health Care, 33*(3/4), 15-32.

Giannone, V., Medeiros, D., Elliott, J., Perez, C., Carlson, E., & Epstein, I. (2004). Adolescents' self-reported risk factors and desire to talk about family and friends: Implications for practice and research. *Social Work in Mental Health, 3*(1/2), 191-208.

Kirk, S. A. (1999). Good intentions are not enough: Practice guidelines for social work research. *Research in Social Work Practice, 9*(3), 283-301.

Labor, N., Medeiros, D., Carlson, E., Pullo N., Seehaus, M., Peake, K.,& Epstein, I. (2004). Adolescents' need to talk to a about sex and sexuality in an urban mental health setting. *Social Work in Mental Health, 3*(1/2), 135-154.

Medeiros, D., Carlson. E., Surko, M., Munoz, N., Castillo, M., & Epstein, I. (2004). Adolescents self-reported substance risks and their need to talk about them in mental health counseling. *Social Work in Mental Health, 3*(1/2), 171-190.

Medeiros, D., Kramnick, L., Diaz-Cruz, E., Surko, M., & Diaz, A. (2004). Adolescents seeking mental health services: Self-reported health risks and the need to talk. *Social Work in Mental Health, 3*(1/2), 121-134.

Peake, K., Epstein, I., Mirabito, D., & Surko, M. (2004) Development and utilization of a practice-based, adolescent intake questionnaire (Adquest): Surveying what risks, worries, and concerns urban youth want to talk about. *Social Work in Mental Health, 3*(1/2), 55-82.

Peake, K., Mirabito, D., Epstein, I., & Giannone, V. (2004). Creating and sustaining a practice-based research group in an urban adolescent mental health program. *Social Work in Mental Health, 3*(1/2) 39-54.

Peake, K., Surko, M., Epstein, I., & Medeiros, D. (2005). Data-mining client concerns in adolescent mental health services: Clinical and program implications. *Social Work in Mental Health, 3*(3), 287-304.

Pruett, R., Shea, T., Zimmerman, J., & Parish, G. (1991). The beginning development of a model for joint research between a hospital social work department and a school of social work. *Social Work in Health Care, 15*(3), 63-75.

Surko, M., Ciro, D., Blackwood, C., Nembhard, M., & Peake, K. (2005). Experience of racism as a correlate of developmental and health outcomes among urban adolescent mental health clients. *Social Work in Mental Health, 3*(3), 235-260.

Surko, M., Ciro, D., Carlson, E., Labor, N., Giannone, V., Diaz-Cruz, E., Peake, K., & Epstein, I. (2004). Which adolescents need to talk about safety and violence? *Social Work in Mental Health, 3*(1/2), 103-120.

Surko, M., Peake, K., Epstein, I., & Medeiros, D. (2005) Multiple Risks, Multiple Worries and Adolescent Coping: What Clinicians Need to Ask About. *Social Work in Mental Health, 3*(3), 261-285.

Rehr, H. (2001). Forward. *Social Work in Health Care, 33* (3/4), xxi-xxx.

Reid, W. J. (1997). Long term trends in social work. *Social Service Review, 71*(2), 200-213.

Sidell, N., Barnhart, L., Bowman, N., Fitzpatrick, V., Full, M., Hillock, L., & Setoff, J. (1996). The challenge of practice based research: A group approach. *Social Work in Health Care, 23*(2), 99-111.

SPSS Inc. (2003). Statistical Package for the Social Sciences (Version 11.5) [Computer software]. Chicago IL: SPSS Inc.

Subramian, K., Siegel, E., & Garcia, C. (1994). Case study of an agency-university research partnership between a school of social work and a medical center. *Journal of Social Service Research, 19*(3/4), 145-161.

Weinbach, R. W. (1985). The agency and professional contexts of research. In R. M. Grinnel (Ed.), *Social Work Research and Evaluation.* Itasca, IL: Peacock.

Young, C. (1986). Social work roles in collaborative research. *Social Work in Health Care, 11*(4), 71-81.

Index

Academic failure, 156
Accountability, 85
Acculturation theory, 237,238-239
Adolescence
　myths about, 5-6,8-9
　as professional opportunity, 9
　sexual orientation and, 214
Adolescent development
　health care systems and, 19
　healthy, 19
　theories of, 193-194
Adolescent Health Center (AHC). *See*
　　Mount Sinai Adolescent
　　Health Center (AHC)
Adolescent intake questionnaire
　　(Adquest). *See* Adquest
　　(adolescent intake
　　questionnaire)
Adolescents. *See also* Lesbian, gay,
　　bisexual, and questioning
　　(LGBQ) adolescents
　building trust with, 94-95
　critical transition period of, 167
　demographics for, 4-5
　desire to talk and, 205-208
　effects of part-time employment on,
　　157
　health risks and, 167-168
　interpersonal relationships and, 192
　myths about, 5-6,8-9
　opportunities for health care
　　systems and, 9
　permission to talk and, 14-15
　ratings of schools by, 167
　role of friends for, 194-195
　sleep and, 130
　substance use and, 183-185
Adolescent Self-Esteem Questionnaire,
　　63

Adquest (adolescent intake
　　questionnaire), 48-49,84-85,
　　122,193,266-267
　as bridge to engagement, 90
　for building trust with adolescents,
　　94-95
　as clinical data-mining resource, 61
　clinical mining approach of,
　　266-268
　conceptualization of safety items in,
　　107
　contents of, 60-61
　evolving organizational context of,
　　58-59
　for exploratory research purposes,
　　72-73
　forced-choice questions in, 69-71
　as forum for self-reflection for
　　young people, 92
　giving children permission to talk
　　and, 90-91
　giving practitioners permission to
　　ask and, 91-92
　implementation of, 60-61,87-89
　as instrument for studying violence,
　　106
　as internal form for self-reflection
　　for adolescents, 92
　as intervention, 66-67
　for keeping conversations open,
　　95-97
　objectives of, 56-57,59-60
　piloting process for, 68-69
　practice-based contributions to
　　development of, 61-62
　as practice-based research tool, 86
　practitioner-led reflective practice
　　inquiry into clinical uses of,
　　89

© 2005 by The Haworth Press, Inc. All rights reserved.

providing structure to treatment
    planning process and, 97-98
questions about families and friends
    in, 197-198
questions asked in, 76-82
race/racism items in, 241-242,260
reliability of, 63-64
research-based contributions to
    development of, 62-63
as research protocol, 65
Safety Risk Scale for, 107-108
sample size for, 71-72
scanning for "trigger items" and, 99
school questions in, 158-160
as second set of eyes, 98-99
as second voice for adolescents,
    93-94
substance use section of, 174-176
theoretical assumptions underlying,
    195-196
as tool for clinicians, 263-264
validity of, 64
work questions in, 158-160
Age
    adolescents' desire to talk about sex
        and, 144-145
    education issues and, 162-163
    mental health services and Adquest
        questions for, 126-127
    safety risk indicators and,
        110-111,115
    substance use and, 179-180
    work issues and, 162-163
AHC. See Mount Sinai Adolescent
    Health Center (AHC)
Alcohol use. See also Substance use
    conduct disorders and, 172
    depression and, 172
Assessment instruments, 56-57. See
    also Adquest (adolescent
    intake questionnaire)
    in social work practice, 85-86

Beck Depression Inventory, 63

Behavioral risks
    defined, 138
    desire to talk and, 145-146
    desire to talk and, about friends and
        family, 203-205
    by gender and stage of adolescents,
        sex and, 142-143
Bingeing, 125
Bisexual adolescents. See Lesbian,
    gay, bisexual, and
    questioning (LGBQ)
    adolescents

CDM. See Clinical data-mining
    (CDM)
Child Behavior Checklist (CBCL),
    63,88
Client involvement, at AHC, 16
Clients
    distinguishing "wants" from
        "needs" of, 69-71
    organizations as, 29
Clinical data-mining (CDM), 288-289.
    See also Practice-based
    research (PBR)
    Adquest as resource for, 61
    at AHC, 306-307
    implementation strategy for, at
        AHC, 291-294
    lessons from implementing,
        296-301
Clinical engagement, model of,
    264-267
Clinicians. See also Practitioners
    experiences of, PBR and, 309-312
    lessons learned by, 312-313
    pointers for, PBR and, 315
    practice-based research and,
        307-309
    results of participation in PBR for,
        313-315
Conduct disorders
    alcohol use and, 172
    substance use and, 172

Coping. *See also* Desire to talk
  Adquest findings for, 275
  clinical significance, 281-282
  defined, 138
  with friends and families, and
    desire to talk, 202-203

Data mining. *See* Clinical data-mining
  (CDM)
Depression, alcohol use and, 172
Desire to talk, 268-270
  about school, 163-164
  about sex, by gender, 144-145
  about substance use, 180-182
  about work, 163-164
  adolescents and, 205-208
  behavioral risks and, 145-146
  behavior risk and, about friends and
    family, 203-205
  clinical significance of, 275-278
  coping with friends and family and,
    202-203
  LGBQ adolescents and, 230-232
  research on
    discussion of findings for,
      275-282
    findings for, 268-275
    methodology for, 266-268
    practice implications for,
      282-284
  stages of adolescence and, about
    friends and family, 199-200
  worry and, 201
Development, adolescent
  health care systems and, 19
  healthy, 19
  theories of, 193-194

Eating disorders, 130

Education. *See* School
Effects management, 24
Employment. *See* Work, adolescents
  and
Engagement
  conceptual model of, for
    adolescents, 264-266
  using Adquest as bridge to, 90
Environmental risks, defined, 138
Ethnic identity, theories of, 237-239
Ethnicity. *See* Race/racism
Ethnic pride, 252-253

Families, adolescents and
  behavior risk and desire to talk
    about, 203-205
  coping with, and desire to talk,
    202-203
  research on
    discussion of findings for,
      205-208
    findings for, 198-205
    methodology for, 196-198
  stages of adolescence and desire to
    talk about, 199-200
  worries about, gender and, 199
Forced-choice questions, in Adquest,
  69-71
Forced sex, 146-147
Friends, adolescents and
  behavior risk and desire to talk
    about, 203-205
  coping with, and desire to talk,
    202-203
  research on
    discussion of findings for,
      205-208
    findings for, 198-205
    methodology for, 196-198
  role of, for adolescents, 194-195

stages of adolescence and desire to talk about, 199-200
worries about, gender and, 199

Gateway theory, 7,185
Gay adolescents. *See* Lesbian, gay, bisexual, and questioning (LGBQ) adolescents
Gender
    adolescents' desire to talk about sex and, 144-145
    behavioral risks and worries by, sex and, 142-144
    differences in, for needing to talk, 130-131
    education issues and, 162
    mental health services and Adquest questions for, 125-126
    safety risk indicators and, 110-111,115
    substance use and, 177-179
    work issues and, 162
    worries about friends and family and, 199
    worry and desire to talk and, 201-202
Global Assessment of Functioning scale (GAF), 88
Grade level, education risk factors and, 161-162

Health care, myths about adolescents and, 5-6
Health care systems. *See also* Mental health systems
    external challenges for, 24-26
    healthy adolescent development and, 19
    opportunities for, adolescents and, 9
    practice-research challenges for, 30
    reflective cultures for, 24-26
Health risks, for adolescents, 167-168

Home life. *See* Families
Homicide, 104

Instruments. *See also* Adquest (adolescent intake questionnaire); Assessment instruments
Interpersonal relationships, adolescents and, 192. *See also* Families; Friends
Interventions
    Adquest as, 66-67
    standardization in, 86
Invulnerability, adolescent, knowledge *vs.* myths about, 8-9. *See also* Vulnerability

Lesbian, gay, bisexual, and questioning (LGBQ) adolescents, 227-230. *See also* Adolescents
    coming out and, 214-215
    desire to talk and, 230-232
    emotional distress and, 215
    findings of, 218-227
    gender, sexual identity and risk for, 223-225
    gender and sexual identity for, 218-219
    practice principles for, 215-216
    research on
        discussion of findings for, 227-232
        findings for, 218-227
        methodology for, 216-218
    sexual identity and, 215,218
    sexual identity and desire to talk for, 225-227
    sexual identity and risk for, 219-223
    sexual orientation and, 214

stages of adolescent development and sexual identity for, 218

Managers, program and policy challenges for, 29
Medical care systems. *See* Health care systems
Mental health problems, substance use and, 172-173
Mental health services
for children, 122
desire to talk and, 127-128
at Mount Sinai Adolescent Health Center, 122
research on, at AHC
age trends for, 126-127
discussion of findings for, 130-131
findings for, 124-125
methodology for, 123-124
trends by gender for, 125-126
Mental health systems. *See also* Health care systems
external challenges for, 24-26
practice-research challenges for, 30
reflective cultures for, 24-26
Mount Sinai Adolescent Health Center (AHC), 4,106,137-138, 173-174,263
adolescent involvement and governance of, 16
client involvement and, 16
communities of concern for, 11-12
creating havens for adolescents at, 14-15
experience of PBR at, 294-301
flexible programming and, 16-17
flexible programming at, 16-17
implementation strategy for CDM at, 291-294
innovation at, 16-17
mental health services at, 122
philosophy and service design of, 12-13

as place to talk, 14-15
practice-based research at
benefits for practitioners and, 50-52
challenges and opportunities for, 42-43
committee process for, 44-45
evolution of model for, 43-44
examples of, 45-49
lessons learned about, 50-52
origins of, 40-41
stabilizing, 50
Practice-Based Research Group of, 58
as practice setting, 87
practice standards and competencies at, 18-19
reflective practice at, 27
service approach of, 13-14
staffing at, 17-19
youth development perspective at, 11-12
Myths, about adolescence, 5-6,8-9

Organizations
as clients, 29
reflective social work, 28-29

Part-time employment, effects of, on adolescents, 157-158
PBR. *See* Practice-based research (PBR)
Peers. *See* Friends
Permission to ask, Adquest and, 91-92
Permission to talk, adolescents and, 14-15, 90-91. *See also* Desire to talk
Practice-Based Research Group (PBRG), 58

challenges and opportunities for,
42-43
contributions to practice-based
research by, 52-53
evolution of model of, 43-44
lessons learned by members of,
50-52
Practice-based research (PBR),
17,236,288. *See also* Clinical
data-mining (CDM);
Research-based practices
(RBPs)
benefits of, to organizations, 52-53
defined, 40
as dialectical continuum, 65-66
experiences of clinicians and,
307-309
lessons from, at AHC, 294-301
at Mount Sinai Adolescent Health
Center
benefits for practitioners and,
50-52
challenges and opportunities for,
42-43
committee process for, 44-45
evolution of model, 43-44
examples of, 45-49
lessons learned about, 50-52
origins of, 40-41
stabilizing PBR efforts at, 50
reasons for undertaking, 289
vs. research-based practice, 31-33
resources and constraints for,
290-291
Practices. *See also* Health care systems
challenges facing, 29
models of research-practice
integration for, 30-31
reflective, 26-27,40
research challenges facing, 30
Practitioners. *See also* Clinicians
Adquest, and permission to ask
questions by, 91-92
benefits of practice-based
research and, 50-52

program and policy challenges
for, 29
reflective social work
organizations and, 29
views held by, instruments and,
86
Problem behavior theory, 7
Programming, flexible, 16-17
Purging, 125

Questioning adolescents. *See*
Lesbian,gay, bisexual, and
questioning (LGBQ)
Questionnaires, self-reporting, 85. *See
also* Adquest (adolescent
intake questionnaire);
Assessment instruments
Questions, permission to ask, Adquest
and, 91-92

Race/racism, adolescents and
ethnic pride and, 252-253
experience of, 253-255
impacts of, 239-240
levels of, 239-240
practice implications of, 255-258
as presenting problem, 236
research on
discussion of findings for,
251-258
findings for, 242-251
methodology for, 240-242,260
risk exposure and, 251-252
Rapid Assessment Instruments (RAIs),
57,88
RBPs. *See* Research-based practices
(RBPs)
Reflection-in-action, 17,27-28
Reflective cultures, creating, 24-26
Reflective organizations, 27-28,289
Reflective practice
defined, 26-27,40

at Mount Sinai Adolescent Health
Center, 27
Reflective social work organizations
defined, 28-29
practitioners and, 29
Relationships, interpersonal,
adolescents and, 192. *See
also* Families; Friends
Research-based practices (RBPs),
30-31. *See also*
Practice-based research
(PBR)
as dialectical continuum, 65-66
vs. practice-based research, 31-33
Research challenges, for health and
mental health systems, 30
Research-practice models, 30-31
Risks, adolescent, 4. *See also*
Behavioral risks; Health risks
Adquest findings for, 270-275
clinical significance of, 278-281
theories of, 7-8

Safety, adolescents and, 104-106. *See
also* Violence, adolescents
and research on
discussion of results for, 113-117
methodology for, 106-108
results for, 108-113
Safety risk indicators. *See also*
Violence, adolescents and
age and, 111-112
desire to talk about safety and,
112-113
gender and, 110-111
Safety Risk Scale (SRS), 107-108
School, adolescents and, 156-157
desire to talk about, 163-164
grade level and risk factors for,
161-162
health risks and, 164-166
research on
discussion of findings for,
166-168

findings for, 160-161
methodology for, 158-160
risk factors for, grade level and,
161-162
Screening tools, 85
Self-reporting questionnaires, 85
Serial risk behavior theory, 7
Sex and sexuality, adolescent, 136
Adquest questions related to,
138-140
behavioral risks and worries for, by
gender and stage of
adolescence, 142-144
desire to talk and, 144-145
potential negative consequences of,
136-137
research on
discussion of findings for,
147-151
findings for, 140-147
methodology for, 137-140
substance use and, 183
Sexual orientation. *See also* Lesbian,
gay, bisexual, and
questioning (LGBQ)
adolescents
adolescence and, 214
defined, 214
Skipping school. *See* Truancy
Sleep, adolescents and, 125,130
Social identity theory, 237,238
Social workers. *See* Clinicians;
Practitioners
Social work organizations, reflective,
28-29
Social work practice, assessment
instruments in, 85-86
Staffing, for vulnerable adolescents,
17-19
Standardization, in interventions, 86
Substance use, adolescents and,
183-186
conduct disorders and, 172
desire to talk about, 180-182

mental health problems and,
    172-173
research on
    age trends for, 179-180
    discussion of findings for,
        185-186
    findings for, 176-177
    gender trends for, 177-179
    methodology for, 173-176
sex and, 183
vulnerability and, 182-183
Suicide, 104

Talk, AHC as place to, 14-15. *See also*
    Desire to talk
Treatment planning process, Adquest
    and, 97-98
Trigger items, in Adquest, 99
Truancy, 156-157,166
Trust, Adquest as means for building,
    94-95

Violence, adolescents and, 104-106.
        See also Safety, adolescents
        and
    research on
        discussion for, 113-117
        methodology for, 106-108
        results for, 108-113
Vulnerability, adolescent, 4,6-8
    adolescent self-perceptions of, 8-9
    age differences in, 129-130
    gender and age trends regarding,
        and substance use, 182-183
    gender differences in, 128-129

Work, adolescents and
    desire to talk about, 163-164
    effects of part-time, on adolescents,
        157
    health risks and, 164-166
    research on
        discussion of findings for,
            166-168
        findings for, 160-166
        methodology for, 158-160
Worries. *See also* Desire to talk
    about sex, desire to talk and,
        145-146
    Adquest findings for, 270-275
    clinical significance of, 278-281
    defined, 138
    desire to talk about, 201
    by gender and stage of adolescent,
        sex and, 142-144

Young people. *See* Adolescents
Youth Development perspective, 4
    adolescent involvement and, 15-16
    at Mt. Sinai Adolescent Health
        Center, 11-12
    overview of, 10-11
Youth Risk Behavior Survey (YRBS),
    62-63

For Product Safety Concerns and Information please contact our EU
representative GPSR@taylorandfrancis.com Taylor & Francis Verlag GmbH,
Kaufingerstraße 24, 80331 München, Germany

Printed and bound by CPI Group (UK) Ltd, Croydon, CR0 4YY
08/06/2025
01896977-0016